10-8-10

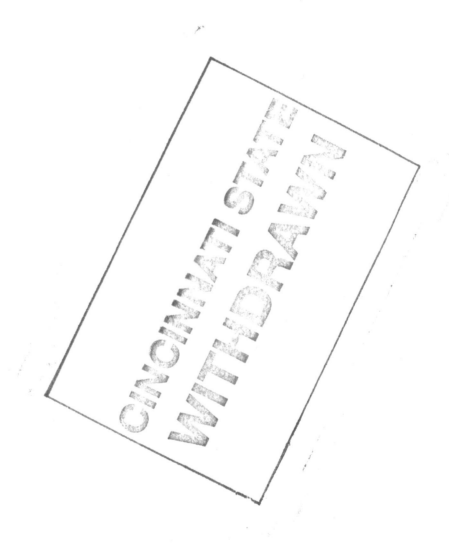

Communication

Core Interpersonal Skills for
Health Professionals

Communication
Core Interpersonal Skills for Health Professionals

Gjyn O'Toole

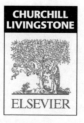

CHURCHILL
LIVINGSTONE

ELSEVIER

Sydney Edinburgh London New York Philadelphia St Louis Toronto

Churchill Livingstone
is an imprint of Elsevier

Elsevier Australia. ACN 001 002 357
(a division of Reed International Books Australia Pty Ltd)
ELSEVIER Tower 1, 475 Victoria Avenue, Chatswood, NSW 2067

National Library of Australia Cataloguing-in-Publication Data

O'Toole, Gjyn.

Communication : core interpersonal skills for health
           professionals / Gjyn O'Toole

ISBN: 9780729538596 (pbk.)

Includes index.
Bibliography.

Communication in medicine
Medical personnel and patient
Interpersonal communication

610.696

Publisher: Heidi Allen
Developmental Editor: Samantha McCulloch
Publishing Services Manager: Helena Klijn
Editorial Coordinator: Eleanor Cant
Edited by Alexandra Holliday
Proofread by Gabrielle Challis
Internal design and typesetting by Midland Typesetters
Cover design by Trina McDonald
Index by Master Indexing
Printed by Ligare Pty Ltd

It is the policy of Elsevier Australia to use vegetable-based inks on paper manufactured from sustainable forests
wherever possible.

Contents

Acknowledgements   x
Preface   xi
Reviewers   xii

SECTION ONE – THE SIGNIFICANCE OF INTERPERSONAL COMMUNICATION IN THE HEALTH PROFESSIONS   1

1 Defining communication for health professionals   3
Why learn how to communicate? – Everyone can communicate!   3
Defining communication   4
Effective communication requires mutual understanding   4
Factors contributing to effective communication   5
Chapter summary   7
References   8

2 The overall goal of communication for health professionals   9
A model demonstrating the importance of communication   9
The general purpose of communication for the health professions   10
Chapter summary   14
References   15

3 The specific goals of communication for health professionals: 1   16
Making verbal introductions   17
Providing information: A two-way process   20
Chapter summary   22
References   23

4 The specific goals of communication for health professionals: 2   24
Gathering information   24
Comforting: Encouraging versus discouraging   29
Confronting unhelpful attitudes or beliefs   32
Chapter summary   33
References   35

SECTION TWO – DEVELOPING AWARENESS TO ACHIEVE EFFECTIVE COMMUNICATION IN THE HEALTH PROFESSIONS   37

5 Awareness of and need for reflective practice   39
The 'what' of reflection: A definition   39
The result of reflection: Achieving self-awareness   41
The 'why' of reflection: Reasons for reflecting   42

The 'how' of reflection: Models of reflection   45
Reflection upon barriers to experiencing, accepting and resolving emotions   48
Chapter summary   51
References   53

6   Awareness of self   **55**
Self-awareness: An essential tool   55
The benefits of achieving self-awareness   56
Beginning the journey of self-awareness   56
Individual values   58
Is a health profession an appropriate choice?   59
Values of a health professional   59
Characteristics and abilities that enhance the practice of a health professional 60
Personal unconscious needs   61
Conflict between values and needs   63
Perfectionism as a value   64
Self-awareness of personal communication skills   65
Self-awareness of skills for effective listening   66
Barriers to listening   67
Self-awareness about skills for effective speaking   69
Preferences for managing information and resultant communicative behaviours   70
Personality typology and resultant communicative behaviours   72
Humour   72
Chapter summary   74
References   76

7   Awareness of the 'other'   **78**
The *whole* 'other'   78
Who are the 'others'?   79
What information will assist the health professional in relating to the 'other'? 80
The purpose and benefit of respect   81
Defining respect   81
Demonstrating respect   82
Physical aspects of the 'other'   84
Emotional aspects of the 'other'   84
Sexual aspects of the 'other'   92
Cognitive aspects of the 'other'   93
Social needs of the 'other'   96
Spiritual needs of the 'other'   96
Chapter summary   98
References   99

8   Awareness of different environments   **101**
The physical environment   102
The emotional environment   108
The cultural environment   111
The sexual environment   113
The social environment   114
The spiritual environment   115

Chapter summary 116
References 117

SECTION THREE – DEVELOPING CORE SKILLS IN COMMUNICATION 119

9 Communication with the whole person 121
Defining the whole person 121
Holistic care 122
Holistic communication 125
Chapter summary 127
References 128

10 'Other'-centred communication 130
Benefits of active listening 131
Barriers to listening 131
Preparing to listen 132
Characteristics of effective listening 133
Disengagement 133
Chapter summary 135
References 137

11 Ethical communication 138
Respect regardless of differences 139
Honesty 140
Clarification of expectations 141
Consent 142
Confidentiality 143
Boundaries 145
Ethical codes of behaviour/conduct 147
Chapter summary 147
References 149
Further reading 150
Informed consent 152

12 Non-verbal communication 154
The significance of non-verbal communication 155
The benefits of non-verbal communication 155
The effects of non-verbal communication 155
The components of non-verbal communication 155
Chapter summary 162
References 164

13 Stereotypes, judgement and communication 166
Reasons to avoid stereotypical judgement when communicating 167
Stereotypical judgement that relates to roles 168
Developing attitudes that avoid stereotypical judgement 170
Overcoming the power imbalance: Ways to demonstrate equality in a relationship 172
Chapter summary 172
References 174

14 Conflict and communication 176

Conflict during communication 176
Resolving negative attitudes and emotions towards another 178
Patterns of relating during conflict 179
How to communicate assertively 181
Chapter summary 183
References 184

15 Culturally appropriate communication 185

Defining culturally appropriate communication 186
Why consider cultural differences? 187
Factors affecting culturally appropriate communication 187
Managing personal cultural assumptions and expectations 190
Strategies for demonstrating culturally appropriate communication 192
Using an interpreter 194
The culture of each health profession 196
The culture of disease or ill-health 196
Chapter summary 197
References 198

16 Communicating with indigenous peoples 200

Correct use of terms 200
The complexity of cultural identity 201
Principles of practice for health professionals when working with indigenous
peoples 202
Chapter summary 211
References 213
Further reading 213

17 Misunderstandings and communication 215

Communication that produces misunderstanding 215
Factors affecting mutual understanding 216
Causes of misunderstandings 217
Strategies to avoid misunderstandings 220
Resolving misunderstandings 221
Chapter summary 223
References 224

18 Remote communication 225

Characteristics of remote forms of communication for the health professional 226
Principles that govern professional remote communication 228
Chapter summary 233
References 235

SECTION FOUR – THE FOCUS OF COMMUNICATION IN THE HEALTH PROFESSIONS: PEOPLE — 237

Introduction — 238

19 People experiencing strong emotions — 241
A person who behaves aggressively — 242
A person who experiences extreme distress — 245
A person who is reluctant to engage or be involved in communication or intervention — 248

20 People in particular stages of the lifespan — 252
A child — 253
An adolescent — 256
A person who is older — 260

21 People in particular roles — 263
A person who fulfils the role of carer for a person seeking assistance — 264
A person who fulfils the role of a colleague — 267
A person who fulfils the role of parent to a child requiring assistance — 270
A person who fulfils the role of single parent to a child requiring assistance — 273
A person who fulfils the role of a student — 276
Groups in the health professions — 279
References — 283
Further reading — 283

22 People with particular conditions — 284
A person who has decreased cognitive function — 286
A person who experiences a life-limiting illness and their family — 290
A person experiencing a mental illness — 294
A person experiencing a hearing impairment — 297
A person experiencing a visual impairment — 301
References — 304
Further reading — 304

23 People in particular contexts — 306
A person who experiences an emergency — 307
A person who experiences domestic abuse — 311
A person who speaks a different language to the health professional — 315

Glossary — 319
Index — 325

Acknowledgements

Thanks to Deirdre Heitmeyer from the Birabahn Indigenous Education Unit at the University of Newcastle, Newcastle, NSW, Australia, and Ailsa Haxell for their invaluable evaluation of the details found in Chapter 16.

The people who assisted with compilation of Section Four (Chs 19–23) include Esther Brooks (teacher extraordinaire), Matt Peters (talented health professional) and Nell Harrison (creative and reliable health professional) – all phenomenal people. To say thanks is not enough.

I especially thank three people: Mitch, a wonderful model of a communicator in many forms; Esther, author, communicator and editor extraordinaire; and Jasen, an interested and invaluable communicator. The encouragement and support I receive from the three of you makes it all possible.

I also have students, colleagues, friends and other family members to thank for their commitment to both challenging and encouraging me in my journey towards becoming an effective communicator.

I am, however, most in debt to the Creator and Sustainer of the Universe, God.

Preface

Development of skills in communication is an ongoing journey for each person. It requires awareness of personal biases and prejudice, awareness of the needs of the 'other', awareness of the effects of environment and background, as well as reflection about communicative practice. Even the best communicators have times when they experience unsatisfactory communicative acts and regret the effects of an interaction. The journey for a health professional in developing communication skills is often eventful and sometimes difficult. However, commitment to perseverance in overcoming the barriers to effective communication is a beneficial and rewarding process for any person, but especially for a health professional.

This book contains four sections that focus on particular elements of communication. Section One examines the significance of communication in the health professions. Section Two highlights the importance of reflection and increased awareness when communicating as a health professional. It indicates this awareness must be of 'self' as well as the 'other' and the environment. Section Three emphasises the specific characteristics of and skills required for effective communication in the health professions.

Section Four presents forty-one scenarios that illustrate typical situations and people a health professional might encounter during their working week. This section challenges readers to consider in depth the circumstances and needs of the people in the scenarios. Section Four encourages readers to validate the information found in the first three sections of the book, thus promoting application of the information learnt and consolidation of the skills developed in these sections.

All sections include presentation of information and opportunity for reflection and discussion. They provide opportunities to communicate with both 'self' and 'others' in an attempt to promote awareness of the major factors contributing to effective communication.

Reviewers

Katherine Bathgate, BSc, GradDipDiet, GradCertTeach, MPH
Lecturer, School of Public Health
Curtin University of Technology, Perth, WA, Australia

Ailsa Haxell, RN, MHSc (Hons)
Senior Lecturer, School of Health Care Practice
Auckland University of Technology, Auckland, New Zealand

Steve Parker, RN, RPN, DipT (NurseEd), BEd, PhD
Senior Lecturer, School of Nursing & Midwifery
Flinders University, Adelaide, SA, Australia

Erika Gisel, PhD (Biol), MSc, BSc (Occ Ther), BA (Ed)
Professor, Faculty of Medicine; Head of School of Physical & Occupational Therapy
McGill University, Montreal, Quebec, Canada

ONE

THE SIGNIFICANCE OF INTERPERSONAL COMMUNICATION IN THE HEALTH PROFESSIONS

Defining communication for health professionals

1

CHAPTER OBJECTIVES
Upon completing this chapter, students should be able to
- Explain why it is essential to learn about effective communication
- Define effective communication
- Understand the importance of effective communication
- Identify factors contributing to effective communication
- Understand the importance of the 'audience' when communicating.

Why learn how to communicate? – Everyone can communicate!

Communication occurs constantly throughout the world and most individuals participate in acts of communication every day regardless of their nationality, age or interests. Most people would agree that communication is unavoidable and usually essential for satisfactory daily life. Every person communicates, even those who are unable to produce speech. If everyone communicates in daily life, however, then you may think it unnecessary to learn how to communicate in healthcare settings, because everyone can communicate already. While it is true that almost everyone communicates, in most healthcare settings there are specific required characteristics of communication and particular situations that test the communication skills of any communicator. **Effective communication** in a healthcare setting requires particular understanding of others and oneself, as well as highly-developed communication skills. Individuals do not usually acquire such awareness or skill in daily life and thus it is beneficial to learn about communication if preparing to be an effective health professional. Higgs et al (2005) indicate that effective communication is an essential core skill that ensures positive outcomes for individuals seeking the assistance of any health professional. If effective communication skills are vital for successful practice in the health professions, it is crucial to understand both communication and effective communication.

Defining communication

Many dictionaries indicate that communication involves the sending and receiving of messages. They state that communication can take place through auditory/verbal, visual and non-verbal forms. This understanding of communication suggests that the act of communicating resembles a game of tennis. In the same way that tennis players hit a ball to each other, communicators send and receive a message. A message is sent and the receiver responds by returning a message. Initially this metaphor seems appropriate, but tennis players only connect with the ball; they normally do not connect with each other. As communication requires a connection between two or more people, there appear to be limitations if comparing tennis and communication.

REFLECTION

- When considering the health professions, what are the similarities and differences between tennis and communication?
- Does communicating in the health professions require more than voice, ears and eyes? If so, what does it require?

Effective communication involves more than sending and receiving words through producing and receiving sound. Effective communication occurs in many forms including vocalising without words (e.g. laughing or crying), non-verbal cues (e.g. eye contact, facial expressions, gestures and signing) and material forms (e.g. pictures, photographs, picture symbols, logos and written words) (Crystal 2007).

Effective communication requires mutual understanding

Each communicative act or interaction is unique, with unique requirements and constraints. These requirements and constraints influence the effectiveness of the interaction within the particular context at the time. The combination of these factors along with ongoing negotiation determines whether the outcome is one of **mutual understanding**. Successfully negotiating mutual understanding will encourage those communicating to trust their ability to communicate effectively (Stein-Parbury 2006) and thus they will continue to communicate. Every communication act requires all communicators to be actively involved, to connect with and understand each other, and to understand the factors affecting the communication act (Brill & Levine 2005). Effective communication requires the communicating parties to have some basic knowledge about each other and their individual goals when communicating (Devito 2007).

Without a sharing of meaning, communication is ineffective. Therefore, the sending and receiving of a message achieves nothing unless there is mutual understanding. The specific purpose of communication among health professionals (see Chs 3 & 4) is to share information and fulfil needs. If mutual understanding is not negotiated through words and non-verbal messages (Gietzelt & Jones 2002), there is no appropriate information to guide an intervention and potentially limited fulfilment of needs. For example, if there is no connection and mutual understanding when there is a need for a toilet or something in which to vomit, the results can be messy and, more importantly, time-consuming.

Effective communication in the health professions occurs when the sender and receiver connect with each other for a common purpose and negotiate mutual understanding. It is necessary for health professionals to negotiate during their interactions until achieving shared understanding.

Factors contributing to effective communication

Effective communication requires two or more people to have a topic of mutual interest, a mutual desire, intent or need to communicate about the topic, the opportunity to communicate and the means of communicating. If there is no common language or way of communicating there will be no mutual understanding and thus no effective communication (Nunan 2007).

Mutual understanding is essential for effective communication. However, many underlying factors influence the comprehension of a message. These factors may either facilitate or restrict communication.

REFLECTION

- Consider the different meanings of the following words: file, stand, form, compress, bracing, and 'a simple case'.
- Can you think of other words or combinations of words that might cause miscommunication?
- What factors change the meaning an individual might assign to a word or combination of words?

Factors external to the sender

The words in the box above (file, stand etc) have meanings that might vary within the **context** of a specific sentence. In the context of the question *Is that bracing working?* it is obvious the word 'bracing' does not refer to the temperature or energy levels, but rather to something that is supporting or strengthening. The receiver of the message in this case assumes the meaning of the word 'bracing' from the other words in the sentence (i.e. possibly after a fleeting thought about the weather conditions or a workout at the gym the receiver assumes that the question refers to an engineering or therapeutic context).

The meaning assigned to words can also vary according to the **situational** and **environmental** context (Nunan 2007). Thus, if asked for a 'file' (e.g. *Pass that file please*) when there is no obvious folder with pieces of paper inside, the receiver of the request might search for other meanings of the word. They might see an implement used to file nails in the environment and assume that is the required file. In this case the receiver of the message assumes the meaning because of factors in the environment.

There are other external factors that affect the meaning an individual might assign to a word. Someone who comes from a particular **background** or who has particular life **experiences** might assign a particular meaning to one word. For example, someone with a scientific or nursing background might assume that the word 'stand' means a structure used to hold or support something, while someone with a political background might assume it means to run for election. Someone with a military background might assume it means to resist an onslaught without being harmed, while someone with another background or experience might assume it means to stay in one place without moving. In this case it is the background and experience of the individuals communicating that affect the understanding of the particular word. The background or experience might be particular to a family, socioeconomic group or culture; all of these factors and more can affect and vary the meaning of messages. It is important when communicating in the health professions, therefore, to consider any related factors that might influence the effectiveness of communication.

Factors within the sender

Senders of messages often express their messages according to their own thoughts, agenda, needs or feelings at a given time. For example, senders often communicate their intended meaning through **emphasis** or stress on a particular word, rather than the actual words they use (Crystal 2007). Consider

- *It **is** time we had those ATOs in the store* means *Can you do it now?*
- *Have **you** seen that splinting material?* means *I have asked everyone else – do you know?*

It is often the emphasis on a particular word that changes the intended meaning of an entire sentence. Compare

- *I **want** a drink of water.*
- ***I** want a drink of water.*
- *I want a drink of **water**.*

The emphasis changes the meaning of each statement. The first is a statement of a desire to have a drink of water. The second suggests a focus upon the speaker; thereby implying the desires of others are irrelevant. The third indicates that the desired drink is water and nothing else. In each case the emphasis indicates the particular desire of the person sending the message. If the receiver fails to note the emphasis in the last sentence, for example, the sender of the message may not receive the desired drink.

Factors within the receivers or 'audience'

In every communicative event someone receives a message or information. The **audience** is the person or group of people who receive the message or information. In the health professions there are many people who constitute the audience.

There are a multitude of factors that influence the effectiveness of communication and some of these factors are within the receiver or audience. The potential impact of these audience factors upon communication makes it important for health professionals to consider these factors when communicating.

ACTIVITY

- List all the people with whom a health professional might communicate.
- For each person or group of people list factors specific to that person or group that might affect their ability to understand a sent message.

Every person has particular **knowledge** and associated levels of **understanding** that affect their ability to comprehend particular messages (Milliken & Honeycutt 2004). Thus, when practising as a health professional it is important to communicate in ways that acknowledge the level of understanding and/or knowledge of the audience.

The **age** of the person is one factor that can influence the knowledge or level of understanding. Therefore, when talking to a young child it is appropriate to adjust the communication style by using less complex words or sentences. This adjustment of communication style assists the mutual understanding of both the speaker and the child. Using the same simplicity of language when talking to an adolescent or adult, however, may cause offence. Another factor that requires adjustment of language is the **cultural/language background** of the audience (see Chs 13 & 15 and Section Four).

A further factor that requires consideration is whether or not to use **professional jargon**. The decision of how and when to use professional jargon requires the health professional to consider the experience and background of the person (Purtilo & Haddad 2002). The use of medical terminology may be appropriate if the person has a medical background and understanding of the particular field of medicine. It may also be appropriate if they have previous experience with such terminology, but may cause confusion if they do not have the knowledge, understanding or experience of such terminology. When communicating with health professional colleagues about medically-related topics, use of non-medical terminology may cause confusion! In order to avoid confusion it is important to consider and sometimes request information about the knowledge and experience of the audience when communicating as a health professional.

A particular **disorder** affecting an individual may also influence the success of the communicative event. In some circumstances it may be essential to communicate only one idea or step at a time. For example, individuals with limited cognitive ability and reduced affect require adjustments in the communication style of the health professional and their manner of constructing and delivering a message.

It is not only the age, background and experiences of the receiver that can affect their level of understanding. Receivers of messages often interpret messages according to their own **thoughts**, **ideas**, **needs** or **emotions** at that given time, which may assist or adversely affect their understanding of the messages (see Chs 5 & 6 and Section Four). Effective communication between a health professional and those seeking their assistance should be an exchange of thoughts, ideas, needs and emotions that has a therapeutic outcome (Paré & Lysack 2004, Seikkula & Trimble 2005). A health professional who considers and appropriately adjusts to the thoughts, ideas, needs and emotions of the receiver will usually promote mutual understanding and thus achieve effective communication.

ACTIVITY

- List at least six factors that facilitate effective communication.
- State whether these factors are external or internal to the sender or receiver.

Chapter summary

Effective communication requires

- Mutual understanding of the interaction
- Understanding and consideration of the various external and internal factors that affect mutual understanding
- Understanding of the specific characteristics of the 'audience'.

References

Brill N I, Levine J 2005 Working with people: the helping process, 8th edn. Pearson, Boston

Crystal D 2007 How language works. Penguin Books, London

Devito J A 2007 The interpersonal communication book, 11th edn. Pearson, Boston

Gietzelt D, Jones G 2002 Importance of language – single words don't communicate all that is necessary. In: Bergland C, Saltman D (eds) Communication for healthcare. Oxford University Press, Melbourne, p 18–32

Higgs J, Sefton A, Street A et al 2005 Communicating in the health and social sciences. Oxford University Press, Melbourne

Milliken M A, Honeycutt A 2004 Understanding human behavior: a guide for healthcare providers, 7th edn. Thomson Delmar, New York

Nunan D 2007 What is this thing called language? Palgrave Macmillan, Basingstoke

Paré D, Lysack M 2004 The willow and the oak: from monologue to dialogue in the scaffolding of therapeutic conversations. Journal of Systemic Therapies 23:6–20

Purtilo R B, Haddad A 2002 Health professional and patient interaction, 6th edn. Saunders, Philadelphia

Seikkula J, Trimble D 2005 Healing elements of therapeutic conversations: dialogue as an embodiment of love. Family Process 44:461–473

Stein-Parbury J 2006 Patient and person: interpersonal skills in nursing, 3rd edn. Elsevier, Sydney (Original work published 2005)

The overall goal of communication for health professionals

2

CHAPTER OBJECTIVES

Upon completing this chapter, students should be able to

- Understand the relevance of the WHO ICF model when communicating with a person seeking their assistance
- Understand the overall purpose of communication for the health professions
- Recognise the steps required to fulfil the overall purpose of communication in the health professions
- Understand and recognise the characteristics of each step.

While the purpose of communication in the health professions is ultimately to facilitate the delivery of a service, the overall goal of communication for health professionals should be to communicate in a manner that makes the delivery of the service a positive experience for all. This chapter describes the means of achieving this goal to ensure optimum health and wellbeing for all people seeking the services of a health professional.

A model demonstrating the importance of communication

The International Classification of Functioning (ICF) shown in Figure 2.1 (World Health Organization [WHO] 2001) is a biopsychosocial model that highlights the complex and multidimensional nature of health and the factors affecting health and functioning (Allan et al 2006). It provides a common language for multidisciplinary or interdisciplinary communication. The ICF classifies the 'components of health' and places health on a continuum where any limitation in functioning can disrupt health.

The ICF also describes the importance of participation in six interrelated domains or life situations (Ewert et al 2004, Weigl et al 2004), including

- Communication
- Movement
- Learning and applying knowledge

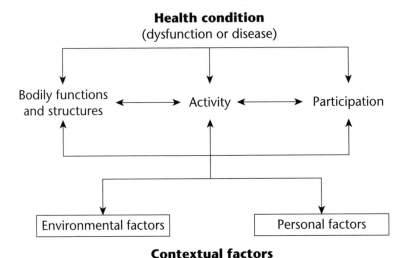

FIGURE 2.1 International Classification of Functioning. Adapted from WHO ICF 2001, p 18.

- Participation in general tasks and the demands of those tasks
- Self-care and interpersonal interactions
- Major life areas associated with work, school and family life.

The ICF model encourages health professionals to consider the factors that affect function and participation. It directs health professionals to collaborate *with the person* to overcome the challenges that restrict participation in a chosen activity, because participation contributes to health. It directs health professionals to develop holistic goals that are person-centred and thus unique to the needs of the individual (Brown et al 2003).

The ICF model indicates that communication is an important domain that facilitates participation and functioning and thus significantly affects health. It reminds health professionals to acknowledge the importance of communication for health and a sense of wellbeing, and therefore to encourage the individual to engage in the act of communicating.

The general purpose of communication for the health professions

Health professions exist to provide specific services to individuals seeking their assistance. Regardless of the particular health profession, communication is a vital activity within that service. Mutual understanding between the individual seeking the service and the health professional is vital to ensure positive outcomes; it is a characteristic of any meaningful interaction. Mutual understanding provides the foundation for the development of a therapeutic relationship between the individual and the health professional. Similarly, this therapeutic relationship ensures that the individual or group is at the centre of the goals and interventions, thereby facilitating family-centred, client-centred or person-centred practice (Parker 2006, Harms 2007, Higgs et al 2005, Purtilo & Haddad 2002, Rini & Grace 1999, Stein-Parbury 2006) (see Figure 2.2).

The concept of **family/person-centred practice** is the focus of discussion and publication in some health professions. In other health professions it is an underlying assumption but rarely discussed, while in others it is neither an assumption nor a topic of discussion.

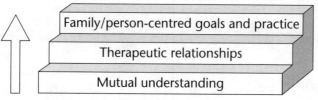

FIGURE 2.2 Mutual understanding is the first step.

Family/person-centred practice is a partnership between the health professional and the person/people seeking their services. This **collaborative partnership** exists to establish the needs of the person (Unsworth 2004) and enable them to achieve their goals through the assistance of the health professional (Duncan 2006). Achievement of these goals **empowers** the individual to experience participation and fulfilment in their daily lives.

Mutual understanding

Mutual understanding means that those communicating share a common meaning – all parties comprehend the verbal and non-verbal signals used during the interaction. In the health professions, mutual understanding must mean more than simply understanding words (see Ch 1).

A foundation factor that builds mutual understanding and appropriate results in any health profession is **respect** (Egan 2007). Respect of self and the other is a fundamental value of all health professions. It affects the views that individuals have of themselves and of others. It requires unconditional regard for self and the other regardless of weaknesses or failures, position or status, beliefs and values, material possessions and socioeconomic level (Purtilo & Haddad 2002). Respect demonstrates that the health professional values every individual. It is the basis of empathic reactions in a health professional.

As a health professional it is imperative to understand that every person seeking assistance feels disconnected and vulnerable. The individual often feels inadequate to meet the demands of their situation (Stein-Parbury 2006) and may be afraid of the unknown elements of the situation. Vulnerable individuals want to know that the health professionals around them care about them and want to understand their experiences (Milliken & Honeycutt 2004). It is the responsibility of the health professional to demonstrate this care and facilitate understanding of the vulnerability of each individual. Direct, clear and accurate understanding of the **emotions** of the individual and expression of this understanding is known as **empathy** (Stein-Parbury 2006). Davis (2006) states that expressing empathy to the vulnerable individual enables the health professional to communicate both 'humanistically and therapeutically'. This manner of communicating has a positive effect (Ley 1998) upon the participation of the individual in all activities associated with seeking assistance from the health professional (see Figure 2.3).

REFLECTION

- If you are feeling vulnerable, how do you feel when someone indicates they are interested in what you are feeling and attempts to understand your experiences and feelings?
- What actions demonstrate that someone is interested?
- How might expressing such interest and care affect communication?

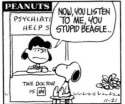
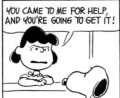
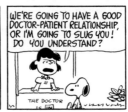
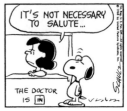

FIGURE 2.3 The doctor is IN. COPYRIGHT: UNITED FEATURES SYNDICATE INC. Distributed by Auspac Media.

It requires personal and professional skill to appropriately express empathy. Such skill requires reflection about self (Pendleton & Schultz-Krohn 2006), practice in expressing empathy, making time to practise, commitment to the expression of empathy and in many cases self-control on the part of the health professional. It requires awareness of and respect for the feelings of the individual – being able to see the world from the viewpoint of the other and respecting that viewpoint. Appropriate expressions of empathy require the health professional to make responsible choices about what, how and when they communicate. The health professional needs also to be aware of and able to control, express or resolve their own negative emotions, without allowing them to have an effect upon vulnerable individuals (see Chs 5 & 6). Appropriate expressions of empathy take little time or effort and they can have the individual believe they are the only person in the world for that time. While expressions of empathy are beneficial in all areas of life, they are essential when practising as a health professional (Egan 2007, Harms 2007, Milliken & Honeycutt 2004, Stein-Parbury 2006).

REFLECTION

- How do negative emotions affect your ability to send, receive or understand messages?
- Why are positive feelings and reactions essential when communicating as a health professional?

ACTIVITY

From the perspective of the person receiving the service, list the possible consequences of negative emotions either in you or in them.

Health professionals must consider whether they will validate and acknowledge the experience and associated needs of the individual and, if so, at which point (Davis 2006). While such choices require skill, health professionals must take every appropriate opportunity to express empathy with those around them because this indicates acceptance and validation of the emotions associated with the experience. Such acceptance and validation indicates respect. Respect is something that all individuals appreciate and it produces positive feelings that facilitate the development of **trust**. If the health professional is worthy of trust their behaviour will be predictable and reliable.

A therapeutic relationship

Mutual understanding and the characteristics it expresses facilitate the development of a therapeutic relationship. Therapeutic relationships require collaboration between health professionals and those they serve. A collaborative relationship promotes a real connection between the professional and the person. This connection is known as **rapport**. Rapport develops as trust develops and can empower individuals to persevere with achieving their health-related goals.

A therapeutic relationship requires independence not dependence. It demands a focus on the needs of the person, not fulfilment of the needs of the health professional. There may be expression of strong and deep emotions along with genuine distress with the individual, but this expression is *always* focused on the needs of the individual not the needs of the health professional (Purtilo & Haddad 2002). A therapeutic relationship desires neither to manipulate nor to be manipulated. In a therapeutic relationship the health professional desires to share their knowledge, skill and, where required, comfort and support to facilitate function and participation in the activities of life. Such a relationship empowers an individual to continue to face challenges that restrict participation and function. The support characteristic of a therapeutic relationship enables the individual to overcome situations that initially may seem overwhelming.

A Chinese scholar Lao Tsu (700 BC) when answering the question *What should a therapist do?* (they did not have health professionals in 700 BC!) said

> Go to the people   Work with them
> Learn from them   Respect them
> Start with what they know   Build with what they are
> And when the work is done   The task accomplished
> The people will say
> 'We have done this ourselves'.

A therapeutic relationship encourages a collaborative partnership. A collaborative partnership is one in which the contribution of each person is essential to achieve a satisfactory and appropriate outcome. It facilitates involvement from the individual who is intimately aware of their own needs. It also requires input from the health professional who has the knowledge, understanding and skill to assist. This collaboration enables the individual to face and overcome the relevant challenges. It gives them strength to achieve their own goals. It provides the mutual knowledge and understanding that is required to consider all relevant factors and resolve any areas of dysfunction. Collaboration allows people to be agents of change in their own circumstances, ultimately empowering them to increase their levels of function and participation in meaningful activities.

Family/person-centred goals and practice

The abovementioned steps contribute to a focus on the person. The characteristic of each step mandates that the health professional should not put their own desires or values consciously or unconsciously upon the person. Instead, these steps require investigation of the abilities, feelings, needs and desires of the person, in order to establish and prioritise their individual goals for participation in their chosen daily activities (Unsworth 2004). Such efforts will maintain the levels of motivation, effort and satisfaction in the person seeking assistance (Gilkeson 1997). They will give the individual **control** and thus increase **positive emotional responses**.

While each step has particular characteristics, one skill necessary for successful completion of each step and the overall purpose of interpersonal communication in the health professions is **effective listening** (see Ch 10). The health professional must invest the time to listen, validate and confirm understanding in every situation. These communication events contribute to and increase positive outcomes.

While the ultimate purpose of communication in the health professions may be the facilitation of the delivery of a service, it is the three steps of mutual understanding, developing a therapeutic relationship and family/person-centred goals and practice that make the delivery of any health service a positive experience for all. These steps create an experience that facilitates function, empowers people to participate and thus positively affects health and wellbeing.

Chapter summary

Family/person-centred practice is built upon therapeutic relationships, which depend on the presence of mutual understanding. Each step has a number of components that facilitate the achievement of the overall goal of communication among health professionals. The health professional can contribute to the establishment of each component directly, and thus can achieve effective communication and positive experiences that facilitate participation and functioning in activities that have meaning and produce fulfilment.

The steps leading to the overall goal of communication for health professionals are summarised in Figure 2.4.

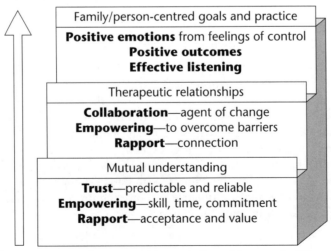

FIGURE 2.4 The components of movement towards the achievement of the overall goal of every health professional.

References

Allan C M, Campbell W N, Guptill C A et al 2006 A conceptual model for interprofessional education: the international classification of functioning, disability and health (ICF). Journal of Interprofessional Care 20:235–245

Brown G, Esdaile S A, Ryan S 2003 Becoming an advanced healthcare professional. Butterworth-Heineman, London

Davis C M 2006 Patient practitioner interaction. An experiential manual for developing the art of healthcare, 4th edn. Slack, Thorofare NJ

Duncan E A S 2006 Skills and process in occupational therapy. In: Duncan E A S (ed) Foundations for practice in occupational therapy, 4th edn. Elsevier, London, p 43–57

Egan G 2007 The skilled helper, 8th edn. Thomson, Belmont CA

Ewert T, Fuessl M, Cieza A et al 2004 Identification of the most common patient problems with chronic conditions using the ICF checklist. Journal of Rehabilitation Medicine 44(suppl):22–29

Gilkeson GE 1997 Occupational therapy leadership. Davis, Philadelphia

Harms D 2007 Working with people: communication skills for reflective practice. Oxford University Press, Melbourne

Higgs J, Sefton A, Street A et al 2005 Communicating in the health and social sciences. Oxford University Press, Melbourne

Ley P 1998 Communicating with patients. Improving communication satisfaction and compliance. Chapman and Hall, London

Milliken M A, Honeycutt A 2004 Understanding human behavior: a guide for healthcare providers, 7th edn. Thomson Delmar, New York

Parker D 2006 The client-centred frame of reference. In: Duncan E A S (ed) Foundations for practice in occupational therapy, 4th edn. Elsevier, London, p 193–215

Pendleton H M, Schultz-Krohn W (eds) 2006 Pedretti's occupational therapy. Practice for physical dysfunction, 6th edn. Mosby, St Louis MO

Purtilo R B, Haddad A 2002 Health professional and patient interaction, 6th edn. Saunders, Philadelphia

Rini D L, Grace A C 1999 Family-centered practice for children with communication disorders. Child and Adolescent Psychiatric Clinics of North-America 8(1):153–174

Stein-Parbury J 2006 Patient and person: interpersonal skills in nursing, 3rd edn. Elsevier, Sydney (Original work published 2005)

Unsworth C A 2004 How do pragmatic reasoning, worldview and client-centredness fit? British Journal of Occupational Therapy 67(1):10–19

Weigl M, Cieza A, Anderson C et al 2004 Identification of relevant ICF categories in patients with chronic health conditions: a Delphi exercise. Journal of Rehabilitation Medicine 44(suppl):12–21

World Health Organization 2001 International Classification of Functioning, Disability and Health. WHO, Geneva

The specific goals of communication for health professionals: 1

3

CHAPTER OBJECTIVES

Upon completing this chapter, students should be able to

- Understand the difference between the overall goal and specific goals of communication for health professionals
- State the role and purpose of introductions
- Understand the characteristics of a good introduction
- Demonstrate skills in introductions
- Recognise the scope of introductions
- Understand the importance of skills in providing information, specifically informing, instructing and explaining
- Demonstrate understanding that providing information is a two-way process that requires organisation, appropriate ordering and timing, and summarising.

The overall goal of all health professionals is to provide family/person-centred practice, which requires mutual understanding and a therapeutic relationship (see Ch 2). This goal should guide every interaction between health professionals and those seeking their assistance. There are, however, specific goals that also guide communication for health professionals. These specific goals may vary from one interaction to another. The first part of this discussion (Ch 3) examines the two major goals of

- Making verbal introductions
- Providing information.

Making introductions and providing information are two specific goals for communicating in the health professions. Many other goals for communicating fall within these two areas. The second part of the discussion relating to the specific goals of communication in the health professions examines the skills of i) gathering information (through interviewing and the related skill of questioning); ii) comforting; and iii) confronting. These skills require specific management to ensure appropriate outcomes for all individuals involved in an interaction, and it is for this reason that they are considered separately in Chapter 4.

Making verbal introductions

In family/person-centred services, the initial purpose of every health professional is to introduce themself, their role and their workplace environment. Introductions are a form of giving information, and many overlook their significance and potential impact. Introductions can establish a precedent for any future interactions with the individual; they 'set the tone and the scene' (Harms 2007). Through introductions, the person listening learns about the person introducing themself – this establishes the reliability and trustworthiness of the health professional. Introductions also demonstrate interest in the listening person and in the circumstances surrounding that person. Introductions should reassure the listening person, allowing them to decide whether they will continue listening. They should produce a sense of confidence that means the listening person will willingly invest in any future interactions.

In the health professions, the person listening – whether the person seeking assistance or a related person – is often vulnerable (Milliken & Honeycutt 2004). People often feel unsure of and overwhelmed by their circumstances and the generally unknown environment surrounding the health professions. This may be the case for new colleagues (including colleagues unfamiliar with the particular context) and students, in addition to individuals seeking the specific assistance of a health professional (Higgs et al 2005).

REFLECTION

Every introduction should reflect the essential characteristics that demonstrate family/person-centred practice.

- What generally occurs during an introduction?
- What constitutes a good introduction when you are in a new environment and do not know anyone?
- What makes introductions different for a health professional?
- What should the health professional introduce?

Remember: The people you are assisting are vulnerable and may feel disconnected. Consider what you might need to know if you were in their place.

Introductions generally provide information that allows the speaker and listener to achieve mutual understanding and establish whether they share a common experience or intent. The vulnerable person listening to a health professional is certainly listening for answers. In their mind, they have often-unconscious questions they want answered about the health professional talking to them (Harms 2007), for example, *Who is this person?, What do they want?, What can they do to help me?, Do they really want to help me?, Can I trust them?, Will they listen to me?, Will they understand me and therefore help me?, Will they really want the best for me?, Will they want what I want?, Are they worth listening to?, Do I want to keep listening?*

The verbal message or actual words used may contribute to the answers of only two or three of the questions in the listener's mind. In fact, during their first introduction the manner and non-verbal messages (see Ch 12) sent by the health professional will provide the most powerful message to the person seeking their assistance (Devito 2007). Both verbal and non-verbal messages influence future interactions and future collaboration between the person and the health professional.

Introducing yourself and your role

Introducing oneself is simple; it is a statement of a name. *Hi, I'm.....* is easy to say many times a day. Introducing the role of a health profession, however, can be challenging. A well-known and well-understood health profession in the public mind may seem easy to introduce. It may even be tempting to omit an introduction of such a health profession. However, possible preconceptions may cause confusion. If the role is not clearly understood in the particular context or setting this confusion requires clarification through questioning or a verbal or written explanation.

Some health professions are unknown or commonly misconstrued in the public mind. In such cases, preconceptions are equally challenging. It is important to use a clear and easy-to-understand explanation of the role of the profession. The use of professional jargon and potentially confusing descriptions must be avoided in this explanation. It may be useful to include specific examples of the role of the particular health profession in the specific setting or context. It may be important when explaining a role to understand the role of other health professions, because this may assist in dispelling confusion about the role of the profession in question compared with that of the other health professions. A written explanation can be helpful when working with adults and may address any misconceptions concerning the role of a particular health profession (Johnson & Stanford 2005).

Failure to introduce a particular role, or at least to question and clarify their understanding of the role, may result in a misunderstanding that is difficult to correct. More importantly, the people who require assistance may not receive the appropriate service. This certainly limits the possible outcomes for those who seek assistance.

REFLECTIVE ACTIVITY

- Write down the role of your health profession.
- Introduce yourself and explain your role to
  - Someone from your health profession. Do they understand you? Do they agree?
  - Someone from another health profession. Do they understand you? Do they agree? Discuss their perception of your health profession.
- Do you need to adjust your explanation because of the above responses?

Introducing the unfamiliar environment

There is usually an element of uncertainty and anxiety for an individual entering an unfamiliar environment (Purtilo & Haddad 2002). New environments create questions about a number of things – the physical layout of the environment, the people in the environment, the emotional safety and predictability of the environment, the possible events that will occur within the environment and, for some, survival within the new environment.

These questions and the overall goal of a health professional determine the order of an environmental introduction. Thus, the first part of an environmental introduction is usually introducing the physical environment. Essential information for all newcomers to an unfamiliar environment includes the location of the toilet! Introducing the physical environment does not merely assist in the orientation of the person but also allows the health professional and the person to begin progressing through the steps that facilitate family/person-centred practice.

Further information required for an environmental introduction will depend on the needs of the newcomer. If they indicate a need to know more about the events they can expect in the environment then a verbal or written description of the typical events should follow the physical introduction. It may be more appropriate to provide a deeper explanation of possible events as they occur, rather than when a person is new to an environment. Remember that the person is vulnerable and too much information in a new environment may be lost. When people feel vulnerable what they remember is often selective.

If the person demonstrates an interest in the people around them then a verbal or written introduction of the other people or professionals in the environment should follow the initial environmental introduction. This may be a suitable time to introduce these people or at least arrange a time for such an introduction. A written description of the people they might encounter and their respective roles may be beneficial. Allowing a person to read such a document at their leisure ensures understanding and may stimulate questions for future interactions.

If the newcomer exhibits anxiety of any kind, it may be necessary to demonstrate particular interest in their emotional safety. This demonstrates empathy (Davis 2006) and respect. Emotional safety is achieved by answering their questions or indicating interest in and care about their concerns. This behaviour indicates to the person that the health professional is willing to consider and address their concerns. Physical concerns are often easy to address, for example, a cup of something or a blanket. Emotional concerns take more thought and time to address. It is important at this early stage to spend time acknowledging their concerns and fears, and reassuring them with information to allay their fears (Stein-Parbury 2006). Statements such as *You'll be all right* and *You don't need to worry – we'll look after you here* will not reassure and they do not demonstrate empathy or respect. It is sometimes helpful to introduce a concerned and fearful person to another person with similar difficulties who has positive experiences associated with assistance from the particular health profession. Consideration of emotional concerns during an initial introduction is important because it establishes the new, unfamiliar environment as a safe and caring environment for future interactions.

CASE STUDIES

Person 1 (age 24) has pain in the lower back. They have been to lots of health services and do not have much confidence in this one to care about their needs or assist with their particular difficulties.

Person 2 (age 72) has never accessed any healthcare services – they have always been very healthy and active. They have had a fall while walking to their car after doing some grocery shopping and are experiencing extreme pain in their left hip. Suddenly finding themself at your health service they are worried about everything – they have no idea what is wrong, the pain is terrible, they are worried about their future, are afraid they may not be able to return home, they have no idea what happened to their shopping or the cat food, and what about the cat?... who will feed the cat?... pain and anxiety make it difficult to think.

ACTIVITY

This is the first time you have met the person described in each case study. Decide how best to demonstrate empathy, respect and behaviour worthy of trust using introductions. List what needs to be said and done to develop a therapeutic relationship and ensure family/person-centred practice.

Whether the health professional first provides or gathers information in their relationship with the person seeking assistance varies according to the needs of the person and the context. It is essential to consider the factors that affect both providing and gathering information. The order chosen in this book reflects the reality that introductions provide information. It is not intended to suggest that one has greater significance than the other or that one should occur before the other. In reality, when attempting to understand the perspective of the vulnerable individual, the health professional provides and gathers information simultaneously.

Providing information: A two-way process

A health professional provides information to various people throughout the working day. This information takes two main forms – verbal or written – and generally has the purpose of **informing**, **instructing** or **explaining**. When a health professional informs, they provide information about people, possible events or situations – usually about what to expect. This information may empower the person to act and react appropriately (Egan 2007). Instructions are directions about ways to successfully complete tasks or required procedures. Information or instructions will reassure the person and/or create questions. If the information creates questions then the health professional responds with more information in the form of answers that inform, instruct or explain. The health professional must respond to the needs of the person by providing the required information and ensuring it has been understood. The provision of information is a two-way process requiring mutual understanding.

REFLECTION

Understanding information
Consider a specific time when you received information (e.g. listening to the person next to you introduce themself or listening to the news). What made it easy to understand? What limited your understanding?

ACTIVITY

- Divide a page into two, top to bottom. On one side, list the factors that assisted your understanding and on the other side list those that limited your understanding.
- Using the information in this list, create a list of ways to effectively organise and present information to ensure understanding.

Regardless of the reason for providing information, it is important to consider the factors that facilitate understanding. These factors fall into three main categories: environmental, presentational and organisational. The environmental factors affecting understanding are described in Chapter 8.

Before presenting information it is important to **prepare the listener**. Preparing the listener involves asking permission to provide the information at that time. It requires a clear statement of the purpose and significance of the information. This simple, respectful preparation potentially relaxes the person and ensures that they listen to and focus upon understanding the information. It is important to establish if they know anything about the particular topic, event or procedure. Establishing their existing knowledge can be an appropriate point at which to begin presenting the information. This not only demonstrates respect and can develop trust, but also provides an opportunity to establish the accuracy of their previous knowledge. Discussion of their existing knowledge may also develop interest and enhance concentration.

The presentation of information must be clear and take into consideration the language needs (see Ch 15 and Section Four) and the physical, emotional and cognitive needs (see Ch 7) of the person. It is important to ensure the person is feeling well and able to concentrate, because if unwell or tired they will understand and retain less. In such circumstances, making another time to provide the information will be beneficial for all and is more likely to achieve effective communication.

To ensure effective communication it is important to avoid overlaying the information with opinion, bias or uncertainty (Mohan et al 2004). For example, *I think you should....*, *It is obvious you must...*, *Have you thought about doing...?*, *Maybe the procedure will be tomorrow* and so on. While presenting information it is important to avoid distractions. Present and explain one point at a time. State each point clearly and succinctly using precise language, and avoid using words such as *here, there, thing* etc. A long, complicated and wordy presentation of each point is time-consuming and often results in the listener losing concentration (Devito 2007).

When presenting each point health professionals should focus on that point until they are sure that the person understands. It is often helpful to provide examples to illustrate or explain each point because examples can facilitate comprehension. If instructing it may be beneficial to demonstrate the task while explaining each point. Reporting the experiences of other people receiving assistance from the specific service or health profession may also facilitate understanding, but maintaining confidentiality is imperative (see Ch 11). Repeating the important points can be appropriate and may enhance understanding. Take care, however, because repeating information may not be necessary and may negatively affect the receipt of the information.

Seeking indication of their understanding may be more beneficial than repetition, and the use of specific questions will confirm their actual understanding. Careful observation of the non-verbal responses of the person may also indicate their interest and understanding. When completing the presentation of the information it is important to provide an opportunity for the person to express their perception of the information, explore issues relevant to them and to ask questions. If giving instructions, close observation of the person performing the task will demonstrate their understanding and ensure safe performance of the task.

Organising the information is equally important. Compiling the information into points assists in achieving understanding, as does the order of each point. It may be appropriate to begin with areas of information that stimulate the most interest and then move to related but less motivating areas (Holli et al 2003). Initially it is helpful to introduce the main point of the information and then to present the detail of each connected point. Using language appropriate to the audience (see Ch 1) is important. When each point has been explained it is important to finish with either a summary of the main point(s) or questions that establish their understanding of each point. This repetition provides an opportunity to further process the information and ask questions that clarify meaning.

Organising the information includes consideration of the **timing** of the information provision. Giving detailed information about something that is 4 weeks away has limited relevance and meaning. Providing information about something that is immediate, however, will be both relevant and meaningful. Providing information in both verbal and written forms allows processing, answering of relevant questions and thus understanding. Research indicates that providing written information enhances retention and application levels (Johnson & Stanford 2005). The written form of any information must consider the abovementioned factors.

ACTIVITY

- Choose a procedure or routine typical to your health profession.
- Compile a clear and easy-to-understand written form about that procedure and all relevant information.
- Verbally present this information to someone who knows nothing about the procedure. Respond to any questions or comments until they clearly understand.
- If necessary adjust your verbal or written information to make it easier to understand.
- Present your form to people from your health profession. Discuss ways of refining and improving it.

Chapter summary

Introductions are crucial in establishing the quality and thus success of future interactions. Introducing oneself, the role of the particular health profession and the environment is important for family/person-centred practice and positive outcomes. The manner of presenting, organising and sequencing the relevant information (whether informing, instructing or explaining) has equal significance for positive outcomes in all health professions.

Complete the following:
1. The ultimate goal of health professions is

   _____

2. Introductions establish the quality of future interventions and include introducing
   i. _____
   ii. _____
   iii. _____

3. Providing information about a health profession can take two main forms:
   i. _____
   ii. _____

4. Providing information requires mutual understanding and may inform, instruct or explain. The manner of providing information should result in
   i. _____
   ii. _____

5. When providing information there are important principles to follow, including consideration of at least seven points. List the points below.
   i. _____
   ii. _____
   iii. _____
   iv. _____
   v. _____
   vi. _____
   vii. _____

6. Achieving mutual understanding when providing information requires

    i. _____

    ii. _____

References

Davis C M 2006 Patient practitioner interaction. An experiential manual for developing the art of healthcare, 4th edn. Slack, Thorofare NJ

Devito J A 2007 The interpersonal communication book, 11th edn. Pearson, Boston

Egan G 2007 The skilled helper, 8th edn. Thomson, Belmont CA

Harms D 2007 Working with people: communication skills for reflective practice. Oxford University Press, Melbourne

Higgs J, Sefton A, Street A et al 2005 Communicating in the health and social sciences. Oxford University Press, Melbourne

Holli B B, Calabrese R J, O'Sullivan Mailett J 2003 Communication and education skills for dietetics professionals, 4th edn. Lippincott, Williams & Wilkins, Philadelphia

Johnson A, Stanford J 2005 Written and verbal information versus verbal information only for patients being discharged from acute hospital settings to home: systematic review. Health Education Research: Theory and Practice 20:423–429

Milliken M A, Honeycutt A 2004 Understanding human behavior: a guide for healthcare providers, 7th edn. Thomson Delmar, New York

Mohan T, McGregor H, Saunders S et al 2004 Communicating as professionals. Thomson, Melbourne

Purtilo R B, Haddad A 2002 Health professional and patient interaction, 6th edn. Saunders, Philadelphia

Stein-Parbury J 2006 Patient and person: interpersonal skills in nursing, 3rd edn. Elsevier, Sydney (Original work published 2005)

The specific goals of communication for health professionals: 2

4

CHAPTER OBJECTIVES

Upon completing this chapter, students should be able to
- Identify the role of gathering information
- Outline the appropriate manner of gathering information
- List the different types of questions, their purpose and their effect
- Use questions to gather information
- Understand the significance of comforting
- Understand that every response can encourage or discourage
- State the significance and characteristics of encouragement versus discouragement
- State the basis of, role of and reasons for confronting.

The overall purpose of providing family/person-centred practice should guide every interaction between health professionals and those seeking their assistance (see Ch 2). The specific purpose of communication for health professionals is outlined in this book in two parts. The first part of the discussion (see Ch 3) describes introductions and providing information. The second part of the discussion comprises Chapter 4 and examines the specific purposes of

- Gathering information – interviewing and questioning
- Comforting – encouraging versus discouraging
- Confronting unhelpful attitudes and beliefs.

Gathering information

A health professional gathers various types of information from many sources throughout the working day. When gathering information it is important to consider the possible responses of the person providing the information, the effect of the environment (see Ch 8) and the possibly sensitive nature of the required information.

ACTIVITY

Ask the person next to you
- Their name
- Their health profession
- Where they were born
- How they travelled today
- Do they have a tattoo? If so, where is it?

REFLECTION

- How easy was it to obtain the information about the person next to you?
- Were there any difficulties? If so, what were they? What caused the difficulties?
- How did the interviewee feel?

The most common method of gathering information through personal interaction is the interview (Mohan et al 2004), whether formal or informal. The interviewing process in the health professions usually begins (although not always) with a more formal setting – the initial interview. This type of interview seeks to gather both general and specific information about the person and the factors affecting the person. Whether the interview is an initial interview or not it is reassuring for the person (the interviewee) to know the purpose of the interview (Holli et al 2003). Therefore, taking the time to explain the reason for each interview is a way of demonstrating respect and care for the interviewee(s). Regardless of the particular health profession or the purpose of the interview, the major tool used in any interview is the question.

Questioning: The tool

A question is a tool and, in common with most tools, it requires skill to use questions successfully. The skill of asking questions that gather the maximum amount of desired information in the required time is valuable in all resource-stretched health professions. It is important to know the purpose of questioning, what types of questions exist, the information they typically gather and the effect that particular questions may elicit in the listener. This knowledge assists health professionals when deciding exactly what question types to use or avoid when gathering information.

Why use questions?

A health professional does not use questions only to gather information. Questions serve several purposes that contribute to family/person-centred practice. Initially, questions assist the health professional to develop trust and rapport (Mohan et al 2004, Tyler et al 2005). The right question at the right time encourages the person seeking assistance to relax and develop confidence in the health professional, and may assist them in recognising a person who is interested in them (Devito 2007). Secondly, the right question can encourage the person to communicate, either verbally or non-verbally (Milliken & Honeycutt 2004). Questions can facilitate exploration of and elaboration about particular areas and thus provide additional relevant information (Davis 2006). Questions also establish mutual understanding – they clarify whether the person understands the health professional and whether the health professional understands them. Finally, regardless of the type of question, the ultimate goal of questioning is to gather information. It is this information that will create a clear understanding of the person and thus allow the health professional to act appropriately to establish and fulfil goals relevant to that person.

Types of questions and the information they gather

There are two main types of questions – closed and open questions.

Closed questions

Closed questions elicit discreet information that is short and definite (Harms 2007, Mohan et al 2004, Tyler et al 2005). They are often recognised as questions that have a yes or no answer. For example, *Is the pain sharp? Did you use the splint? Have you kept to your diet? Is your workstation comfortable?*

In family/person-centred practice, after an introduction, the first question should be a closed one that seeks the permission of the person to ask some questions. For example, *Is it all right if I ask you some questions?* Such a question demonstrates respect, a desire to empathise (Davis 2006) and an indication that the person seeking assistance from this particular health professional may have control over the events directly relating to them. After asking this initial question it is best to use open questions until there is trust and adequate levels of rapport.

When communicating with people who do not have English as their native language it is important to remember that there are different ways of answering particular kinds of closed questions that can cause confusion. In English, the question *It doesn't hurt, does it?* requires a yes if it hurts or a no if it does not hurt. In some languages such a question requires the opposite answer – yes indicates it does not hurt while no indicates it does hurt. This difference in responses provides a warning for health professionals; it indicates that the use of particular types of closed questions with individuals from non-English-speaking backgrounds requires careful clarification and negotiation to establish mutual understanding. It may be tempting to use closed questions with such people because they require minimal spoken language, however, confining the use of closed questions to simple questions may avoid confusion.

When communicating with people from a non-English-speaking background it may also be tempting to rely on movements of the head to indicate yes or no. This can also create confusion, however, because different cultures use shaking and nodding the head to mean different things. Thus, it is important for health professionals to be aware that the use of this type of non-verbal communication may also create confusion when attempting to establish mutual understanding with such individuals.

Some closed questions require specific and discreet information rather than yes or no (Mohan et al 2004). For example, *Where is the pain most severe? For how long did you wear the splint? How many days did you keep to your diet? What is it about your workstation (e.g. desk, chair, computer) that causes the most discomfort or pain?*

Another form of closed questioning that requires discreet or specific information is the multiple-choice question. Multiple-choice questions can be useful if people are unable to express themselves specifically. Instead, the health professional uses their knowledge of the specific situation to provide possible answers. These answers can assist the person to clarify their thoughts and thus provide an appropriate answer (Stein-Parbury 2006). *Would you describe the pain as burning, sharp, dull, gripping, pressing, in a particular place or moving?* is one example of a multiple-choice question.

- Think of an issue specific to your health profession and create a multiple-choice question about this issue. (If relevant you may use the questions above re pain, splinting, diet or workstation; if not, devise a relevant and appropriate question.)
- Use the question with a friend to test its clarity and effect. Explain any terms specific to your profession if necessary.

In all closed questions there is only one answer, which is short, definite and clear. The question does not require elaboration or descriptive detail. Closed questions can be useful when the health professional requires particular types of information. They demand little of the person, can save time and provide the exact answer without the complications of too much thought or too many words.

Open questions

Open questions are the other main type of question. There is no wrong or right answer to an open question. These questions give the person answering control over the interview and allow the health professional to listen, observe and learn (Harms 2007, Tyler et al 2005). Open questions are useful when the required information is not discreet and may need thoughtful use of memory, elaboration, opinion, detail and sometimes sharing of experiences and feelings. Open questions can be less threatening because they allow the person answering to control the information they give and, therefore, are best used at the beginning of an interaction. Open questions are useful when there is a need to explore or elaborate on a particular subject (Devito 2007). They are also useful when changing the subject or when gathering information from a sensitive or defensive person. Open questions may begin with *How…?* and *What…?*, but can also begin with phrases such as *Tell me about….*

ACTIVITY

Change the following closed questions into open ones.
- Do you feel angry?
- How many children do you have?
- Did you keep to your diet this week?
- Did you follow your exercise regimen carefully?
- Is your workstation comfortable?

Questions that probe

Questions that probe usually seek more information about a particular topic (Stein-Parbury 2006). They should encourage the person to provide more detail about the information already provided (Tyler et al 2005). The subject of probing questions usually arises from information provided during the interaction and begins with phrases such as *Can you tell me more about…? What happened before…? What were you thinking when …… happened? How did you feel about…?* The answers to probing questions provide specific detail about situations, people, events, thoughts and feelings. They can provide deeper insight into the person, their supports and needs and, often, their feelings.

Probing questions can also change the focus or return the focus to an earlier point in the conversation (Stein-Parbury 2006). A probing question is useful if the health professional requires information about something different to the current focus, or if the health professional thinks of something more they need to know about a previous point. Overuse of probing questions may create a negative response in the person seeking the assistance, however, because probing questions can produce the feeling of interrogation (Harms 2007). It is important to be aware of the responses of the person (see Ch 7) and react in a manner that fulfils both the general and specific goals of communication in the health professions.

Questions that clarify

Questions that clarify usually seek understanding rather than information (Stein-Parbury 2006). If the person gives information that is unclear or may be interpreted several ways, the health professional can ask for clarification or an explanation (Devito 2007, Mohan et al 2004), for example, *What did you mean when you said…? Can you explain what happened…? Do you mean…?* Questions that clarify can be used by either the person or the health professional. Such questions are important in order to avoid misunderstandings (Purtilo & Haddad 2002) and achieve mutual understanding. Any incomplete meaning or lack of understanding may result in assumptions that limit the possible outcomes of the interventions.

Overuse of questions that clarify meaning may have a negative effect on the interaction. They may suggest the health professional is not able to understand or make themself understood to the person. It is important in such situations to listen effectively and to demonstrate respect and empathy rather than frustration while attempting to establish mutual understanding.

Questions that 'lead'

Leading questions direct the response of the listener. They are not person-centred, do not give the person control and usually do not provide honest responses. A vulnerable person will answer a leading question according to the cues in the question that indicate the desired answer. For example, *It's a beautiful day, isn't it?* leads the listener to agree and say *Yes, beautiful*; or *Oh it's a bit hot isn't it?* leads the listener to agree that it is indeed hot, regardless of what they really feel. Leading questions such as these do not necessarily have a negative effect (Purtilo & Haddad 2002). If the subject of a leading question is external to the person, their actions and needs, then the effect can be positive, creating a link between the health professional and the person. Such questions do not ask for important information and thus are not threatening; they are a verbal recognition of the presence of the person.

Leading questions are not always positive, however. A health professional who uses leading questions will limit the development of trust and the accuracy of the gathered information. For example, questions such as *You weren't drinking while you were on this medication were you? You're all right aren't you? That didn't hurt so much did it? We covered how to care for your back and I know you understand the importance of caring for your back, so I know you didn't try to move furniture did you?* usually direct the person to the required answer – *No I was not drinking, Yes I'm all right, No that was OK* and *No I did not move furniture* – regardless of the truth. It is best to avoid leading questions (Mohan et al 2004) if the health professional seeks to encourage an honest relationship based on trust, respect and non-judgement, as well as relevant and appropriate outcomes.

Think back to the earlier activity: 'Ask the person next to you'.
• What did you want to know more about? List questions that would gather this information.
• Was there anything that was not necessarily clear? List the questions that would clarify your understanding.
• Can you think of a leading question you might ask?
• Now, if possible, ask the same person a question that probes for more information, one that clarifies your understanding and maybe even a leading question.
• Discuss what feeling each question created in the interviewee. Note the different feelings experienced, if any, and relate them to the different types of questions.

The skill of questioning depends upon another beneficial skill – listening (see Ch 10). However, a successful interview involves more than skill in questioning and listening. It also involves appropriate timing of questions, the use of appropriate non-verbal messages (see Ch 12), the use of silences and, most importantly, a focus on the vulnerable person who requires the assistance of the health professional (see Chs 7 & 8).

Comforting: Encouraging versus discouraging

The vulnerable and sometimes disconnected people seeking the assistance of health professionals often share their anxieties and negative emotions with those health professionals. The health professional has knowledge of their particular health service and understands exactly what that service offers while the people they assist do not have that knowledge or understanding. The health professional also possesses knowledge about conditions and the consequences of those conditions which the people seeking assistance may not possess (Higgs et al 2005). This knowledge may make it difficult for the health professional to understand the concerns, anxieties and negative emotions of vulnerable individuals. However, this very knowledge dictates careful and respectful management of all interactions between the health professional and the people seeking assistance (Egan 2007). The health professional is responsible for ensuring that people are comforted in a manner that encourages, affirms and empowers them to continue with meaning, purpose and quality in their life. Remember that such people may also include a colleague new to the service or a student.

• Consider a time when you were feeling anxious or negative about something – perhaps an examination or a job interview, or feedback from an assignment.
• Did you share your feelings with anyone? How did they respond? How did you feel after they responded? Was it the way they responded that created your feelings?

The way in which a health professional responds to expressions of anxiety or negative emotions either encourages, affirms and empowers or discourages, trivialises and dismisses that person and their anxieties or emotions (Devito 2007).

Characteristics of encouragement and discouragement

The characteristics of encouraging and discouraging responses to expressions of negative emotions are outlined in Table 4.1.

Characteristics of encouraging versus discouraging responses to expressions of negative emotions	
Encouraging responses	**Discouraging responses**
• Focus attention on the person and acknowledge their emotions • Indicate that in this situation such emotions are common • Indicate (without a detailed description) that the health professional has some understanding because of a similar experience • Ask for clarification of the emotions and the cause.	• State that there is no need to feel the emotions • Acknowledge the emotions but change the subject • Interrupt, to avoid hearing the expression of such emotions • Totally ignore the expressions of emotions.

TABLE 4.1

ACTIVITY

Classifying responses to negative emotions
Consider each response to the following expressions of anxiety and decide whether it is encouraging or discouraging.

1. *Person: I am really worried about this surgery.*
   Health professional (HP): You don't need to worry. Dr Super is a great surgeon and the procedure is routine.

2. *Person: I don't know how I will cope at home.*
   HP: Don't worry, you'll be OK. There's lots of help available.

3. *Person: I don't like hospitals – my Dad died in one.*
   HP: No wonder you don't like hospitals! That must have been difficult. Can you tell me about it?

4. *Person: Boy we are busy today. Two new people have just arrived. I don't think I will get everything done.*
   HP: The quicker you get over that feeling the better. It is always the same here – busy, busy!

5. *Person: I am just not coping here – I can't do this.*
   HP: You're feeling overwhelmed. Mmm (watching as the person struggles to complete a task and then gives up) ... that can be difficult. What are you struggling with most?

6. *Person: I am angry. I need that report for the appointment tomorrow and it's not ready.*
   HP: I understand your anger. I am not too impressed either – it was supposed to be ready today. What time is the appointment? Maybe it can be delivered there tomorrow before the appointment.   ↳

↳ How would you typically respond to each of these statements? Change the discouraging, trivialising and dismissive responses to encouraging, affirming and empowering responses. Create other ways of responding to each statement that are affirming and encouraging.

It is obvious from the examples above that the easiest and shortest way to respond to negative emotions has a discouraging effect. It may seem appropriate to the health professional because they have both relevant knowledge and previous experience but such responses do not meet the needs of the anxious or negative individual. Health professionals are often busy and thus it is easy to respond in a manner that requires minimal time or effort. When communicating with an anxious or negative person, however, it is important to respond in a manner that indicates interest, respect and empathy. Such a response is an investment that ultimately saves time. Responding in this manner is not always easy when the health professional has knowledge and understanding that overrides the negative emotions. It is important, however, to respond in a non-judgemental way that indicates the equality of the vulnerable person. People often feel vulnerable when in an unknown area of expertise. Responses that demonstrate a superiority of knowledge without sharing that knowledge will only discourage and may appear dismissive. A dismissive response does not acknowledge the emotions – whether logical or illogical – of any person seeking assistance from a health professional. Producing encouraging, affirming and empowering responses is sometimes difficult but is essential to maintain family/person-centred practice.

ROLE PLAYS

Practising encouraging responses

Role-play each scenario in pairs, taking turns to play the health professional (who responds encouragingly) and the person. Compare the responses and note the different effects of the responses. List the responses that were encouraging, affirming and empowering.

Person 1: You are worried about your family because you are the person who always organises their meals and now you have a broken shoulder.

Person 2: You are angry and frustrated because you have not improved in the way the doctor said you would after the surgery on your back. The doctor has not answered your questions nor given any explanation for your lack of improvement.

Person 3: Your child is in the final stages of leukaemia. You are emotionally exhausted and are worried about being able to remain emotionally calm and supportive to your spouse and family as you watch him die.

Person 4: You have had your leg amputated because of a car accident. You cannot see how you can go back to work – you are a roof tiler. You are worried about your finances.

Person 5: You are a national sports star and you have recently had a relatively minor knee injury. You are worried that your coach will replace you while you are recovering.

Person 6: You are frustrated and desperate because your 79-year-old husband fell more than 20 hours ago – he is in extreme pain, has been left to lie on a trolley for all that time and no-one seems interested in examining him.

In the busy life of a health professional it is important that any words are comforting and that they encourage and empower those seeking assistance.

Confronting unhelpful attitudes or beliefs

Many individuals who seek the assistance of health professionals express attitudes and beliefs that restrict their communication, recovery and participation. The health professional can challenge the person to examine these attitudes and beliefs by confronting and, in some cases, disagreeing with the person (Milliken & Honeycutt 2004). If expressed with empathy, confrontation or challenge can facilitate new perspectives, thoughts and behaviours in many individuals (Ellis et al 2004, Stein-Parbury 2006), thereby improving the effectiveness of communication. Confrontation provides an opportunity to highlight the discrepancies or inconsistencies apparent in the life or environment of the individual (Holli et al 2003). It can empower individuals to face those discrepancies, patterns of thought and actions that require change and adjust them to facilitate improved communication, recovery and increased participation (Brill & Levine 2005).

Only experienced health professionals should attempt to confront attitudes or beliefs. If an inexperienced health professional is concerned about the attitudes and beliefs of a particular individual seeking their assistance it is advisable to develop a therapeutic relationship with that person and discuss any action with a health professional experienced in confronting or challenging. Egan (2007) states that the health professional must 'earn the right to challenge'. This statement indicates the significance of the therapeutic relationship when confronting. Any confrontation or challenge must arise from a developed therapeutic relationship that demonstrates respect and rapport. If there is genuine mutual understanding and freedom from judgement, confrontation may increase the likelihood of positive communication and outcomes.

Brill & Levine (2005) and Egan (2007) agree that any confrontation or challenge must be specific and relate to a particular attitude or belief. General confrontation that judges and intimidates a person will damage rather than empower. Statements such as *You are your own worst enemy – you depress yourself* will only discourage. However, asking a question relating to a particular belief (e.g. *Do you think it is true that your life is terrible? Can you think of anything that was good yesterday?*) might confront the individual with the belief that is limiting their functioning and perhaps encourage them to think differently about their life. A positive change in thought patterns will increase interest, communication, participation and recovery.

When confronting it is important that the health professional uses non-verbal messages that reinforce rather than contradict the verbal message. If the voice, face or hands of the speaker contradict the spoken words, this inconsistency will produce negative emotions in the listener (Tyler et al 2005) and make the confrontation useless.

Confrontation should not judge or criticise. It should not provide the opportunity for the health professional to express anger or frustration (Brill & Levine 2005). Nor should confrontation or challenge ever be direct and assertive, because strength of expression may become a barrier that disempowers the individual (Egan 2007). Instead, tentative expression will allow the person to confront the attitude or belief and thus potentially facilitate the required changes in thought and actions. Confrontation is about respect and understanding that encourages and strengthens the vulnerable individual to embrace changes in thoughts and behaviours.

CASE STUDY

A young person has failed an assessment task, receiving a third of the possible marks. Very distressed and near to tears they express belief that they just cannot do the course – that they are 'dumb' and cannot learn anyway.

The lecturer has noticed that the general attitude and manner of the student suits the health professions and, while she feels there was limited application to the assessment task, makes a choice about how to respond.

REFLECTION

- What is your response?
- Will you judge? Write down how and why.
- Will you encourage? Write down how and why.
- Will you confront and challenge? Write down how and why.

ROLE PLAYS

In groups of four assign two people to observe and scribe, and two to play the following roles. Continue acting the role play until there is some kind of closure.

Person 1: You are the lecturer. Respond to the distressed student. Choose how you will respond before the role play begins.

Person 2: You are the distressed student. Talk to the lecturer. You feel that the mark for your assignment simply reinforces that you cannot be successful in this health professional course. You did very well during professional placement but you cannot do the academic work.

- Discuss the effect of the communication – the reactions and feelings evoked. How did the lecturer respond? Did the response encourage the student to change their beliefs about themself? Did the non-verbal behaviours support the words?
- Repeat the role play and the discussion with different people in the different roles.

It is challenging for health professionals to confront the attitudes or beliefs of another person but, if performed appropriately, confrontation produces positive outcomes for the individual seeking assistance. The willingness of health professionals to challenge themselves enhances the ability to confront (Egan 2007). If health professionals are comfortable with confronting and challenging their own attitudes and beliefs they will be more able to understand the needs of the individuals they seek to confront. Confrontation in the health professions is not something that necessarily occurs every day. When used appropriately, however, confrontation enhances and produces effective communication, participation and recovery.

Chapter summary

Health professionals commonly gather information through interviewing. Questions assist the development of trust and rapport, and establish mutual understanding. A person seeking the assistance of a health professional often feels vulnerable. The health professional is responsible for responding to negative emotions by comforting the person in a manner that encourages and empowers them. Confronting attitudes that restrict the participation of the person can facilitate improved participation and recovery.

Complete the following:

1. When gathering information, the health professional must consider three major factors:

    i. _____

    ii. _____

    iii. _____

2. Health professionals gather information by interviewing. When interviewing it is important to

    i. _____

    ii. _____

3. Questions can achieve much, but five main achievements are noted in this chapter:

    i. _____

    ii. _____

    iii. _____

    iv. _____

    v. _____

4. There are two main types of questions.
    • List five features of closed questions.

        i. _____

        ii. _____

        iii. _____

        iv. _____

        v. _____

    • List five features of open questions.

        i. _____

        ii. _____

        iii. _____

        iv. _____

        v. _____

5. Vulnerable people do not usually have the required k_____ or u_____ to feel comfortable.

6. Responding to expressions of emotion can e_____ or d_____.

7. Encouraging and discouraging responses have particular characteristics. List three characteristics of encouraging responses.

    i. _____

    ii. _____

    iii. _____

8. The health professional should respond with

    _____

9. Confrontation challenges attitudes and beliefs and has positive results. It requires

   i. _____

   ii. _____

   iii. _____

   iv. _____

10. What must a health professional confront in themselves in order to confront effectively?

   _____

   _____

   _____

References

Brill N I, Levine J 2005 Working with people: the helping process, 8th edn. Pearson, Boston

Davis C M 2006 Patient practitioner interaction. An experiential manual for developing the art of healthcare, 4th edn. Slack, Thorofare NJ

Devito J A 2007 The interpersonal communication book, 11th edn. Pearson, Boston

Egan G 2007 The skilled helper, 8th edn. Thomson, Belmont CA

Ellis R B, Gates B, Kenworthy N 2004 Interpersonal communication in nursing, 2nd edn. Churchill Livingstone, London

Harms D 2007 Working with people: communication skills for reflective practice. Oxford University Press, Melbourne

Higgs J, Sefton A, Street A et al 2005 Communicating in the health and social sciences. Oxford University Press, Melbourne

Holli B B, Calabrese R J, O'Sullivan Mailett J 2003 Communication and education skills for dietetics professionals, 4th edn. Lippincott, Williams & Wilkins, Philadelphia

Milliken M A, Honeycutt A 2004 Understanding human behavior: a guide for healthcare providers, 7th edn. Thomson Delmar, New York

Mohan T, McGregor H, Saunders S et al 2004 Communicating as professionals. Thomson, Melbourne

Purtilo R B, Haddad A 2002 Health professional and patient interaction, 6th edn. Saunders, Philadelphia

Stein-Parbury J 2006 Patient and person: interpersonal skills in nursing, 3rd edn. Elsevier, Sydney (Original work published 2005)

Tyler S, Kossen C, Ryan C 2005 Communication: a foundation course, 2nd edn. Pearson, Prentice Hall, Frenchs Forest, Sydney

TWO

DEVELOPING AWARENESS TO ACHIEVE EFFECTIVE COMMUNICATION IN THE HEALTH PROFESSIONS

Awareness of and need for reflective practice

5

CHAPTER OBJECTIVES

Upon completing this chapter, students should be able to

- Recognise the importance of reflection for effective communication
- Demonstrate understanding of the importance of reflection for the health professions
- State the difference between reflective and reflexive practice
- Understand the significance of the result of reflection – changes in thoughts and actions
- List their own barriers (defenses) to experiencing and resolving negative emotions
- Reflect about their own functioning and thus their abilities when communicating.

Effective communication requires an understanding of how an individual affects others and how others affect the individual (Higgs et al 2005). It requires awareness of the 'self' and the effects of personality and communication styles upon interactions. Effective communication requires an understanding of how elements of the self, the 'other' and the environment influence the outcomes of interactions. Reflection promotes this understanding.

Reflection is the process through which experience, knowledge and theory are used to guide and inform thoughts, action and practice (Thompson 2002). Reflection ultimately facilitates the transformation of the individual and thus transforms the thoughts and actions of that individual to achieve positive outcomes in practice (Brown & Ryan 2003). Reflection achieves the necessary awareness of those factors that contribute to the self-maintenance essential for health professionals. It also contributes to their effectiveness when communicating. These reasons make reflective practice important for health professionals.

The 'what' of reflection: A definition

Reflection provides connection with and awareness of unconscious emotional processing (Pritchard 2005). Please note that reflection in this context is not synonymous with meditation. Reflection occurs when individuals examine their attitudes and reactions to an interactive experience. It reveals causes of negative emotional responses, which facilitates understanding of these reactions. It allows resolution of these causes and, ultimately, changes in thought and thus behaviour in preparation for more positive responses in similar future interactions. The process of reflection usually makes some parts of an interaction clearer and may allow the fading or removal of other parts (see Figure 5.1).

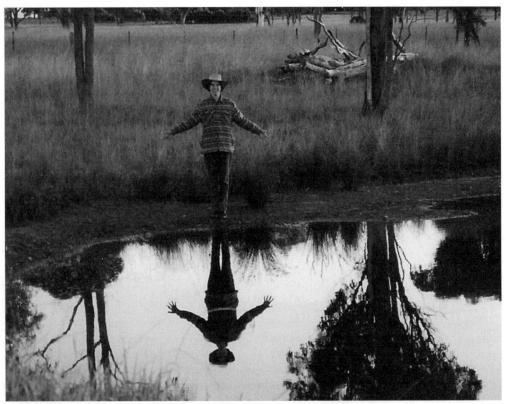

FIGURE 5.1 Some things become clearer when reflecting and others fade.

Boud & Walker (1991) suggest that reflection is the basis of knowledge. Reflection for the health professional is certainly the basis of self-knowledge. Payne (2006) describes reflection as being the bridge between theory and practice. Reflection can certainly form the theoretical basis of effective communication, because effective communication is not possible without reflection. Some view reflection as the process of revisiting experiences in order to understand them. When reflection results in changes in behaviour over time to manage similar situations with greater satisfaction, this is known as reflective practice (Gustafson & Fagerberg 2004, Stein-Parbury 2006). Others see reflection as a consideration of the way in which the self affects and is affected by particular events; this is known as reflexivity (Finlay & Gough 2003). Perhaps the best health professionals are both reflective and reflexive.

Reflection for a health professional consists of thoughtful and often critical consideration of events and reactions occurring during previous interactions or times of decision-making (Harms 2007). Such reflection promotes understanding of the thoughts, attitudes and associated reactions that occurred during those interactions or while making those decisions. It facilitates clearer understanding of the causes of the negative reactions that can occur during interactions. Reflection highlights areas needing conscious attention and further exploration, and can result in acceptance and resolution of the causes of negative reactions. Resolution facilitates behavioural change and thus positive outcomes during future interactions. Note that reflection here is not about 'reflecting back' the perceptions of the feelings of the 'other'.

For health professionals, reflection is about careful, deliberate and critical consideration of events that take place during communicative interactions. It does not provide a formula for thoughts or behaviours, or a 'one-answer-fits-all' solution, but it does provide insight and understanding upon which to base behaviour during future interactions (Thompson 2002).

The result of reflection: Achieving self-awareness

Reflection is the primary method of achieving **self-awareness**. Reflection reveals the reality of the unique nature of each individual and promotes understanding of self and others (Miller 2003). Reflection has the potential to create a new awareness of self. It provides direction for constructive use of that knowledge to establish the truth about the self and related events (Plack 2006). This truth allows the individual to institute different methods of relating, reacting and being (Backus & Chapian 2000). This reflection promotes change in actions and reactions.

REFLECTION

- How have the comments of others about your abilities affected your performance in particular activities? Think about the positive or negative comments of a parent, teacher, friend, acquaintance or fellow worker.
- Does it enhance or erode your motivation and performance when someone does or does not believe in your abilities despite the reality of the situation?
- How important are the opinions of others to you?

Reflection is a process through which the individual considers and learns from positive and negative experiences. The individual considers the meaning of their experiences and why the experiences have that particular meaning (Andrews 2000, Roberts 2002). This consideration facilitates understanding of the inadequacy, fear or vulnerability of the inner-self that manipulates and directs thoughts and responses during interactive events (Ben-Arye et al 2007). These inadequacies and fears often cause negative and regrettable events during interactions. Reflection is the process that facilitates understanding of the action required to overcome the inadequacies, fears or vulnerabilities that manipulate the reactions of individuals when communicating.

Particular individuals react differently to reflecting, and factors such as personality, age and gender affect interest in and commitment to reflection. Because reflection promotes informed and controlled thought and thus action, practising reflection has potential benefit for all health professionals regardless of personality, age or gender.

REFLECTION

- Do you usually 'reflect' about interactive events?
- Do you replay positive interactions or simply savour the emotions associated with those interactions?
- Do you replay unpleasant and uncomfortable interactions?
- Think of interactions you have had in which there were negative feelings.
  - *In situations where you cause the reason for bad feelings*, what do you usually do after the interaction? Do you regret your actions? Do you replay the interaction while thinking of different ways to react next time? Do you feel guilty? Do you think the other person deserved the bad feelings? Do you try to think of how you can redeem the situation and/or relationship? Do you feel OK about admitting you were inappropriate and apologising? Do you simply forget it and move on? Can you describe your typical reaction if it is none of the above? Does your reaction depend on the closeness of the relationship? Why do you think this is so? Should the closeness of a relationship be relevant when practising as a health professional?
  - Consider each reaction listed above.
    - Which are unproductive? How can *you* avoid these reactions?
    - Which are productive and an investment for future interactions? How can *you* ensure such productive reactions in the future?
  - *In situations where another person provides the reason for discomfort*, how do you usually react after the interaction? Do you feel hurt and continue 'licking your wounds' for some time? Do you think about it often and avoid seeing the other person if you can do so? Do you minimise interacting with them if you have to see them? Do you find it difficult to understand how anyone could treat you that way? Do you feel angry and resentful towards the person? Do you try to understand their behaviour and thus forgive them? Do you talk about their behaviour to other friends to try to discourage others from relating to that person? Do you reflect upon why you feel hurt, explore the reasons and resolve them? Do you place 'walls' around your emotions so you never feel hurt in an interaction? Do you think the reaction of the other person tells you more about them than it does about you and therefore understand that you do not need to feel hurt (i.e. do you have control of your emotional 'button')? Do you think life is too short and move on?
  - Consider each reaction listed above.
    - Which are unproductive? How can *you* avoid these reactions?
    - Which are productive and an investment for future interactions? How can *you* ensure such productive reactions in the future?

The 'why' of reflection: Reasons for reflecting

Reflection is an important means of learning about attitudes, experiences and self (Mohan et al 2004, O'Toole 2007, Plack 2006). It provides information that promotes improved performance when communicating with others, allowing health professionals to repeat actions and reactions that achieve positive outcomes and to change them when they have a negative effect. Reflection provides health professionals with awareness about their individual abilities (Jack & Smith 2007, Kinsella 2001) and also highlights abilities and skills that are lacking. Thus, through reflection health professionals can focus on improving those skills that will increase their emotional control and therefore facilitate family/person-centred practice.

REFLECTIVE ACTIVITY

- List at least five things you know you perform well.
- List five things in which you would like to improve your performance.
- Ask someone who knows you well to make a similar list.
- Ask this person *Do you know how I will react to your list?* Was their expectation of your reaction correct?
- Compare both lists. Are they similar? Consider the other person's list and explore why you might agree or disagree with their list.

Reflection allows health professionals to understand the 'chaos' sometimes evident during interactions (Purtilo & Haddad 2002, Stein-Parbury 2006). It indicates that individuals are responsible for their own reactions and emotions, whether the individual is the health professional or the person seeking assistance. Reflection reveals that no-one can actually make another person feel particular emotions or make them react in a particular way. It indicates that feelings and emotional responses come from within the individual and usually originate from previous life experiences. Reflection releases the health professional to understand that they are not the cause of emotional responses in others and that the other person is not the cause of the emotional responses of the health professional. It provides the understanding that individuals behave and respond in particular ways because of underlying, usually internal causes. This realisation encourages the tolerance and understanding that promotes unconditional positive regard of individuals regardless of the situation (Purtilo & Haddad 2002, Rogers 1967).

REFLECTION

- When you have a negative emotional response to an interactive event, what is your usual reaction? Do you say or think *They/It made me feel really bad?* Is this your typical response?
- If so, have you ever explored the reasons why you respond in this manner in particular circumstances?
- Have you ever thought that negative emotions are your responsibility?
- Have you ever thought *I make a choice about how I will feel* during an interaction?
- Have you ever wondered about the other person and what caused them to relate in that particular way?
- Can you see the benefit of considering the above perspectives? That is, that
  - Your attitudes and reactions are your responsibility and you may need to explore your reactions and resolve the causes.
  - A negative interaction reveals more about the other person than it does about you and thus their reactions are not your responsibility.
- Reflect on the benefits of understanding that you are responsible for your own reactions to situations – that you cannot make anyone feel a particular emotion and nor can others make you feel emotions. You alone control your responses; you alone can choose how you will feel and react.

Reflection offers the individual an understanding of their primary need (see Ch 6), allowing them the opportunity to fulfil that need outside of their work environment. If health professionals seek fulfilment of their driving need within their professional life, not only will they experience disappointment but they will fail to provide family/person-centred practice. All individuals are responsible for their emotional responses and for how they fulfil their driving need.

Reflection provides understanding that the value of an individual does not come from what people think of that individual, the role the individual has in society, the car they drive or the clothes they wear. Individual value comes from within through understanding and respecting the self.

REFLECTION

- What do you feel gives you value?
- What do you feel gives other people value?
- From the perspective of a health professional, consider the benefits and limitations of believing that individual value comes from achievements or external factors (e.g. social status, colour, race, sporting skill or musical skill etc).

Reflection provides understanding that not only increases self-control, but also promotes self-honesty, self-awareness, self-acceptance and ultimately self-respect. If health professionals are able to practise these they will be more able to demonstrate awareness, honesty, acceptance and respect towards the vulnerable individuals seeking assistance (Purtilo & Haddad 2002). Demonstration of self-awareness promotes the overall goal of every health profession – family/person-centred practice.

REFLECTION

- How comfortable are you with considering your emotional responses? Do you find it easy or do you prefer to avoid experiencing emotions?
- Do you think that feeling emotions is a sign of weakness? If so, why?
- Do you think *your* emotional responses are never important? If so, why are the feelings of others more important than your feelings?
- Do you find that your emotions dominate your actions? If so, why is this?
- Do you think you really do not have emotional responses? If so, it is important to remember that everyone feels; why do you block yourself from feeling your emotions?
- Are the thoughts isolated through answering these questions true? For example, is it true that the feelings of others are more important than your feelings? Where do these thoughts originate?

Rudduck & Turner (2007) indicate that reflection is important when learning about previously unknown cultural contexts. It provides an understanding about the culture of the health professional compared with the previously unknown culture. This understanding can facilitate appropriate behaviour and communicative interactions to ensure effective communication with people from other cultures.

Health professionals who reflect are able to identify the reasons for their negative reactions during interactions and, as a result, resolve the causes of these reactions. They are able to improve their skills in managing emotional responses (of themselves and others) that control and negatively influence communication with the 'other'. Such health professionals are able to use their skills of reflecting to observe and recognise emotions in those around them and thus validate and clarify these emotions and their possible causes.

The 'how' of reflection: Models of reflection

So how does one reflect? It is not difficult to consider some past interactions – the more pleasant ones usually do not pose questions, just happiness and pleasure. However, the uncomfortable ones often leave an individual wondering how and why. To remove any guilt associated with such interactions an individual will often wish to re-experience the events for an opportunity to react differently. Alternatively, individuals may feel hurt and resentment because of the actions or words of another during an uncomfortable interaction. The purpose of reflection is to provide information that empowers the health professional to react appropriately and thus i) avoid regret and guilt; or ii) understand, accept and forgive rather than feel hurt and resentment.

A model of reflection is a helpful tool when attempting to answer the question of how to reflect. A model guides an individual through a process. It explains the way to complete a process. Some may think that the process of reflection does not require directions or a plan because it simply requires the individual to ask and answer questions (Mohan et al 2004). While this may be true, some people find it difficult to establish which questions to ask and to determine the exact focus of those questions. Sometimes thoughts lack clarity when uncomfortable emotions are being experienced and thus a model can bring clarity and resolution to those emotions by providing a focus for possible questions. Such focus facilitates appropriate and adequate answers for any communicative interaction, but is particularly useful when considering uncomfortable interactions. The information in the following paragraphs is adapted from an article by Boud & Walker (1990).

Reflection upon an interaction requires returning to the interaction through either thought, verbal word, written word or some combination of all three (Ellis et al 2004). Consideration should be given to the individuals involved in the interaction and *all* the known information about each person (e.g. knowledge of and past experience in relating to these individuals). Examining the process leading to the outcome of previous interactions can guide the health professional to understand this outcome. This understanding, together with other information (e.g. whether they appear happy, tired, hurried, preoccupied etc), is something most people relate to and absorb unconsciously when beginning an interaction. The appearance of the person or their non-verbal behaviour or perhaps an environmental factor (e.g. the threat of rain can cause preoccupation) provides this information. Consciously considering such information assists when reflecting about an interaction.

GROUP ACTIVITY

- List the factors and skills relating to the 'person' that require consideration when reflecting about interacting (e.g. age, knowledge, experience, emotional state etc). First consider the health professional, then the person seeking their assistance and then a colleague. Refer to the previous chapters of this book when compiling the list.
- What other factors might be included in *all* in the above paragraph?

Reflection should also involve consideration of the intent of each interacting person. It should establish whether the intent of each person was clear initially and throughout the interaction, and whether everyone in the interaction had the same intent or purpose. If there were differences in the intent of each person, consideration could be given to the way in which this variation influenced the outcome of the interaction. Reflection should involve consideration of a method for clarifying intent in future interactions. Consideration of how an individual was feeling before the interaction (i.e. were there related or unrelated events causing negative emotions before the interaction that may have adversely affected their intent unconsciously?) is important and may explain differences in purpose or intent.

CASE STUDY

Edith is a 76-year-old mother of three. She has been falling regularly lately, and her last fall caused her to fracture her neck of femur. As Edith has indicated she feels unsafe living alone, a family meeting to discuss her future living arrangements is organised for today. One of her daughters has been happy to talk about Edith living with her, so the team is confident that this meeting will be positive with an agreeable outcome for all family members. The daughter who is happy to have Edith live with her arrives a little earlier to spend time with her mother and during that time Edith experiences bowel incontinence. Because of Edith's embarrassment she has been successfully hiding this problem from her daughter. The daughter, while not showing her mother, has a strong emotional reaction to this event. A nurse cleans up the floor and Edith just in time for the meeting. The other children arrive feeling confident because they know their sister is happy to have their mother live with her; they have no idea of the 'accident' before the meeting.

GROUP ACTIVITY

- Suggest the possible team members to be present for such a meeting.
- Decide how the negative emotion of the daughter might unconsciously affect her responses in the meeting. Remember that her intent was positive, but she has had no time to process the event or her emotions, nor does she have any idea of the support services available for her mother, herself and her immediate family.
- Discuss the possible effects this negative emotion might have on the events during the meeting and on the people interacting throughout the meeting. Remember that all members of the family are present, including Edith.

Reflection should involve consideration of the events occurring during the interaction, including actions, words, non-verbal behaviour and environmental factors. A person who is effective at reflecting considers the reason for each event, the outcome of each event and the overall result of the interaction. Sometimes the overall outcome is positive despite negative events during the interaction and – while answers to questions relating to each 'event' within an interaction are important – it is the overall result that must guide future interactions. Reflection should include decisions about whether or not each event was necessary or appropriate. While some negative events are necessary to produce positive outcomes, they require skilful management and experienced personnel. Discussion with significant others can result in expression of strong emotions that initially appear negative; however, the expression of these emotions may result in positive interventions and resolution of emotions.

When the health professional is responsible for negative events they should reflect on the causes of these events and, if appropriate, how to avoid unnecessary events in future interactions. It is important to examine the causes and reactions of all the interacting individuals including the health professional to avoid the repetition of negative events during similar interactions.

Reflection should consider the emotional responses of all interacting individuals. Emotional responses may or may not be expressed verbally during an interaction. They may simply be non-verbal responses that require understanding to guide future interactions and, perhaps, intervention. The cause of these responses should be considered and support or suggestions provided for resolution of these responses. Sometimes this support takes the form of referral to an appropriate health professional. No health professional has *all* the answers for every person seeking assistance and this reality should guide health professionals in their communication with all people involved in the health professions.

REFLECTION

- When events become unsatisfactory what questions are beneficial? Consider an uncomfortable event you remember – preferably a recent one (e.g. with teachers, family members, fellow workers, an accident, in a parking lot). Use the following questions to guide your reflection about that event.
  - What was the purpose of the communicative interaction?
  - What was I feeling before the interaction?
  - Was I preoccupied? Was I focused?
  - Do I have a fundamental bias relating to this person or situation? Do I have a past negative history when communicating with the person or in similar situations? If so, why?
  - When did this interaction start to go wrong?
  - What was the trigger?
    - Something that was said?
    - Something that happened before?
    - Something the person was already feeling?
    - Non-verbal? From who?
  - How do I feel in response to this event? What is the cause(s) of these emotions?
  - What could I have done differently?
  - What do I do now?
  - What do I need to do in relation to the other person?
  - What do I need to do within myself to ensure positive interactions in the future?
- Do these questions assist you to isolate and highlight those factors that could promote a more comfortable and satisfactory interaction next time?
- What other questions could assist you to change your patterns of thought and action to ensure positive reactions and outcomes that produce effective communication?

Johns (1993) provides a model to assist in the process of reflection. Although similar to Boud & Walker's (1990) model, Johns expresses the steps differently and includes additional possible factors for consideration:

1. Describe the experience – what actually happened.
2. Consider the possible causes of the reactions, including the abovementioned contributing factors and any others.
3. Consider the significant background information relating to the environment and each individual in the interaction.

4. Consider the aims of each action and the possible reasons for the actions.
5. Consider the consequences of the actions including the feelings of each individual.
6. Consider why possible alternative actions were not chosen and the possible consequences of such actions.
7. Consider the resultant learning and how to change reactions in the future.

These seven points provide a sound basis for reflection about interactive experiences while practising as a health professional or in daily life.

Reflection is a process that although challenging does not have to be tedious. It takes commitment and varying amounts of time – the time decreases as experience increases. Writing in a journal and sipping an enjoyable drink may be helpful in the process of reflecting. Other individuals can also assist if they are willing to journey in honesty into the realm of the reasons for negative responses when communicating. The benefits of reflective and reflexive practice are many for the person seeking assistance and for the health professional.

Reflection upon barriers to experiencing, accepting and resolving emotions

There is some controversy and discussion about the definition, name and use of unintentional or unconscious barriers to experiencing, accepting and resolving the reality of emotions (Blackman 2004, Cramer 2000, Cramer 2005, Cramer 2006, Egan 2007, Hentschel et al 2004). There is also a long-standing argument about the reality of the effects and role of the unconscious in determining behaviour. The concept of an unconscious mind with power to influence behaviour can cause discomfort and thus some people prefer to avoid discussion about the possible role of a subconscious. The idea that there are processes of which an individual is unaware seems unnerving; however, currently psychologists do suggest that there are mental processes occurring outside the awareness of the individual that affect behaviour (Murphy 2001). Some of these processes are called defenses or defense mechanisms.

Defenses (DSM-IV 1994), adaptive mental mechanisms (Vaillant 2000) or defense mechanisms assist the individual to unconsciously avoid uncomfortable emotions, thoughts, information or wishes by removing them from the conscious mind. They are a method of managing thoughts and emotions that would otherwise be unmanageable (Giroux et al 2002). Every individual unconsciously uses defenses to avoid experiencing negative or anxiety-provoking emotions. Some defenses are a form of deception (Smith 2004); they allow the individual to continue behaving in a particular way regardless of the outcome of that behaviour. Others are simply ways of 'coping with life' at a particular time; they maintain self-esteem and self-respect and as such are successful coping mechanisms that encourage mature functioning. Overuse of defense mechanisms, however, limits self-awareness and awareness of negative emotions, restricts the harmony within the individual and protects individuals from change (Egan 2007).

REFLECTIVE GROUP ACTIVITY

- List reasons why health professionals should be aware of commonly used defenses (defense mechanisms).
- Discuss possible reasons why health professionals should be aware of the defense mechanisms they habitually use.

Defenses can be important for survival in particular situations – they may allow a person to continue functioning in extremely difficult circumstances. Continual use of defense mechanisms by individuals will, however, habitually disconnect them from reality, sometimes distort reality and limit their ability to achieve effective communication. Over-reliance on particular defenses reduces the ability to consider and choose appropriate options or responses during difficult interactions. Recognition of the defenses an individual commonly uses assists the individual to understand their behaviour and allows them to exercise choice and control during difficult interactions.

While description and categorisation of defenses has occurred for many years, a more recent discussion suggests that defenses occur on a continuum of maturity (Cramer 2000). The ability of the individual to function as a mature adult indicates the use of the **mature defenses**. These include altruism, sublimation, suppression, anticipation and humour, and are essential to positive mental health (Vaillant 2000). Children often demonstrate use of the **immature defenses**, which are projection, fantasy, hypochondriasis, passive aggression and acting out. The use of immature defenses usually decreases as people develop into adulthood. The movement along the continuum usually indicates less self-deception.

Consistent and prolonged use of defenses typical of immature functioning is the cause of maladaptive behaviour and the individual may demonstrate psychotic disturbances (Giroux Bruce et al 2002). While this is true from one perspective, from another it seems problematic because it suggests that only maladjusted individuals employ defenses from the immature end of the continuum. This is not necessarily true. For example, individuals experiencing grief may use denial for a time to facilitate adjustment and acceptance. While coping with grief does not usually require prolonged use of denial, denial in the short-term is an important defense for many individuals and does not demonstrate maladaptive behaviour or psychotic disturbance. The **neurotic defenses** – displacement, isolation of affect (intellectualisation), repression and reaction formation – usually require relatively less self-deception than the immature and **psychotic defenses**, and may be used in times of stress.

The commonly used defenses and their definitions are outlined in Table 5.1.

Every individual uses defenses in some form at some time to continue functioning (Milliken & Honeycutt 2004). Habitual use of the defenses causes maladaptive behaviour. Individuals who demonstrate obvious maladaptive behaviour (i.e. some forms of psychosis) usually employ either psychotic or immature defenses.

REFLECTIVE ACTIVITY

- Consider each of the commonly used defenses individually. List behaviours that indicate use of each. Can you think of someone you know who regularly uses any of these? How do you recognise these defenses? Can you explain their use?
- Consider those defenses you have used. Why did you use those defenses? Why did you stop using them?
- If you still use defenses, how will this affect your communication as a health professional? Do you need to seek assistance from a psychologist or counsellor to reduce the use of defenses that block your ability to experience, accept and resolve particular emotions?

Consideration of the defenses individuals regularly employ can assist the health professional or the 'other' to overcome barriers to experiencing particular emotions, thus facilitating change in thoughts and actions. Awareness of defenses can empower individuals to face the reality of their situation and negotiate required changes in the use of defenses

Commonly used defense mechanisms		
Category	**Defense mechanism**	**Description**
Psychotic	Denial	The person refuses to accept the truth about something (e.g. refuses to believe particular news).
Immature	Projection	Unacceptable feelings, thoughts and inadequacies, unwanted characteristics and inappropriate desires are attributed to another person (e.g. I am unconsciously angry with you, but I convince myself you are angry with me – that it is your fault, not my emotion). Such individuals always blame others for uncomfortable situations.
	Fantasy	The person ignores the real world and retreats into an imaginary world that fulfils the needs that reality has not met. The fantasy relieves the discomfort of life. The individual does not usually insist on or act on the fantasy. Children may have a special imaginary friend.
Neurotic	Displacement	Strong feelings about one person are unhealthily redirected onto another (e.g. after a disagreement with a supervisor, the person goes home and shouts at their roommate or kicks the dog).
	Repression	Painful or anxious memories are forced into the unconscious. This usually occurs during childhood. Repression has a powerful influence on behaviour and is often very destructive.
	Reaction formation	Conscious thoughts and emotions are the opposite of the actual unconscious wishes and emotions (e.g. the person really likes another person but consciously thinks they do not like them).
	Isolation of affect (intellectualisation)	Intellectual processes are used excessively in order to avoid uncomfortable emotions. The person may focus on details to avoid emotions (e.g. intellectualisation allows someone to organise a funeral without being overwhelmed by emotion).
Mature	Sublimation	Unacceptable impulses are rechannelled into personally and socially acceptable channels (e.g. aggressive impulses are channelled into a game of squash).
	Suppression	The person makes a semiconscious decision to ignore a thought, idea or wish momentarily. They return to it later.
	Humour	This subtle and elegant defense occurs when least expected and permits the expression of emotions without discomfort or paralysis. It does not deny pain or seriousness – it simply allows expression and improves life.

TABLE 5.1 Adapted from Vaillant 1995, p 36.

and thus in behaviour. With such awareness health professionals can learn to appropriately manage both expected and unexpected difficult situations in order to provide consistent family/person-centred practice.

Chapter summary

Reflection promotes awareness of unconscious emotional processes. Thus, reflection facilitates transformation of the thoughts and actions of the health professional to achieve effective communication and positive outcomes in practice. It is important for health professionals to be aware of their own barriers (defenses) to resolving negative emotions.

Complete the following:
1. What is reflexive practice?

    _____

    _____

    _____

2. Reflection is thoughtful exploration and consideration of the _____ of events and _____ during events.

3. Reflection achieves ten possible outcomes – list at least eight of these.

    i.   _____

    ii. _____

    iii. _____

    iv. _____

    v.   _____

    vi. _____

    vii. _____

    viii. _____

4. What is the purpose of a model of reflection?

    _____

    _____

    _____

5. What do most models of reflection encourage?

    _____

    _____

    _____

6. What five major behaviours are required for reflection regardless of the particular model of reflection?

    i.   _____

    ii. _____

    iii. _____

    iv. _____

    v.   _____

7. What does reflection encourage when considering future events within interactions?

    _____

    _____

    _____

8. Reflection requires commitment and time, and perhaps a journal, a glass of your favourite drink and a good honest friend to join in the journey of self-awareness, acceptance and respect. Devise a plan or strategy that will encourage and develop your skills in reflection.

    _____

    _____

    _____

9. In everyday language, state a definition of defenses.

    _____

    _____

    _____

10. State three reasons why everyone uses defenses.
    i.   _____

    ii. _____

    iii. _____

11. Defenses include the following four categories (Vaillant 1995, p 36). When might they be seen?
    i.   Psychotic:
    ii. Immature:
    iii. Neurotic:
    iv. Mature:

12. Organise the following list into the appropriate type of defense mechanism: Projection, humour, fantasy, displacement, altruism, denial, acting out, hypochondriasis, repression, isolation of affect, sublimation, reaction formation, suppression, anticipation, passive aggression.

Psychotic	Immature	Neurotic	Mature

References

American Psychiatric Association 1994 Diagnostic and statistical manual of mental disorders, 4th edn (DSM-IV). APA, Washington DC

Andrews J 2000 The value of reflective practice: a student case study. British Journal of Occupational Therapy 63:396–398

Backus W, Chapian M 2000 Telling yourself the truth. Bethany, Minneapolis MN

Ben-Arye E, Lear A, Mermoni D et al 2007 Promoting lifestyle awareness among the medical team by the use of an integrated teaching approach: a primary care experience. The Journal of Alternative and Complementary Medicine 13(4):461–469

Blackman J S 2004 101 Defenses: how the mind shields itself. Brunner-Routledge, New York

Boud D, Keogh R, Walker D 1985 Reflection: turning experience into learning. Kogan Page, London

Boud D J, Walker D 1990 Making the most of experience. Studies in Continuing Education 12(2):61–80

Boud D J, Walker D 1991 Experience and learning: reflection at work. Deakin University, Melbourne

Brown G, Ryan S 2003 Enhancing reflective abilities: interweaving reflection into practice. In: Brown G, Esdaile S A, Ryan S (eds) Becoming an advanced health care professional. Butterworth-Heineman, London, p 118–144

Cramer P 2000 Defense mechanisms in psychology today. American Psychologist 55:637–646

Cramer P 2005 A new look at defense mechanisms. Guildford Press, New York

Cramer P 2006 Protecting the self: defense mechanisms in action. Guildford Press, New York

Egan G 2007 The skilled helper, 8th edn. Thomson, Belmont CA

Ellis R B, Gates B, Kenworthy N (eds) 2004 Interpersonal communication in nursing: theory and practice. Churchill Livingstone, London (Original work published 2003)

Finlay L, Gough B 2003 Reflexivity: a practical guide for researchers in health and social sciences. Blackwell, Oxford

Giroux Bruce M A, Borg B 2002 Psychosocial frames of reference: core for occupation-based practice, 3rd edn. Slack, Thorofare NJ

Gustafson C, Fagerberg I 2004 Reflection: the way to professional development? Journal of Clinical Nursing 13:271–280

Harms L 2007 Working with people: communication skills for reflective practice. Oxford University Press, Melbourne

Hentschel U, Smith G, Draguns JG et al (eds) 2004 Defense mechanisms: theoretical, research and clinical perspectives. Elsevier, Amsterdam

Higgs J, Sefton A, Street A et al 2005 Communicating in the health and social sciences. Oxford University Press, Melbourne

Jack K, Smith A 2007 Promoting self-awareness in nurses: to improve nursing practice. Nursing Standard 21(32):47–52

Johns C 1993 Professional supervision. Journal of Nursing Management 1:9–18

Kinsella EA 2001 Reflections on reflective practice. The Canadian Journal of Occupational Therapy 68:195–198

Kondrat ME 1999 Who is the 'self' in self-aware: professional self-awareness from a critical theory perspective. Social Service Review 10:302–317

Miller L 2003 Understanding and managing human nature on the job. Public Personnel Management 32(3):419–434

Milliken M E, Honeycutt A 2004 Understanding human behavior: a guide for health care providers, 7th edn. Thomson Delmar, New York

Mohan T, McGregor H, Saunders S et al 2004 Communicating as professionals. Thomson, Melbourne

Murphy J 2001 The power of your subconscious mind. Bantam, New York (Revised by McMahan I; original work published 2000 by Reward)

O'Toole G 2007 Can assessment of attitudes assist both the teaching and learning process as well as ultimate performance in professional practice? In: Frankland S (ed) Enhancing teaching and learning through assessment. Springer, The Netherlands

Payne M 2006 What is professional social work? 2nd edn. Policy Press, Bristol

Plack M M 2006 The development of communication skills, interpersonal skills and a professional identity within a community of practice. Journal of Physical Therapy Education 20(1):37–46

Pritchard A 2005 Ways of learning: learning theories and learning styles in the classroom. David Fulton, London

Purtilo R B, Haddad A 2002 Health professional and patient interaction, 6th edn. Saunders, Philadelphia

Roberts A 2002 Advancing practice through continuing professional education: the case for reflection. British Journal of Occupational Therapy 65:237–241

Rogers C 1967 On becoming a person. Constable, London

Rudduck H C, Turner D S 2007 Developing cultural sensitivity: nursing students' experiences of a study abroad programme. Journal of Advanced Nursing 59(4):361–369

Smith D L 2004 Why we lie: the evolutionary roots of deception and the unconscious mind. St Martin's Press, New York

Stein-Parbury J 2006 Patient and person: interpersonal skills in nursing, 3rd edn. Elsevier, Sydney (Original work published 2005)

Thompson N 2002 People skills, 2nd edn. Palgrave Macmillan, Basingstoke

Vaillant G E 1995 The wisdom of the ego. Harvard University Press, Cambridge MA (Original work published 1993)

Vaillant G E 2000 Adaptive mental mechanisms: their role in a positive psychology. American Psychologist 55:89–98

Awareness of self

6

CHAPTER OBJECTIVES

Upon completing this chapter, students should be able to
- Recognise the importance and benefits of self-awareness for a health professional
- Demonstrate awareness of their abilities and 'inabilities'
- State some of their own values, characteristics and abilities
- List the values, characteristics and abilities that benefit a health professional
- Demonstrate understanding of their own basic dominant need(s)
- Recognise the effect of conflict between needs and values
- Understand the concept of listening barriers and their effect on communication
- Listen and speak more effectively
- Recognise differences in learning and processing preferences
- Understand their own learning and processing preferences.

Self-awareness: An essential tool

Self-awareness equips individuals for life. It also equips relevant individuals for an effective career as a health professional. Self-awareness allows a person to know and understand themself. It allows a person to know how they will react in any situation and assists them to understand why they react as they do in those situations (Egan 2007). Self-awareness increases self-understanding and results in increased control of thoughts and behaviours (Devito 2003). The information resulting from self-awareness helps health professionals achieve effective practice for those seeking their assistance. Self-awareness potentially enables the individual to use this information to relate positively. Schore (2005) suggests that awareness of personal emotional states increases the ability of health professionals to recognise and respond appropriately to the needs of others. Stein-Parbury (2006) states that self-awareness is essential for developing a therapeutic relationship and promotes open, honest and genuine health professionals who are not afraid to be caring human beings. Self-awareness potentially facilitates unconditional positive regard for others without prejudice, judgement or negativity (Rogers 1967). Health professionals who seek to achieve positive outcomes in every interaction will increasingly reach this goal through the practice of self-awareness.

Becoming self-aware is a life-long journey that requires commitment and perseverance (Taylor 2000). When embarking on the journey towards self-awareness it is important to remember that even the most self-aware individuals sometimes interact inappropriately; even in these individuals the level of self-awareness varies and thus they may experience negative outcomes when interacting. Such times are inevitable and should motivate those committed to self-awareness to persevere in their attempts to achieve self-awareness. Self-awareness allows health professionals to respond to the needs of the person seeking assistance, rather than responding to their own needs. This response ultimately facilitates family/person-centred practice, the desired outcome of any interaction with a health professional.

The benefits of achieving self-awareness

While achieving self-awareness is sometimes uncomfortable, there are many resultant benefits. Self-awareness allows health professionals to recognise, know, understand and resolve their emotional needs. It frees health professionals to choose how to react rather than reacting to fulfil unconscious emotional needs at any given time. Self-awareness provides understanding of the inadequacies and fears that unconsciously manipulate and direct thoughts and responses while interacting (Ben-Arye et al 2007). This understanding facilitates greater control while relating and decreases regrets after interactions. The greatest benefit of self-awareness is self-acceptance and valuing of self. Self-acceptance empowers health professionals to value and respect others regardless of the situation (Davis 2006). Reflection is a key component for achieving self-awareness (see Ch 5). In this chapter (Ch 6) the reader is encouraged to begin the journey of practising self-awareness. Chapter 6 seeks to demonstrate the benefits of being self-aware for both the health professional and those around them.

Beginning the journey of self-awareness

A journal is a helpful learning tool when developing self-awareness. Recording answers to questions and thoughts while reflecting assists in highlighting information and learning about self (Ellis et al 2004, Mohan et al 2004). It is helpful to revisit a journal at later times as a reminder of the growth and change achieved through a commitment to self-awareness.

Answering questions about 'self' is essential for achieving self-awareness. Honest answers to such questions inform individuals and empower them to choose appropriate responses and behaviours when communicating. Answering questions about personal characteristics and related abilities begins the process of self-awareness.

REFLECTIVE ACTIVITY

This is an extension of the reflective activity on page 43 of Chapter 5.
Part 1
- Make a list of things you enjoy doing. Of those things, what do you do well? What do you not do well?
- Make a list of things you dislike doing. Of those things, what do you do well? What do you not do well?
- Do you like the things you naturally perform well?
- Do you dislike the ones you perform badly?

↳

⮡
- List the characteristics and abilities that assist your performance in these activities.
- List the characteristics and abilities that limit your performance in these activities.

Part 2
- Make a list of all the things you feel you do well and those you feel you do not do well, whether you enjoy doing them or not.
- Share this list with someone who knows you well and ask if they agree. If they disagree, ask them for examples to demonstrate their understanding of what you do well and what you do not do well.
- Does this interaction change the way you see your abilities?
- Are you able to believe the other person's understanding of you?
- Why or why not?

Sometimes an individual has the characteristics and abilities to perform an activity well but experiences have clouded their accurate knowledge about and understanding of those characteristics and abilities.

CASE STUDY

During the process of learning to read, a 6-year-old child changes schools. The new teacher notices that the report from the previous school states the child reads well. The teacher asks the new child to read to the whole class from a reader (booklet) considered an advanced reader for that class. The new child – presented with an unfamiliar reader and a sea of unfamiliar faces – stands in horror staring at the book. The words are so unfamiliar that the child really is not sure that the book is not upside down. Several attempts to pronounce words find the child standing alone, in silence. The teacher says *Well obviously you can't read – sit down.*

GROUP DISCUSSION

- Discuss how the child is likely to react.
- Discuss how each member of the group would react if this had been them.
- Discuss any similar experiences that group members are willing to share and the effect of such negative experiences on the ability to perform the activity.

It took several years after that experience for the child to enjoy reading. Now an adult, that 'bad' reader is today a successful author of readers for children who do not enjoy reading!

REFLECTION

- What do you think facilitated this person to become an author of readers (booklets) for children?
- Could this have resulted from unresolved emotions or does this require resolved emotions concerning the incident years ago?
- Do you like any of the activities you listed in Part 2 of the previous reflective activity because you were encouraged in doing them? Are there any you dislike because you had negative experiences that made you feel unable to do them successfully?

REFLECTIVE ACTIVITY

- Make a list of those things you perform well because of encouragement.
- Make a list of those things you perform well because you have persevered despite discouraging feedback.
  - Do you agree with the negative feedback you received in the past?
  - Have you proved to yourself that you can do these activities well?
  - What did you do to prove your abilities in these activities?
- Make a list of activities you do not do well because you have experienced discouraging feedback.
  - Have you stopped doing these as a result?
  - Do you think you could ever attempt them again? Why or why not?
  - Is there any skill you feel you could never perform well?
  - What might you do to develop your skills in this area?

When told they do not perform an activity well, some people decide to practise that activity until they do perform it well. Many activities can be conquered with practice (e.g. playing basketball; creating a chair from timber; writing assignments, presentations and reports; teaching; managing others; providing leadership; and communicating). Other people, when told they cannot perform something well, withdraw from performing that activity and never conquer it. Such decisions might not be significant where the ability is something that is not essential to quality of life (e.g. knitting or washing a car). Some abilities (e.g. communication and self-control) are necessary for daily life, however, and thus perseverance is required to improve skills in those activities. There are particular characteristics that individuals develop because of personality and experience that promote the development of abilities. An awareness of self provides information about those characteristics and allows thoughtful control to enhance communication.

REFLECTION

- Is there a characteristic that you do not demonstrate well that you feel you need to develop to become an excellent health professional (e.g. patience or confidence when communicating with strangers)?
- What can you do to develop this characteristic and the associated abilities?

Individual values

All people have values that influence their thoughts and actions. A value is the measure of worth, importance or usefulness of something or someone (Banks 2006). Values develop as an individual experiences life. They originate from families, friends, teachers, the media, religious leaders and caregivers (Purtilo & Haddad 2002). Values influence thoughts, desires, dreams, decisions and actions. They contribute to the development of particular characteristics and thus abilities or inabilities. If an individual values hand-made garments, they may persevere to learn knitting. If they do not they may never begin the process of testing their abilities in knitting. If a person values respect of self and others when interacting they will take action to both demonstrate and expect respect (Harms 2007).

Is a health profession an appropriate choice?

There are particular values, characteristics and abilities that facilitate effective practice in the health professions. It is important to be aware of these values, characteristics and abilities because this awareness assists in verifying the choice to become a health professional. Some individuals pursue a career in a health profession because someone they admire is a health professional. These individuals may be seeking a career that does not suit their interests, values or abilities. Other individuals pursue a career in a health profession because they are aware of the role, the values and the required characteristics and abilities of the profession and feel they meet the necessary requirements. Others may not pursue a career in the health professions because they are unaware that their interests, values, characteristics and abilities are well suited to such a career. Still others do not pursue a career in the health professions because it does not provide the economic return they desire or because it is too consuming of time and emotions. The reasons for the choice about whether or not to become a health professional usually indicate the values of the individual.

Values of a health professional

The overall purpose of the health professions centres on people (see Ch 2). Sometimes this overall purpose focuses on individuals and at other times on individuals within the context of a family. If people are the central focus of all health professions, it seems appropriate to assume that all health professionals must value and appreciate people. If health professionals do not value and appreciate people and their associated needs, the outcome of their intervention may be inappropriate and ineffective.

It is important that health professionals value both themselves and others. A health professional must have a desire to understand and assist people with their needs through expressions of empathy, demonstrations of respect and development of trust. It is important that health professionals value a therapeutic relationship that collaborates, empowers and develops rapport. This value promotes family/person-centred practice and is essential for all health professionals. It is also essential that health professionals value the knowledge and skills specific to their profession and those of other health professions. If these values are not important to an individual, that individual should not consider a career as a health professional.

Characteristics and abilities that enhance the practice of a health professional

While particular health professions require specific interests and abilities, there are characteristics and associated abilities that benefit individuals in all health professions. The following questions highlight some of these characteristics and abilities.

Personal unconscious needs

There are needs every individual has that contribute to 'inabilities' or limitations in relationships (Stein-Parbury 2006). These unconscious needs create typical ways of relating and affect the characteristics and outcomes of relationships. This reality indicates that health professionals must be aware of the basic needs that dominate their expectations of relationships and ways of relating. There are three basic human relationship needs:

1. The need to be accepted and valued – to have a 'place', feel special and know that others care (Brill & Levine 2005, Milliken & Honeycutt 2004)
2. The need to be in control
3. The need for affection and affirmation (Stein-Parbury 2006).

All humans have these needs. At different times individuals long to feel valued for who they are – to feel accepted and special. This need expresses itself through relationships in which the person is always fulfilling the needs of others and doing for others, regardless of whether the other can do for themself. These people find it difficult to say no when asked to assist. Some people have a predominant need for control and thus will limit involvement in relationships and situations that are unpredictable. This need expresses itself in relationships with others who are happy to do exactly what the person demands, in the exact manner. These people find it difficult to enter situations that involve change or risk-taking. Other individuals predominantly seek affection and affirmation. This need expresses itself through the seeking of relationships that protect them and affirm whatever they do. These people may also find it difficult to say no, because they crave affirmation and fear rejection. While everyone experiences these needs, some people have a consistently dominant area of need that influences all their relationships and interactions. The dominant need of individuals may vary according to the events in their lives at a particular time. It is important for individuals who choose a career in a health profession to be aware of which of these needs dominate their relationships.

GROUP ACTIVITY

- Discuss each basic human relationship need and decide the effects of each need on the communication and relationships of health professionals.
- For each need, state specific actions that reflect the basic need. Consider your particular health profession when stating the specific actions.

Awareness of the dominant area of personal need(s) allows the health professional to make choices that fulfil the needs of the person seeking their assistance rather than fulfilling their own needs. Answering the following questions may assist in highlighting which basic human relationship needs typically dominate an individual's way of relating.

REFLECTIVE ACTIVITY

- Answer each question with *yes, no* or *sometimes*. In reality the three basic human relationship needs will be true for everyone some of the time (Stein-Parbury 2006). However, these questions ask for the *usual* tendency you experience. Remember that honest answers will increase your self-awareness and potentially empower you to overcome the 'inabilities' or limitations associated with relating because of a predominant need.
  - Do I have a well-defined comfort zone that I do not enjoy leaving?
  - Do I usually feel there is only one answer to a problem and one way to do tasks? Or that there is only one place to keep certain things?
  - Do I usually feel I must have the answer to every situation and problem?
  - Do I only enjoy relating to people who need my help?
  - Do I often feel I am the only person who can solve certain problems?
  - Do I define myself by doing things for other people who need me?
  - Do I often feel I must fix a problem?
  - Do I often feel I must do something to make things better and to rescue people?
  - Do I only feel OK if I am helping people?
  - Do I usually respond strongly to any critical comment about me?
  - Do I find that other people often act in ways that are inappropriate or annoying?
  - Do I find it easy to see the negative rather than the positive aspects of a person?
  - Do I find it easy to form negative ideas about people who are different to me?
  - Do I find it difficult to say no to requests for help?
  - Do I usually want other people to take care of me?
  - Do I often worry about whether people like me or not?
  - Do I feel most content when people do exactly what I want?
  - Do I feel better when people are telling me I am great?
- Classify each question into the three basic human needs.
- Consider your answers to the questions and decide which basic need(s) typically dominate your way of relating.
- Write down what you could do to control this need(s) in order to ensure that you, as a health professional, are able to meet the needs of others.

Reflecting upon answers to these questions is important for health professionals. Such reflection increases self-awareness and control of thoughts and reactions. It also decreases the fulfilment of personal needs while practising as a health professional thus increasing the ability to focus on fulfilling the needs of others.

Conflict between values and needs

When practising as a health professional it is possible to assist people who demonstrate detrimental habits resulting from conflict between personal values and needs. In such circumstances it is the responsibility of the health professional to provide non-judgemental assistance. Self-awareness of the personal values and needs of the health professional promotes self-control and positive understanding of the individual seeking their assistance. Self-awareness potentially frees the health professional to make the choice to provide non-judgemental assistance. Considering their own experiences of conflict between personal values and needs reminds the health professional of the difficulties associated with this conflict and thus facilitates greater tolerance and genuine understanding of those seeking assistance.

REFLECTION

- Is being healthy one of your values? How do you express this value?
- Do you value your quality of life? How do you express this value?
- Do you generally like to be accepted? How do you express this?
- Do you generally like to be included? How do you express this?
- Does acceptance generally make you feel valued? Why?
- As a health professional, how would you respond to someone who has developed a detrimental habit because their dominant need has overcome their values?

In situations where someone has developed a detrimental habit because their dominant need has overcome their values, the health professional should not express judgement either verbally or non-verbally. It is important to remember that the individual seeking assistance is feeling vulnerable and insecure. The health professional seeks to empower people to achieve change and a judgemental response will only discourage rather than empower. Awareness of personal values and needs and the possible conflict between the two is important for all health professionals. This awareness assists them to understand the results of such conflict, which are usually detrimental habits such as smoking or overeating.

REFLECTION

- What do you feel about smoking? Or overeating? If you smoke or use food as comfort, you understand the desire for a cigarette or for food when stressed and upset. If you do not smoke or overeat, you may have a different addiction (e.g. television, computer games, chocolate, coffee, always being right, feeling resentful, being in control, extreme exercise); experience of any addiction will facilitate understanding of addiction to smoking or overeating.
- As a health professional what is your first response to someone who smokes or overeats?
- If you value health and quality of life, you may have a strong opinion about the habit of smoking or about obesity caused by overeating. How do you temper/control these strong opinions?

Given that initially most people find the act of smoking unpleasant, it is remarkable that individuals continue to smoke. A possible explanation is that many people continue smoking because it gives them a perceived 'place' within a particular 'group'. They may continue smoking to experience acceptance and inclusion despite valuing a healthy life and the associated quality of life. A person who is obese because of overeating experiences the overriding need for comfort above their value of a healthy life.

Perfectionism as a value

The value of 'perfectionism' or always being right in actions and words may override the need for affection and affirmation. Individuals who value perfectionism value being right above everything else. When they experience being wrong, they cannot recognise the presence of affection and affirmation. For such individuals the value of perfectionism overcomes the need for and often the ability to receive affection and affirmation (Backus & Chapian 2000). Individuals who value perfectionism can develop the detrimental habit of constantly telling themselves that whatever they say or do is not good enough, regardless of the often-exceptional quality of the attempt. Consistent affirmation, affection and repeated truth about the quality of the attempts is required to overcome this detrimental habit.

This value of perfectionism results in some individuals finding it difficult to complete and submit something (e.g. a written assignment). It can also result in individuals redoing the same thing repeatedly despite their skill in the task and the adequacy of their initial attempt. Other individuals may perform a task but can only see the imperfections of the performance regardless of the overall quality of the performance. For other individuals, the overriding value of perfectionism can mean they do not complete something as well as they are able to because they feel they will not do it well enough – they will not reach perfection. When individuals refuse to do something because they believe they will not achieve an appropriate level of perfection, they may not be able to admit they feel inadequate.

Negative self-talk can result in an individual refusing to attempt something while another person is present, despite their competence in the activity. Perfectionism may mean that a person is constantly planning future tasks – making lists of things to do and ways to complete those things – in an attempt to remember everything or to mentally prepare to 'perfectly' complete the tasks. It can also mean that people find it difficult to believe or accept any form of affirmation about the quality of their performance.

GROUP ACTIVITY

Negative self-talk: 'I am not good enough'
- How would you recognise evidence of this negative self-talk in a colleague or person seeking your assistance?
- List possible actions of a health professional who believes they are not good enough.
- List possible ways of relating for a person who believes they are not good enough and is seeking the assistance of your particular health profession.
- How might you assist either a colleague or a person seeking your assistance if they exhibit evidence of negative self-talk?

Awareness of the existence and experience of conflict between values and needs can assist health professionals to overcome their own detrimental habits. Such awareness also promotes understanding of people with detrimental habits encountered when working as a health professional.

Self-awareness of personal communication skills

Some individuals are effective communicators from birth, others develop skills through life experiences and others make conscious efforts to become effective communicators. Effective communicators are able to express themselves clearly, listen carefully and observe all non-verbal messages. They are committed to understanding the needs of their 'audience' and producing messages that negotiate mutual understanding (Ellis et al 2004). If the audience does not demonstrate understanding, effective communicators take turns communicating and negotiating with their audience to guarantee effective communication. They listen carefully to their audience and respond in ways that facilitate further positive communication.

REFLECTION

- Do you enjoy communicating verbally? Why do you think this is so?
- Do you usually listen when communicating verbally? Why do you do this?
- Do you usually talk? Why do you do this? What do you usually talk about?
- Which do you prefer – listening or talking? Why is this so?
- Do you ask questions about the other to continue the communication?
- Do you often request clarification?
- Do you let others ask questions or speak rather than you talking?
- Do you usually finish a verbal interaction feeling satisfied?
- Do you often feel dissatisfied after a communicative interaction?
- Do you enjoy communicating if you feel unmotivated to communicate?

In providing the answers to the above questions many people may note that their role when communicating varies depending on the topic and the people communicating. This is often true and may indicate that the person is a good communicator who responds appropriately to the topic, situation and audience. Alternatively, it may indicate an uncertainty when communicating that could benefit from reflection and conscious efforts to develop skills in communicating. If the honest answers to the questions above were predominantly *yes*, this could indicate skill in listening and speaking, while answers of predominantly *no* could indicate lack of skill or confidence in either. A health professional must demonstrate skill and confidence in communicating to facilitate excellence in the achievement of family/person-centred goals and practice (Higgs et al 2005).

Self-awareness of skills for effective listening

Full attention is not always necessary for effective communication in personal situations (Ellis et al 2004). For a health professional, however, effective listening requires full attention, skill and often practice (see Ch 10). Listening must be adapted to the particular individual and the context (Devito 2007). It requires active engagement with the person and their message. The listener indicates active engagement through appropriate non-verbal cues (see Ch 12). Effective listening requires understanding of more than the words being spoken; it also requires understanding of the emotions expressed. Effective listening is an essential skill for a health professional because it demonstrates empathy, respect and trustworthiness. Effective listening is characteristic of a therapeutic relationship and promotes family/person-centred goals and practice. Everyone, however, is guilty of ineffective listening at particular times (Mohan et al 2004). Understanding the reasons for ineffective listening empowers the health professional to overcome those reasons and practice effective listening whenever necessary.

What do you typically do when listening? Answer the following questions honestly.
1. Do you concentrate totally on the person and their messages?
2. Do you allow yourself to think of things you have to do later?
3. Do you attempt to understand everything the person is communicating?
4. Do you sit quietly without responding verbally or non-verbally?
5. Do you attempt to identify the main point of the communication?
6. Do you often interrupt?
7. Do you wait for the person to complete their message before responding?
8. Do you avoid eye contact while listening?
9. Do you keep an open mind and avoid judgement about the person/topic?
10. Do you try to 'double-guess' or read the mind of the person speaking?
11. Do you focus on the other person regardless of how you are feeling?
12. Do you change the subject if the person begins expressing negative emotions?

Listening skills vary according to context and life events at any given time. Certainly everyone needs to 'rest their brain' when listening in order to regain concentration. The above questions are not about those times of rest but rather focus on regularly employed habits that restrict or enhance the effectiveness of listening. Typically answering *yes* to the odd-numbered questions and *no* to the even-numbered questions indicates effective skills in listening. Answering *yes* to any of the even-numbered questions indicates a need to practise listening to ensure more effective communication. Answering *yes* to some odd and some even questions also indicates a need to practise listening.

Barriers to listening

Most individuals at different times use barriers that limit the effectiveness of their listening (Gordon 2004). These barriers may be a protective device used during a particular interaction or they may be a learned habit. The explanation for the use of barriers is irrelevant because if they are used at all they limit the possibility of effective listening. It is important that health professionals are aware of barriers to listening. They must be especially aware of the barriers they typically use themselves in order to limit their use of such barriers when listening to individuals who require their assistance.

Read the following list of barriers to listening and write your definition for each. Agree on a definition for each barrier. Together think of an example of each barrier.

Interrupting	Intimidating
Monopolising	Placating
Rehearsing	Reassuring
Switching off	Breaking confidences
Partial listening	Advising
Mind-reading	Judging
Being right	Interrogating
Changing the subject	

REFLECTIVE ACTIVITY

- Of these barriers, which ones have you experienced when you have been communicating with someone?
- Have you experienced any of them regularly?
- What is the major emotion you experience when someone uses a listening barrier while you are speaking?
- List reasons why people would use these barriers to avoid listening.

Reasons for the use of barriers to listening

There are many reasons for the use of listening barriers, some of which are reasonably positive explanations for the use of a barrier. These might include

- Excitement over something being said
- Preoccupation with a difficult situation
- Busyness
- Tiredness
- Greater knowledge of the situation than the speaker
- Genuine interest in the topic
- A desire to further understand the communication
- A desire to compose words carefully to avoid misunderstanding or hurt
- A need to communicate something urgently (e.g. a spider on the speaker's head!)
- A desire to share knowledge and understanding of the topic.

There are also negative explanations for the use of each listening barrier:

- An individual who finds a topic boring or not personally relevant may interrupt, switch off, listen partially or change the subject.
- An individual who feels insecure and intimidated may monopolise, intimidate or interrogate during an interaction.
- An individual may rehearse a statement in their mind instead of listening because they want to correct the speaker about an error.
- When being right motivates a person they might use several additional listening barriers including attempting to mind-read.
- If mind-reading proves incorrect, an individual who feels they know more than the speaker might use advising as a way of avoiding listening.
- An individual who feels someone is attacking them might respond by judging the person or attempting to intimidate or placate the person to stop them from continuing the perceived attack.
- An individual who finds the expression of negative emotions difficult might placate or reassure without any real attempt to listen and understand the speaker.
- An individual who wishes to change the subject or redirect the attention from the speaker to the listener may share confidential information about someone else.

All of these barriers to listening restrict the possibility of developing real understanding and effective communication.

If health professionals desire to demonstrate honest, open and empathic communication with the people seeking their assistance it is essential that they recognise listening barriers and the circumstances that promote their use.

Self-awareness about skills for effective speaking

Self-awareness can help an individual to identify the characteristics and abilities that enable effective speaking skills. Some people demonstrate interest in others with ease and efficacy. Such individuals demonstrate this interest naturally when communicating, whether speaking or listening. They demonstrate an engaging enthusiasm for their topic and their listeners that promotes understanding. Some individuals have a natural ability to effectively interpret non-verbal cues in messages while others must learn from experience what such cues mean. Some can intuitively understand the abilities and needs of those around them while others must ask for information concerning those abilities and needs. Some people can think quickly and respond appropriately regardless of the situation while others must compensate for lacking this ability with various strategies to achieve effective communication. All these skills assist in achieving effective communication when speaking. It is important that individuals know and understand their abilities with regard to speaking. Such understanding allows the health professional to either practise the skill of speaking or employ strategies to facilitate effective speaking when communicating.

Skills that produce effective speaking include personal abilities; familiarity and comfort with the topic; experience in effective speaking; skill in interpreting non-verbal behaviours; and skill in perceiving and understanding the characteristics of each 'audience'. It is important to be aware of this complexity when developing skills in speaking as a health professional. Effective speaking requires demonstration of interest and enthusiasm for both the topic and the 'audience'. It requires skill in, as well as knowledge and understanding about, the particular topic; studying to become a particular health professional provides this skill, knowledge and understanding. Effective speaking requires understanding of the non-verbal behaviours that affect the presentation and comprehension of spoken words (see Ch 12). It also requires understanding of the individual(s) listening (see Chs 1, 7 & 15 and Section Four).

REFLECTIVE ACTIVITY

Write down your answers to the following questions.
- What factors encourage you to demonstrate interest and enthusiasm for a subject when speaking?
- What do you usually do to indicate this interest and enthusiasm?
- What encourages you to demonstrate interest and enthusiasm towards the person/ people (audience) listening?
- What would you do to demonstrate interest and enthusiasm towards each individual person?
- How do you demonstrate interest and enthusiasm through your words?
- How do you demonstrate interest and enthusiasm through your non-verbal behaviour?

GROUP DISCUSSION

- What can health professionals do to demonstrate interest and enthusiasm?
- What might assist them in this demonstration?
- What factors might limit this demonstration? How could they overcome these factors?

A genuine interest in and enthusiasm for both the topic and the audience is important. Such interest and enthusiasm should produce a desire in the speaker to understand and engage with the listener and the relevant information about them. This desire and the resultant knowledge should promote the use of appropriate words and sentence structures to facilitate listener understanding. The use of appropriate non-verbal behaviour will further facilitate listener understanding and ultimately shared meaning. Interest and enthusiasm on behalf of the speaker in turn creates an interest within the listener. These emotions encourage the listener to engage with the speaker and assist in developing and maintaining consistent concentration. They create a desire to know and understand the presented information.

Preferences for managing information and resultant communicative behaviours

There are many descriptions of and theories relating to individual differences in styles of managing and responding to information (commonly known as learning styles or preferences). Information is taken to mean facts or experiences that change thinking or behaviour. Managing and responding to information involves perception, processing, recall of information and response to information (Reid 2006). Individuals adopt different information management styles and behaviours according to the expectations of different contexts (Pritchard 2005). While individual styles can vary, they represent tendencies not absolute choices (La Motta 2004). Individuals generally have preferred ways of functioning within particular contexts. The context and the personality typology (Briggs & Myers 1975, Jung 1941) influence the particular style of information management at a specific time. In combination, context and personality typology influence the reactions, behaviours and communication styles of every individual. It is therefore important for health professionals to have an awareness of their own particular style, to understand that others may have a different style and to realise that these differences are perfectly acceptable (Woolfolk & Margetts 2007).

Differences in individuals create both variety and diversity. While diversity is a challenge, it is here to stay (La Motta 2004). Conquering this challenge is essential and is one of the rewards of practising as a health professional. It requires awareness, understanding, acceptance and appreciation of such diversity. Such awareness enhances effective communication and contributes to the development of family/person-centred goals and practice.

REFLECTION

What do you do to become aware, to understand, to accept and to appreciate? Each of these actions has an individual meaning that results in different behaviour.

It is beneficial for health professionals to consider, establish and appreciate their own preferences for managing and responding to information before considering the preferences of others. Each particular preference or style of managing information has advantages and disadvantages (La Motta 2004). Awareness of their strengths and weaknesses allows health professionals to compensate for the weaknesses. It also empowers health professionals to recognise who can support them because of similarities and who can challenge them to grow because of differences. Health professionals who understand and accept their individual style will be more able to understand and accept the styles of others. They will also be able to adjust their communication style to accommodate the information-management style of those around them to ensure effective communication.

There are many descriptions of and theories about how individuals manage and respond to information (Dunn et al 1989, Felder 1993, Fleming 2001, Gardner 1983, Given 2002, Honey & Mumford 1986, Kolb 1984, Piaget 1968, Pritchard 2005, Reid 2006, Skinner 1989). Careful consideration of these and others would create volumes; however, the model presented by Honey & Mumford (1986) has value for the health professional and is relatively well known and accessible.

Honey & Mumford (1986) suggest four possible styles of managing information: Activist, Theorist, Pragmatist and Reflector. They state that individuals with mature ways of learning adopt any of the four styles for managing information as appropriate (cited in Pritchard 2005, p 57).

ACTIVITY

Your instructor will provide a handout on matching the four information management styles with the descriptions of likes and dislikes.

- Imagine you are a Theorist and you need to communicate information about your health profession with a Reflector who has not previously had any experience of your health profession. List the differences in your styles of relating to information. What difficulties might you experience? How will you compensate for the differences to minimise the difficulties?
- Continue this exercise until you have imagined yourself to be a Reflector, an Activist and a Pragmatist working with someone who manages information in a different way.
- Decide which style you use most and imagine you are working with someone who employs the same style. What are the advantages of this scenario? What are the disadvantages?

Personality typology and resultant communicative behaviours

In the early twentieth century, Carl Jung (1875–1961) pursued theories of the collective unconscious, archetypes and personality types (Berger 2006). In the 1940s, Isabel Briggs Myers and her mother Katherine Briggs began exploring his theories to explain differences in personality. Their explanations – the Myers-Briggs Type Indicator (MBTI) (Briggs & Myers 1975) – are used in this century for various purposes in a variety of contexts. Some understanding of the four basic personality preferences and combinations thereof to suggest personality types assists health professionals to understand their own communicative behaviour and the behaviour of others. Eight letters represent different descriptors that indicate different preferences for (not definitive ways of) relating or communicating.

Note that administration of the MBTI test to establish personality types requires training. Therefore, it is not possible within the confines of this book to establish a personality type. Knowledge of the typology, however, is beneficial for health professionals.

The MBTI personality descriptors combine to make sixteen possible personality types. Each type suggests particular characteristics that distinguish it from other types. These characteristics predict a preference for relating in a particular manner within particular situations and may predict a different style in other circumstances.

An awareness of the different personality types assists understanding of differences in styles of managing information and thus styles of communication. Some personality types enjoy working with people and are better communicators than others; others are task-oriented and prefer to work alone. With well-developed skills in self-awareness, individuals can in most cases adjust their personality tendencies while communicating. Knowledge and awareness of individual tendencies can assist individuals to make the required adjustments and to recognise, understand and accept tendencies in others. Health professionals can use this knowledge to promote effective communication.

Further information on the Myers-Briggs Type Indicator can be found at www.cpp.com.

Humour

The appropriate use of humour can enhance the quality and effectiveness of communication as well as assist an individual in managing uncomfortable circumstances (see Ch 5). Humour typically increases relaxation and the enjoyment of life (Berger 2006). It potentially has a powerful effect when communicating (Holli et al 2003). Humour can subtly dissolve stress, tension and even fear (Purtilo & Haddad 2002, Sprenger 2003). The use of humour requires health professionals to have an established relationship with the person. If health professionals have an established relationship they will be able to use humour at exactly the right time to achieve a therapeutic outcome. However, inappropriate use of humour can be harmful and destructive. It can remove the possibility of trust and positive communication. If used to avoid uncomfortable emotions or as a substitute for confrontation, humour will cause harm rather than fostering respectful communication. Humour can be used to hide anger or aggression; however, the most appreciated type of humour is often the self-deprecating joke that allows health professionals to laugh at themselves with someone else. Health professionals who do not take themselves too seriously may be more able to develop and sustain a therapeutic relationship with those around them.

REFLECTION

- Do you regularly and deliberately use humour?
- Do you use humour successfully?
- What contributes to the successful use of humour?
- Do you use humour to
  - Diffuse tension
  - Avoid negative emotions
  - Help people relax?
- If you habitually use humour for one of the above, why do you do this?
- Does the above answer indicate you need to learn to manage tension and/or negative emotions? What might you do about this?

Chapter summary

Self-awareness is necessary for all health professionals. It requires commitment, time, reflection and a sense of humour. Self-awareness sometimes feels uncomfortable, but it facilitates positive attitudes and promotes beneficial outcomes for all those involved in the health professions.

Complete the following:

1. What four actions does self-awareness allow the health professional to perform?
   i. _____
   ii. _____
   iii. _____
   iv. _____

2. What three areas of self-knowledge does self-awareness provide?
   i. _____
   ii. _____
   iii. _____

3. Health professionals value, demonstrate and enjoy particular things.
   - State four things that most health professionals value.
   i. _____
   ii. _____
   iii. _____
   iv. _____

- What three characteristics are essential for health professionals to demonstrate?
  i. _____
  ii. _____
  iii. _____
- What should you enjoy if you wish to be a health professional?
  i. _____
  ii. _____
  iii. _____
  iv. _____

4. What are three unconscious primary needs that manipulate people?
   i. _____
   ii. _____
   iii. _____

5. Why is it beneficial for a health professional to understand the existence of conflict between needs and values?

   _____
   _____
   _____
   _____
   _____

6. How does perfectionism affect people?

   _____
   _____
   _____
   _____
   _____

7. What does self-awareness highlight about communication?
   i. _____
   ii. _____
   iii. _____

8. What four styles of learning do Honey & Mumford (1986) suggest?
   i. _____
   ii. _____
   iii. _____
   iv. _____

9. What can the use of humour achieve in an established therapeutic relationship?

_____

_____

_____

_____

References

Banks S 2006 Ethics and values in social work, 3rd edn. Palgrave Macmillan, Basingstoke

Backus W, Chapian M 2000 Telling yourself the truth. Bethany, Minneapolis MN

Ben-Arye E, Lear A, Mermoni D et al 2007 Promoting lifestyle awareness among the medical team by the use of an integrated teaching approach: a primary care experience. The Journal of Alternative and Complementary Medicine 13(4):461–469

Berger A A 2006 50 ways to understand communication. Rowman & Littlefield, Oxford

Briggs K, Myers I B 1975 The Myers-Briggs type indicator. Consulting Psychologist Press, Palo Alto CA

Brill N I, Levine J 2005 Working with people: the helping process, 8th edn. Pearson, Boston

Davis C M 2006 Patient practitioner interaction. An experiential manual for developing the art of healthcare, 4th edn. Slack, Thorofare NJ

Devito J A 2003 Human communication. The basic course, 9th edn. Pearson, Boston

Devito J A 2007 The interpersonal communication book, 11th edn. Pearson, Boston

Dunn R, Dunn K, Price G E 1989 The learning style inventory. Price Systems, Lawrence KS

Egan G 2007 The skilled helper, 8th edn. Thomson, Belmont CA

Ellis R B, Gates B, Kenworthy N (eds) 2004 Interpersonal communication in nursing: theory and practice. Churchill Livingstone, London (Original work published 2003)

Felder R 1993 Reaching the second tier: learning and teaching styles in college science education. Journal of College Science Teaching 23:285–290

Fleming N D 2001 Teaching and learning styles: VARK strategies. VARK-Learn, Honolulu HI

Gardner H 1983 Frames of mind: the theory of multiple intelligences. Harper & Row, New York

Given B K 2002 Teaching to the brain's natural learning system. Association for Supervision and Curriculum Development, Alexandria VA

Gordon J (ed) 2004 Pfeiffer's classic activities for interpersonal communication. Pfeiffer, San Francisco CA

Harms L 2007 Working with people: communication skills for reflective practice. Oxford University Press, Melbourne

Higgs J, Sefton A, Street A et al 2005 Communicating in the health and social sciences. Oxford University Press, Melbourne

Holli B B, Calabrese R J, O'Sullivan Mailett J 2003 Communication and education skills for dietetics professionals, 4th edn. Lippincott, Williams & Wilkins, Philadelphia

Honey P, Mumford A 1986 Manual of learning styles, 2nd edn. Honey P, London

Jung C G 1941 The development of personality. Routledge, London

Kolb D A 1984 The learning style inventory: technical manual. McBer, Boston

La Motta T 2004 Using personality typology to build understanding. In: Gordon J (ed) Pfeiffer's classic activities for interpersonal communication. Pfeiffer, San Francisco CA, p. 53–67

Milliken M E, Honeycutt A 2004 Understanding human behavior: a guide for healthcare providers, 7th edn. Thomson Delmar, New York

Mohan T, McGregor H, Saunders S et al 2004 Communicating as professionals. Thomson, Melbourne

Piaget J 1968 Six psychological studies. Vintage, New York

Pritchard A 2005 Ways of learning: learning theories and learning styles in the classroom. David Fulton, London

Purtilo R B, Haddad A 2002 Health professional and patient interaction, 6th edn. Saunders, Philadelphia

Reid G 2006 Learning styles and inclusion. Paul Chapman, London (Original work published 2005)

Rogers C 1967 On becoming a person. Constable, London

Schore A N 2005 Attachment, affect regulation and the developing right brain: linking developmental neuroscience to pediatrics. Pediatrics in Review 26:204–217

Skinner B F 1989 The origins of cognitive thought. American Psychologist 43:13–18

Sprenger M 2003 Differentiation through learning styles and memory. Corwin Press, Thousand Oaks CA

Stein-Parbury J 2006 Patient and person: interpersonal skills in nursing, 3rd edn. Elsevier, Sydney (Original work published 2005)

Taylor B J 2000 Reflective practice: a guide for nurses and midwives. Allen & Unwin, Crows Nest, Sydney

Woolfolk A, Margetts K 2007 Educational psychology. Pearson, Frenchs Forest, Sydney

Awareness of the 'other'

7

CHAPTER OBJECTIVES
Upon completing this chapter, students should be able to
* Define and demonstrate a holistic awareness of the 'other'
* State and understand who the 'others' are for health professionals
* Demonstrate awareness of necessary information to understand the 'other'
* Appreciate the required elements for effective communication with the 'other', specifically respect, confidentiality and empathy
* Consider the physical aspects and obvious needs of the 'other' when communicating
* Demonstrate awareness of and skills in the use of validation, empathy, touch and silence to relate to the emotional aspects and emotional needs of the 'other'
* Recognise the significance of the sexual aspect and needs of the 'other'
* Understand and describe the impact of the cognitive aspects and skills of the 'other' (see also 'A person who has decreased cognitive function' in Section Four)
* Recognise types of communication for the 'other' who cannot use spoken words
* State the basic requirements for the use of alternative communication devices
* Relate to the possible implications of the social aspects and needs of the 'other'
* Relate to the spiritual aspects and needs of the 'other'.

The *whole* 'other'

The consideration of the 'other' in the health professions requires consideration of the whole person (see Ch 9). The 'whole' person is a dynamic system in which every aspect of the individual affects and interacts with the other aspects simultaneously. The whole person contains five fundamental aspects: the physical; the emotional, including the sexual aspect; the cognitive; the social; and the spiritual (Brill & Levine 2005). It is important for health professionals to consider the needs associated with all aspects of the person. Consideration of the most obvious aspect of the 'other' while neglecting the less obvious aspects limits the potential outcomes of the health service.

The most obvious aspect of an individual is usually the **physical** one, because it is immediately noticeable. However, the other aspects of this dynamic system become obvious as the health professional relates to the 'other'. Ignoring the less obvious aspects of the individual can adversely affect intervention outcomes. The **emotional** side of the vulnerable 'other' may dominate the person seeking the assistance of a health professional but may not be immediately obvious. If the emotional aspect of an individual dominates their functioning, it is important to address the issues causing the emotional distress either directly or by referral to an appropriate health professional. Resolution of emotional distress allows the 'other' to focus on the set goals of the relevant health profession rather than the dominating emotions. Recognition and willingness to relate to the **sexual** aspect of an individual may be essential in some health professions. In some cases, unconditional acceptance of the sexual preference of the individual is important for positive outcomes. As the health professional continues to relate to the 'other', the **cognitive** aspect of the person may become more obvious if there is a disability in processing cognitive information. Lack of ability or desire to collaborate is not always resistance. It may arise from lack of understanding because of decreased cognitive ability or limited language skills. The previous **social** and **cultural** experiences or background of the individual may be the least obvious and often the most significant aspect affecting expectations and outcomes for individuals. Experiences because of previous social interaction may affect the response of the 'other' to particular interactions with health professionals. Cultural norms can also influence interactions and thus awareness of cultural norms is essential when relating to 'others' from different cultures (see Chs 15 & 16). An important aspect that can dominate the 'other' is the **spiritual** aspect of an individual. Many health professionals neglect this aspect but it may influence the motivation and interest of the 'other' and thus the outcomes related to the assistance of the health professional. All the above aspects of an individual contribute to the functioning and performance of the 'other'. Consideration of each aspect by the health professional is potentially beneficial for the individuals seeking their assistance.

Who are the 'others'?

Awareness of 'others' is important in any health profession. 'Others' include those seeking assistance as well as the various health professionals and supporting staff who provide the assistance. Those seeking assistance include the individual who requires direct intervention along with the carers, families, friends and, in some cases, guardians of that individual. Health professional colleagues include individuals from many health professions. Some of these health professionals may form a multidisciplinary team within the particular health organisation while others may contribute to fulfilling the needs of the 'other' from outside the organisation. Supporting staff are found in every health service and provide essential assistance to both health professionals and those they assist. These 'others' include the person who answers the phone and the person who cleans the floors and toilets. Their contribution is vital and it is important to recognise that their contribution is an equal part of the service of any health profession.

ACTIVITY

- List the various health professions that may also provide assistance to any person you might assist. Consider both government and non-government medical and alternative health services. Do not forget that the person might have feet, teeth, joints and various needs that health professionals outside the traditional medical model are best qualified to fulfil.
- List the various support staff that are necessary for the effective practice of your health profession. Remember the maintenance of the building and also the grounds if you use an outside area for intervention.

What information will assist the health professional in relating to the 'other'?

Some types of information will be more relevant to some health professionals than others. For example, knowing the dominant hand of the individual seeking assistance is highly relevant for particular health professions whereas for others it is irrelevant. There are other types of information about the 'other' that are important regardless of the health profession. It is beneficial to know the abilities, age and gender of the person because this guides the expectations, practice and communication style of the health professional. For example, knowing their particular abilities might facilitate adjustment of expectations; knowing the age of a person allows the health professional to adapt their language level; and knowing the gender might guide the topic of conversation.

REFLECTIVE GROUP ACTIVITY

Try to remember a time when the messages you were given were too simple or too complicated, that is, when someone thought you knew less or more about a particular thing. Some examples could be when relating to a tradesman, a doctor, a mechanic or an astrophysicist – an expert in a particular area who continues to use their jargon or simplifies it when you actually understand.
- Discuss the feelings associated with this experience.
- Discuss non-verbal ways of responding to this situation and their possible effects – positive and negative.
- Suggest ways of avoiding inappropriate methods of communicating when practising as a health professional.

When communicating with the 'other' it is important to know the reason why the person is seeking assistance and, where applicable, the cause, condition or diagnosis that explains their need. It is important to know what they expect from the service of the particular health profession and to know the goals they want to achieve through intervention. It may be important to know their previous experience with health professions because this information may explain particular reactions. It may also be important to know their background and perhaps their interests. There are usually standardised forms specific to health services that provide a basis for questions to gather the required information. This type of information, while necessary, is not the focus of this chapter. The major focus of this chapter is the unseen needs of the 'other' particularly their emotional, sexual, cognitive, social and spiritual needs. Although perhaps considered obvious, the noticeable physical needs of a person can affect the reaction of the health professional and thus require brief consideration as well.

The purpose and benefit of respect

The aim of a health profession is to achieve family/person-centred practice and thus positive outcomes. Respect is essential in order to achieve both of these aims. Respect is more than an attitude or a value about viewing people from a particular perspective (Egan 2007). It provides the basis for appropriate ways of relating to the 'other' and requires particular behaviour (Sander et al 1997). The demonstration of respectful behaviour to the 'other' requires health professionals to respect themselves. Respecting the self protects the health and wellbeing of the health professional. It also maintains satisfaction and contributes to the fulfilment of both personal and professional goals (Purtilo & Haddad 2002).

Demonstration of respect requires commitment to competent communicative and interpersonal practice – 'other'-centred practice. While the behaviours associated with demonstrations of respect are usually non-verbal, they are easily recognised as respect.

Defining respect

Respect is an underlying personal value that determines both attitudes and actions; as such, it is difficult to define. The following attempt to define respect combines various definitions of this value. Respect does not respond to a person positively merely because of their status or position/role in society. It is not about liking someone or admiring someone. Respect is an interest in and acknowledgement of the person, their viewpoint and their emotions (Stein-Parbury 2006). It assumes that everyone has innate worth and value (Egan 2007). Respect allows everyone to be themselves and to express themselves honestly without condemnation, ridicule or criticism (Long 1978). It does not impose personal values and thus expresses no judgement (Davis 2006). Respect believes in the potential of each person and provides the basis for action that assists in the fulfilment of this potential. It believes that each person is valuable regardless of appearance or action, past and present (Bergland & Saltman 2002). Respect values a person regardless of age, colour, racial group, position, uniform, state, relationship, social status or other characteristics. It gazes past the negatives and positives to the inherent worth at the core of the person (Purtilo & Haddad 2002) – a worth shared by all human beings.

REFLECTION

- What is your immediate emotional response to
    - Someone who lives on the street wearing one set of torn dirty clothes who has all their personal possessions in a damaged shopping trolley
    - Someone with a different sexual preference to you
    - A local sports star
    - A drunken person who offers you a drink
    - A policeman
    - A 58-year-old slightly overweight woman wearing a tight, short skirt and a singlet top, lots of cheap jewellery and heavy, poorly done make-up whose lipstick is not restricted to her mouth
    - A Salvation Army officer?
- Do you have an experience or particular values that explain your immediate response?

GROUP ACTIVITY

- Compile a list of factors that contribute to negative and positive responses and thus restrict potential demonstrations of respect.
- Suggest ways of overcoming any negative responses in order to demonstrate respect.
- What feelings arise in response to the following?
  - *I say what I think, it doesn't matter what happens as a result.*
  - *No-one tells me what to do. I make my own decisions.*
  - *I don't pay 'board' (contribution for food etc at home). I couldn't buy designer clothes if I paid to live at home.*
  - *I must be true to myself and do what I want to do.*
  - *I do whatever I have to for 'the good life'.*
- Decide what is important to the person making each statement.
- Write responses to the attitudes expressed in the statements that demonstrate respect but do not necessarily agree with the statement.

Demonstrating respect

The following attitudes, characteristics or behaviours demonstrate respect: interest, warmth, friendliness, approachability, active concern, honesty, authenticity, responding to the needs of the 'other' and giving careful attention to those needs (Purtilo & Haddad 2002).

GROUP ACTIVITY

- Have each group member think about someone they do not respect – someone with different values and beliefs.
- While considering that person attempt to act with the following: warmth, friendliness, approachability, interest, active concern, honesty, acceptance, care and understanding.
- How easy is it to demonstrate these attitudes when you do not actually feel them?
- As a group, discuss whether the expression of the above attitudes appeared authentic and honest. What would make them authentic and honest?

It is not always easy to demonstrate respect even when there are shared values, beliefs and positive feelings towards someone. Thus, to demonstrate respect when the 'other' acts contrary to the values and beliefs of the heath professional can be extremely challenging. In such situations it is difficult to recognise the worth of the individual – to believe in the reality of that worth and to act according to that worth.

GROUP ACTIVITY

Discuss possible strategies that would overcome the barrier to demonstrating respect when relating to someone who you find difficult to respect.

The 'other' is vulnerable and thus responsibility lies with the health professional to demonstrate respect. It is imperative that the health professional behaves in a manner that communicates the 'other' is important – worthy of the investment of time and energy. Also important is acceptance of the person and availability for them regardless of their dysfunction, disfigurement or the demands on time. Rogers (1967) suggests it is beneficial to expect or believe that somehow the 'other' will be able to overcome the current challenges; that they will persevere and reach the established goals. In situations where the 'other' appears resistant and uncooperative it is important that the health professional demonstrates understanding of their perspective and feelings, assisting as necessary to achieve collaboration. While challenging, it is also important to demonstrate respect when personal values and expectations are different to those of the 'other'. Respect does not mean that the 'other' can manipulate or avoid responsibility for their actions. Respect requires the health professional to challenge the 'other' to act to achieve the established goals of the intervention (Egan 2007). Respect is a foundation value that is essential for effective and positive communication in all health professions.

Cultural expectations

Demonstrating respect can cause difficulty for health professionals when relating to 'others' from particular cultural groups (see Chs 15 & 16). Different cultures have a variety of expectations related to respectful behaviour and thus may expect particular behaviour in specific situations as a demonstration of respect. Some of these behaviours relate to non-verbal cues (e.g. eye contact; see Ch 12) or the use of particular colours in specific circumstances (Devito 2007). Other behaviours relate to specific actions when first meeting or seeing each other after an initial introduction (e.g. some cultures allow men to embrace and kiss in public, others have particular hand shakes, while others kiss twice or maybe three times on each cheek depending on the situation and the culture). Some cultures demonstrate respect according to gender and/or age and thus expect particular behaviours related to the gender and/or age of either the health professional or the person seeking their assistance. When working with people from different cultural backgrounds it is essential to seek information about attitudes and expected behaviour governed by and relating to respect (see Chs 15 & 16).

Using names

The name of a person has particular meaning and generally identifies the person. Using the name of a person indicates interest and acknowledges the person as separate from other people. It indicates value and thus demonstrates respect. Asking a person the name they prefer is very important when first communicating. Individuals from particular generations or cultures prefer the use of their family name (e.g. Mr Thomas or Mrs Berk), finding the use of their given name offensive. Using the preferred name during subsequent communicative interactions continues to demonstrate respect and contributes to the development of a therapeutic relationship.

REFLECTION
• If you are in an unfamiliar place, how do you feel if someone greets you by using your name? • What does this mean for a practising health professional?

Confidentiality

Confidentiality refers to keeping information within a particular context (Stein-Parbury 2006; see Ch 11). It is another way of demonstrating respect. All information about the person seeking the assistance of a health professional is confidential. Confidentiality involves keeping information private. The information, whether written or verbal, is available only to the people with the right to access that information (Higgs et al 2005). It is important that health professionals avoid sharing any information about the people they are assisting in any context except at work. It requires health professionals to restrict what information they provide, to whom they provide the information and when they provide it. Some of this information is kept in a medical record. Medical records should not leave the health service setting except for legal reasons. Taking a medical record home to complete an entry is never acceptable. Leaving it on a desk overnight may not be acceptable either.

When gathering information it is important to indicate to the person seeking assistance what information will be shared, how it will be shared and with whom it will be shared. Many healthcare services require the person seeking assistance to sign an informed consent form (see Ch 11) before commencement of services. These forms generally indicate who could receive information about the person (Higgs et al 2005).

Physical aspects of the 'other'

A person who is seeking the assistance of a health professional and has obvious physical needs may or may not require specific action from the health professional. Someone in a wheelchair may require a clear passage to a particular destination or may feel more comfortable if the health professional sits to communicate with them rather than standing over them.

There are obvious physical characteristics of the 'other' that communicate particular information and it is important that health professionals be aware of their reactions to these characteristics. It may seem possible to assume the socioeconomic background of an individual by their designer clothing or the amount and type of jewellery they wear. However, it is important to remember that the vulnerable 'other' is seeking to present a particular image and that their clothing may in fact be an attempt to present a reality that does not exist. Assuming the socioeconomic background of a smelly 'other' with dirty and cheap clothing is equally dangerous. It is important that health professionals avoid making assumptions because of the appearance of the 'other' and remember to relate equally to the 'other' regardless of physical characteristics.

It is sometimes possible to assume the cultural and religious background of an individual because of their clothing; once again, however, it is necessary to take care when assuming anything about someone because of their appearance. Respect and professional training in the health professions guide appropriate responses to the physical appearance and physical needs of the 'other', and empower health professionals to respond appropriately to those needs regardless of the physical aspects.

Emotional aspects of the 'other'

Validation

Validation is important for the 'other' who feels vulnerable and uncertain. It confirms the existence of their negative emotions and potentially allows the 'other' to acknowledge and accept the existence of these emotions. Acknowledging the legitimacy of the negative emotions is often difficult for the 'other' because they may feel confused and ungrateful (see the case study about 'Eric' later in this chapter). The process of validation requires the health professional to recognise the emotional cues of the 'other' and accurately name those emotions. This process, if performed sensitively, generally releases the 'other' to acknowledge those emotions with greater acceptance and less confusion. The 'other' often feels more able to express, understand and control the emotions after validation. It is important to note that validation does not indicate whether the emotions are reasonable or appropriate, it simply states the existence of the emotions. Health professionals indicate unconditional positive regard by i) separating themselves from their values and judgements (Rogers 1967); ii) recognising the emotion in the 'other'; and iii) expressing awareness of the emotion – usually by asking a question relating to the particular emotion, but sometimes with non-verbal cues.

GROUP ACTIVITY

- In groups of four or five, choose five of the following emotions: happy, frustrated, excited, sad, devastated, unhappy, disappointed, confused, bored, sleepy, depressed, guilty, embarrassed, rejected, helpless, irritated, angry, ashamed, insecure.
- Have each member of the group simultaneously express the chosen emotion non-verbally.
- Consider the variations in the ways of expressing each emotion.
- Which of the emotions appeared to be expressed in a similar manner to each other? Why is it important to consider this when validating emotions in the 'other'?
- List the different ways each group member used different parts of their body to express each emotion.
- Decide what each of these answers means for a health professional.

Clarification within validation

Bergland & Saltman (2002) state it is important to recognise that each individual has a unique communication style. Recognition and understanding of the communication style of the individual ensures positive communication outcomes. Accurate validation of emotions cannot occur without this recognition of individual communication styles. Different cultures, different social groups and different families multiply the variations in styles of communication. Therefore, in recognition of these variations, health professionals might request clarification of their perceptions rather than assume they have accurately recognised the emotional cues of the 'other'. A request for clarification of the perception of the emotion is appropriate before recognising and validating an emotion. A question indicates the interest of the health professional in the 'other' and allows the 'other' to decide if they will admit or deny the presence of the emotion. If admission of the emotion follows, the health professional has the opportunity to empathise and explore the emotion with the 'other'. If denial of the emotion follows then the health professional has lost nothing and is learning about the communication style of the 'other'. In this situation, another question asking the 'other' to name the current emotion may or may not be appropriate. The health professional can then decide whether to pursue the presence of the emotional cues or to leave the 'other' to consider the question alone. The question may begin the exploration process of the emotions of the 'other' amidst their confusion and fear, and allow verbal exploration later. Strong emotions are inevitable in the lives of health professionals and those around them; denial of these emotions is unwise because the emotional cost is enormous (Davis 2006). Validation of strong emotions is necessary because it begins the journey of acknowledgement and resolution, both of which facilitate understanding and control of often overwhelming emotions.

Accurate validation requires the health professional to request clarification of the perceived emotions to facilitate honest communication. Such communication encourages the 'other' to honestly admit and consider the presence of the emotions. Validation prepares the 'other' for empathic exploration of their emotional responses. It is not always easy to be honest when considering emotions; however, honesty is essential for the achievement of positive outcomes.

Empathy

Empathy is a process (Rogers 1975) that requires a health professional to enter

> '…the private perceptual world of the other and becoming thoroughly at home in it…. It includes communicating your sensing of his world as you look with fresh and unfrightened eyes at elements of which the individual is fearful. It means frequently checking with him for the accuracy of your sensings, and being guided by the responses you receive…. To be with another in this way means that for the time being you lay aside the views and values you hold for yourself in order to enter another's world without prejudice…' (Rogers 1975, p 4)

This definition reveals the reality of the complexity of expressing empathy. Unlike many definitions of empathy, it makes the health professional responsible for their emotional response to the person. It demands that the health professional not only express emotional sensitivity that demonstrates understanding of the emotions (Northouse & Northouse 1992), but also requires them to separate themselves from their values and personal prejudices. The definition requires the health professional to feel with the person and yet be non-judgemental. It requires the health professional to patiently listen and reflect on what they hear in order to respond with empathy. It requires the health professional to avoid giving advice, regardless of their experience or understanding. In addition, it requires the health professional to avoid interrupting, except to either affirm the person without words or to encourage further expression of the emotions. The health professional expresses empathy verbally and non-verbally – by what is said and how it is said. Expressions of empathy require that the health professional makes no assumptions about the accuracy of their perceptions of the feelings in the 'other', but rather that they request verification of those perceptions. It is the seeking of verification that allows the health professional to remain themselves while focusing on the person who requires their assistance.

In contrast to empathy, **sympathy** is the expression of the experiences, feelings and perspectives of the health professional and places the focus upon those experiences, feelings and perspectives rather than those of the 'other'. Experiencing events that are similar to those of the 'other' may assist the health professional when interacting. However, this can also lead the health professional to think they know exactly how the 'other' is feeling. This 'feeling' can assist understanding or it can create an illusion of understanding that limits the expression of empathy. That is, this 'feeling' may communicate either authentic understanding or a nonchalance that is inappropriate, depending on how the health professional communicates the commonality of experience. It is safest to avoid sharing a similar experience of the health professional with the 'other' because this places focus on the health professional instead of the 'other'. When communicating with empathy it is important to focus on the needs and reactions of the 'other'.

CASE STUDY

Eric, a 28-year-old, and Mandy, his wife of 6 months, wait quietly in a private room for someone to tell them the results of Eric's tests. To fill the time and stop thinking the worst, they talk about the work they are doing on the house they have just bought and their future plans to travel and have a family.

The specialist doing the tests was highly recommended so they feel confident. He finally comes into the room reading some papers. He smiles quietly and looks up. The tests are all clear. Eric and Mandy visibly relax. The specialist does not notice this, however, because he is not convinced that the results are accurate. He suggests more tests to be sure of the diagnosis. He feels his hunch is right considering the symptoms Eric has been experiencing and just wants to make sure.

A few weeks later Eric and Mandy sit in the same room with a feeling of déjà vu. This time they are not trying to avoid thinking about anything – they feel tired and afraid.

When the pathology report arrives the doctor and three other health professionals rush into the room. This time the specialist has a big smile on his face. He excitedly says he was right, these tests have confirmed his hunch and Eric does have the condition he has suspected from the symptoms. *I was right!* he says repeatedly.

Eric and Mandy are crushed – they have no idea of the implications of the condition, but they know their plans will need major changes. Their faces express devastation.

The specialist stops smiling and looks at them, surprised. He simply says *You should be happy; it could have been worse – you have at least 10 good years.*

Stunned, Eric and Mandy thank the specialist for his perseverance in the search for a diagnosis. Eric is feeling completely confused and afraid. Mandy is horrified and devastated. Eric does not want to seem ungrateful but this is not his idea of something to celebrate or something to smile about and he is in shock. In the confusion he thinks these feelings must be inappropriate considering the response from the specialist – and then he notices the tears rolling down the face of the health professional who had spent time with them when they first arrived at the health service. The one who knew they were newly married with wonderful plans for the future.

Eric in his mind thanks that health professional because it indicates that his feelings are appropriate – he is allowed to feel terrible – and he bursts into tears.

(Adapted from Northouse & Northouse 1992)

REFLECTION

- Consider this scenario from the perspective of Eric and Mandy.
- Consider this scenario from the perspective of the specialist – remember the times you have been preoccupied with something or excited about something and have not noticed the feelings of the people around you.
- Consider this scenario from the perspective of the health professional who had the courage to cry.
- Whose perspective do you find easiest to understand?
- Does this mean something about your ability to demonstrate empathy?

GROUP DISCUSSION

- Using the above thoughts discuss the responsibility of the health professional to focus on the needs of the 'other' regardless of the feelings of the health professional.
- List the reasons why this is the case.
- What can a health professional do to 'survive' the process of sharing the perspective of hurting and often fearful people in order to express empathy on another occasion?
- List actions or behaviours that will assist the health professional to express empathy when communicating with the 'others' around them.

The importance and result of empathy for the seeker of assistance

Empathy has a positive effect on both the health professional and the person seeking their assistance. The context of the particular health service, while familiar to the health professional, is unfamiliar to the person seeking the assistance of that service. Each person has a reason for seeking assistance and this reason may be creating confusion and fear in the person. There may also be factors and events in the life of the person, past or present, that cause confusion and fear independent of the current reason for seeking assistance. In such circumstances the emotional need for understanding and acceptance becomes the dominant need. The needy and fearful 'other' seeks that understanding and acceptance from anyone who will offer it.

CASE STUDY

John lives alone in a dark, cluttered room. His best friend is a bottle of cheap alcohol. He has recently experienced back pain and has come to an alternative health service for assistance. While he has plenty of clothes, he usually wears the same clothes, which show little evidence of laundering. John rarely showers so people leave the waiting room whenever he attends for treatment! John has money to pay for treatment, but does not feel that anyone cares about him so he does not care about himself.

Sam, the osteopath who treats John, is pleasant but distant. He usually works as quickly as possible and says very little while treating John. He sterilises everything and disinfects his hands well after treating John.

Adrian, the cleaner, has lost the ability to smell and often works close to John when he is there, chatting as he cleans. He regularly asks John how he is going and how he is feeling. John has come for treatment for several weeks and Adrian has learnt a lot about John in that time. Adrian makes it his business to clean the waiting room whenever John is there, regularly expressing empathy towards John, and once bringing him some home-made cooking (Adrian's wife is a great cook).

GROUP DISCUSSION

- Why do you think John looks forward to attending the health service?
- Why do you think Sam reacts the way he does to John?
- What do you think Adrian has learnt about John? Use your imagination.
- Why do you think John is clean and in fresh clothes after he has been attending for several weeks?

Making an effort to enter the perspective of the person without judgement is a sign of respect (Egan 2007). It communicates understanding and acceptance, and allows expression and exploration of sometimes debilitating emotions. It reassures the person that their emotions are not 'crazy' and it potentially facilitates management of the confusion and fear in unfamiliar and sometimes unpleasant situations. Empathy can empower the person to take control in a seemingly out-of-control situation, thereby facilitating a change in the way they manage the situation and the way they relate to themself. This reality indicates that empathy is a central component of family/person-centred practice (Davis 2006).

ROLE PLAY

Person-centred practice and solving the problem

Divide the entire group into pairs. If there is an odd number have that person observe the progress of the pairs. Role-play the following roles:

- *Nancy*: You have not been attending for the intervention you originally sought. You like the health professional who telephones, however, you are reluctant to explain why you have not been attending the mutually agreed time for appointments. (You must decide the reason why you have not been attending – you may discuss your reason with the group facilitator/instructor if you feel that is appropriate. Do not tell the reason to the person playing the part of the health professional [at least initially]. Reasons for not attending might include illness; concern about someone in your family; a sick pet; nausea because of a new liquid medication that smells and tastes horrible, despite the existence of a flavoured variety that is more palatable; pain that makes showering very slow and tedious etc.)
- *Health professional*: You are aware of the number of people waiting for intervention but you are intent on establishing why Nancy has failed to attend over the past 2 weeks. You really want to assist Nancy so you persist when she is reluctant to provide an explanation of her absence. Demonstrate how you communicate both for Nancy-centred practice (using empathic responses) and to gather the information you need to assist Nancy. What will you do to assist Nancy?

GROUP DISCUSSION

- How successful was the health professional?
- Does confidentiality affect this scenario? If so, how?
- Did the person playing the health professional achieve their goals?
- How did Nancy feel?
- What assisted Nancy to trust and disclose?
- What made it difficult for Nancy to trust and disclose?
- Repeat the role play, swapping roles, and discuss any differences.

Empathy is a time-saving tool of the health professional. Willingness to explore the needs and problems of the 'other' allows expression of the feelings associated with those needs and problems (Burnard 1992). The expression of these feelings facilitates a sense of control for the 'other'. The health professional should note and acknowledge the feelings immediately, and should encourage their expression to avoid difficulties and further problems. An immediate empathic approach allows efficient provision of the health service. It usually ensures collaboration with and effective fulfilment of the needs of the 'other'.

Touch

Touch is a powerful, non-verbal form of communication (Mohan et al 2004). The habit of touching to communicate depends on the personal style of communicating and should not be forced if it is not naturally part of the communicative style of the health professional. The reality that different personality types have different communication styles (Houghton 2000, Opt & Loffredo 2003) means that sometimes the 'other' may find it difficult to communicate through touch. However, when there is a connection and resultant rapport, a gentle touch on the shoulder, pat on the arm or squeeze of the hand for many demonstrates awareness of the plight of the 'other'. Such a gentle touch usually communicates a desire to collaborate to fulfil the needs of the 'other' without causing offence (Holli et al 2003), regardless of the personal style of communication. It is important that the health professional carefully observes responses to touching and avoids touching if the 'other' responds negatively. Asking permission to touch the 'other' before doing so may avoid any negative response. If there is already established rapport and the intention of the touch is to comfort and encourage – to indicate support and empathy – the 'other' usually senses this and responds positively.

REFLECTION

- Are you a person who naturally touches others to communicate?
- In what situations do you touch? What part of the body do you touch?
- How do you respond when someone you know touches you?
- How do you respond when a stranger touches you?
- Do these responses depend on where you are touched?
- Do these responses depend on your relationship with the toucher?
- Are these responses a result of your upbringing? Social norms? Bad experiences? Your personal tendency relating to touching?
- Do you need to seek professional assistance if these responses will limit your effectiveness as a health professional?

There are social norms in each culture that govern touch conventions when communicating. Sexual harassment is a reality in many professional workplaces. Awareness of the norms governing sexual behaviour for a particular workplace is essential for all health professionals in order to avoid communicating inappropriately through touch.

GROUP ACTIVITY

- List the social norms governing touching in each culture represented in the group. Consider greeting, introducing, saying goodbye, variations in touching because of age and gender, comforting an upset person who is familiar, comforting an upset person who is a stranger and any other situations that might include communication by touching.
- If there are people from different cultures in the group, compare the differences in the social norms governing touching in different situations.
- If the group is monocultural, discuss any experience of different norms governing touching – even within families.
- List ways in which these differences might guide the practice of a health professional.

Touching can provide feedback about the emotions of the 'other'. A gentle touch may inform the health professional that the 'other' who appears relaxed and in control feels unsure and requires encouragement. This previously unnoticeable information encourages the health professional to communicate empathy by investing time and energy in exploring these upsetting emotions.

Parents and significant others communicate emotions through touch with their children. In families, touch is a powerful form of communication that expresses parental or sibling emotion. Kisses, cuddles, tickles and rumbles are fun and comforting; they communicate ease, acceptance, love and affection (Mohan et al 2004). This manner of touch produces positive emotions in both the person touching and the person receiving the touch. Expressions of anger, frustration and disapproval communicated through either touch or tone of voice produce negative emotions in the child. Various types of touch, whether producing positive or negative emotions, can condition a child to respond in a particular manner when touched by anyone. Health professionals who use touch within their treatment media should consider the reaction of anyone they touch. Careful awareness of the responses and needs of children when touching is essential because this provides information about the touching experiences of that child. Accurate knowledge of the touch experiences of a child, if managed appropriately, has potential to restore and protect the emotional growth of the child and their future ability to both give and receive touch as a way of communicating expressions of concern.

When used appropriately to communicate, touch can be a powerful tool for the health professional who feels comfortable touching others.

Silence

Silence can be a powerful and comforting communication device. Words are sometimes inappropriate. Saying nothing with someone – just being with them – is more appropriate than words in particular circumstances.

REFLECTION

- How comfortable are you with silences in conversations?
- What is your natural tendency when there is a silence in a conversation?
- What does that mean for you as a health professional?

When listening the health professional is silent, but the interaction is not silent because the 'other' is speaking. Refraining from speaking while listening in combination with concentrating and focusing on the speaker demonstrates skills in listening as well as interest and respect (Stein-Parbury 2006). There are occasions while communicating, however, when words are inappropriate or inadequate. In these cases, just being with a person and saying nothing indicates interest, care, respect and even empathy. There are occasions when the person seeking assistance does not seek words but the presence of an interested and caring health professional. A carer or relative found sitting outside the room of their seriously ill or dying family member may not desire verbal communication but the non-verbal, silent presence of a previously known, concerned and interested health professional. This presence communicates care and – even though the health professional may be skilful in verbal expressions of empathic care – simply sitting quietly with the person fulfils the needs of the person at that time.

When the 'other' has difficulty expressing themselves verbally, it is appropriate in some health professions to silently perform an activity with the 'other' in an interested and observant manner to build rapport (Schmid 2005). The possible people with whom a health professional might use this type of silence include children, people with mental health disorders or communication difficulties, people experiencing severe pain and people in palliative care units.

Different cultures have different uses for silence. Some cultures find that silence communicates more effectively than words. When communicating with a vulnerable person from a different culture, it is important to clarify the uses and effects of silence (see Chs 15 & 16).

Silence, when used appropriately, can powerfully communicate interest, regard and a desire to assist if possible.

Sexual aspects of the 'other'

People are sexual beings regardless of their culture or gender. Note that sexuality here is not synonymous with gender. Individuals usually have sexual organs, and while these may determine their gender, they do not necessarily determine their ability to discuss and relate to their sexuality. The sexual aspect of individuals refers to their particular reproductive organs and the responsibilities associated with the use of those organs (Milliken & Honeycutt 2004), as well as their sexual preference. Particular health professions may relate to the sexuality or sexual functioning of the individuals they assist, while others may not. All health professionals, however, may need to respond *without* verbal or non-verbal judgement to possible differences in their sexual preference and the sexual preference of the person seeking their assistance.

CASE STUDY

Amy is 14 years old and has an intellectual disability. She has recently begun menstruating and her mother has found it difficult to teach her how to manage this change in her body from the perspectives of both hygiene and sexual activity.

REFLECTIVE GROUP ACTIVITY

- How would you feel if you were asked to assist Amy to manage the sexual changes in her body and ensure safe sexual activity in the future?
- Write a list of the things you would find difficult in this situation and how you might overcome these difficulties.
- In groups, discuss possible strategies for assisting Amy and her mother to manage the emotional and sexual aspects of this situation.

Some individuals find it difficult to explicitly discuss or consider their own sexuality. Such individuals may or may not find it difficult to relate to the sexual aspect of another person. This is true both for some health professionals and some individuals seeking assistance.

SAME-GENDER GROUP ACTIVITY

Peter/Peta is a 21-year-old with paraplegia. He/she is about to begin sleeping with his/her partner for the first time since his/her accident. You have an excellent relationship with Peter/Peta, with many things in common – similar age and interests, same gender etc. He/she indicates fear about his/her sexual abilities since the accident and asks you for assistance about how to approach having intercourse with his/her partner. The doctor says Peter/Peta should be able to function sexually but has given no other guidance or reassurance.

Discuss the possible ways of responding to empower Peter/Peta.

Certainly some health professionals would not usually expect to consider the sexual aspect of a person within the scope of their practice. However, if a particular health professional develops a safe therapeutic relationship with an 'other', that 'other' may wish to discuss their sexual concerns with that health professional. This discussion may or may not feel comfortable, but if managed appropriately it may empower the 'other' to seek qualified assistance that will fulfil their sexual needs.

Cognitive aspects of the 'other'

Cognitive ability is the ability to process information using reasoning, interpretation, intuition and perception. Cognitive events are conscious thoughts (Holli et al 2003) that a person has in an attempt to process and understand received information. It is important that the health professional and the 'other' possess basic cognitive abilities to negotiate mutual understanding and produce effective and emotionally comfortable interactions.

An important cognitive ability is the ability to **concentrate** or attend throughout the communicative interaction. Understanding the limits of the attention span of the 'other' – whether the 'other' is developing cognitive skills (children) or losing them (ageing adults) – is important because it allows the health professional to adjust their communication as necessary. It is important that all communicating individuals **understand** that the words and non-verbal behaviours they use will produce particular effects and **consequences**. Children (who are still developing their cognitive abilities) and individuals with limited cognitive abilities often find it difficult to understand the idea of cause and effect (Purtilo & Haddad 2002). For example, the individual who thinks they have lost their meal tray because they did not exercise enough care does not understand explanations about the cause and effect that resulted in the removal of the meal tray (i.e. the cleaning up at the end of lunchtime). Health professionals have the responsibility to communicate with such individuals with understanding and skill. It is imperative that health professionals adapt their manner of communicating according to the cognitive ability of the 'other', and that they continue to make adjustments according to their observations of the effects of their communication upon the 'other'.

When communicating with children it is important to remember that children demonstrate particular skills in cognition at different ages (Berk 2006). Jean Piaget (1968) developed an explanation of the stages of cognitive development in childhood. Although there is discussion about the accuracy of the timing of these stages, it does appear that children develop cognitive skills as they grow and experience their world. Variations can occur because individual children may demonstrate highly developed cognition at a particular age while other children may not, despite apparently similar intelligence and experience. Adults with diminishing cognitive skills may revert to demonstrating cognitive abilities typical of some of these earlier stages. It is important to adjust communication styles according to the cognitive abilities of the 'other'.

When communicating with people who have limited cognitive abilities or a disorder affecting their comprehension of language, it is important for health professionals to use short and simple sentences with non-abstract words wherever possible. This will maximise the comprehension of the 'other'. Unless the person also has a hearing impairment, there is no need for a raised volume of voice.

If someone does not understand what is being communicated to them, regardless of the reasons for the lack of comprehension, they will cease listening. In such situations, negotiation of meaning and mutual understanding becomes less possible. Interpreting the non-verbal cues related to potential comprehension is sometimes useful, but may be unreliable in many situations. To check for adequate comprehension the health professional should ask the individual to repeat in their own words the meaning they ascribe to the delivered message.

Remember that emotional states may restrict cognitive functioning regardless of the considered cognitive abilities of the individual. Consideration of and attention to the emotional state of the 'other' may increase their ability to concentrate and thus improve the potential for effective communication.

GROUP ACTIVITY

- Share, list and discuss possible strategies for communicating with people who have limited cognitive abilities.
- Discuss group members' experiences with such strategies.
- List the characteristics of each strategy and discuss the factors that contribute to the success of each strategy.

Some individuals are limited in their cognitive abilities but these abilities are stable – they are not developing or deteriorating. Most of these individuals have reached a particular level of cognitive functioning that is below the typical level of their age. Individuals with an intellectual disability are representative of this group and may require the use of particular methods of communication to communicate effectively. Another group of individuals who may experience difficulty communicating are those who have a disorder related to the Autism Spectrum Disorder (American Psychiatric Association 2000). Other individuals who may experience communication difficulties include those with head injuries, sensory impairments, learning disorders, specific language disorders and some physical disabilities including cerebral palsy.

Individuals with limited verbal skills may communicate through certain behaviours, such as biting, hitting, kicking, pushing, spitting, screaming, crying, laughing, withdrawing, touching, smiling, smelling, reaching, physically guiding, head banging/butting, absconding from a particular situation, cuddling, undressing in public and many more. If an individual has severe difficulties communicating verbally, resorting to such behaviours may be the only manner of expressing their feelings at the time.

REFLECTION

- Consider your response to the behaviours listed in the previous paragraph.
- Have you seen others respond to such behaviours?
- Was their response appropriate? Was it effective? Why or why not?

It is important for the health professional to accommodate and appropriately manage difficult behaviours while implementing strategies to establish appropriate communicative behaviours for such individuals.

Useful types of communication for the 'other' with limited cognitive skills

In some countries there are devices and forms of communication that do not rely on verbal transmission. **Augmentative and alternative communication (AAC)** refers to systems of communication for people who find speaking difficult or are unable to speak. Such communication systems may help reduce frustration levels and thus decrease the use of disturbing behaviours to communicate.

Augmentative and alternative forms of communication include the use of symbols, aids, strategies and techniques to transmit and receive messages through either electronic or non-electronic means (Beukelman & Mirenda 2006). Augmentative communication refers to non-verbal forms of communication that *highlight* the spoken word through simultaneous gestures or signs (e.g. finger spelling, key-word signing [e.g. Makaton], sign language [e.g. Auslan]), or through pointing to objects or pictures. Alternative communication uses forms of communication to *replace* the spoken word (e.g. an electronic device using visual communication software).

Individuals who experience difficulty communicating because of physical or cognitive limitations may rely on AAC to transmit and receive information. The use of AAC will assist such individuals to interact socially and engage in the activities of their choice. Such individuals can use one or a combination of several forms of AAC to process and understand information as well as express themselves. Some individuals use AAC until speech develops, or to supplement attempts at vocalisation. For others AAC is a permanent means of communication that can assist comprehension and self-expression.

Successful use of AAC requires competence in the dominant language of the environment; social competence in the expected norms of communication; competence in operating the particular system; and an ability to compensate for the ignorance of communication partners who are unfamiliar with the particular system. Understanding the norms of personal interaction and communication are necessary for effective communication. They include 'competence as to when to speak, when not, and as to what to talk about, with whom, when, where, in what manner' (Hymes 1972, p 277). Most individuals absorb these norms as they grow up in a particular culture or society and use them skilfully yet unconsciously whenever interacting.

Augmentative and alternative forms of communication are generally visual in nature. (Any individual who finds it difficult to process auditory information may benefit from using visual forms of communication.) Visual forms of communication are useful because they are concrete and do not usually require abstract thought. They are also stable, lasting longer than the spoken word. The use of a symbol or sign that resembles a real object also makes accurate assumptions possible for the person receiving the message.

If possible, it is beneficial for AAC devices to be flexible and portable, allowing the individual to use them in a variety of situations. Such devices are generally individualised to the needs, wants and emotions of the particular individual. Augmentative and alternative forms of communication can function to give directions, provide single-step pictures for completion of activities, or facilitate choices of activities. They can take many forms, for example

- A community request card containing a picture of a particular type of burger and can of drink
- A notice board containing a pictorial representation of the schedule for the day
- A 'chat book' that introduces an individual who communicates regularly with a variety of people; the book might include pictures of their likes and dislikes, family, hobbies, social experiences and the events of the previous week

- A pictorial shopping list displaying pictures of the goods needed for the next week
- An activity choice board or book that allows an individual to choose the activity they would prefer to perform after completion of the current activity.

These are the less technical forms of AAC. However, such systems can also take the form of electronic devices that may provide vocalisation in addition to visual forms of messages.

Health professionals will find AAC systems to be useful when relating to the 'other' who has difficulty communicating verbally. They encourage self-expression and can increase independence. Augmentative and alternative communication creates a connection with those around the individual by increasing the likelihood of communicative exchanges.

Social needs of the 'other'

Humans often seek social interaction. The extent and enjoyment of social interactions may vary according to personality type but most typically-functioning individuals seek the company of other humans some time during every day (Brill & Levine 2005). Individuals who feel vulnerable and fearful may desire the company of people they trust. In such situations the 'other' may not want to actively interact – they may simply desire the presence of a friendly, caring individual. In the busy world of the health professional, this can be a demand the health professional is unable to meet.

ACTIVITY

- How might a health professional fulfil the social need of the 'other' in the situation where the 'other' would like to have someone present? List ways.
- If one of the people seeking your assistance is lonely and often monopolises your time because of this loneliness, how might you assist this 'other'?

Many individuals have their needs for social contact met through the ownership of an animal. Underestimating the significance of the relationship with a long-term pet is unwise when assisting any individual regardless of age or gender. A vulnerable 'other' may feel their pet is their only reliable and supportive social relationship and thus acknowledgement of the pet is essential.

Spiritual needs of the 'other'

Every individual has a spiritual component. The spiritual component of a person determines the focus of their lives and dictates what is valuable and meaningful to them. It determines notions of self and the place of the individual in life. It can refer to the 'things' that renew, the 'things' that bring comfort and lift the spirit as well as the 'things' that inspire and encourage. The spiritual aspect relates to the beliefs and values that motivate and sustain individuals. As such, it is the basis for explanations about the meaning and purpose of the events in life. Consideration of spirituality is an important element of healthcare and can benefit the health and wellbeing of both health professionals and those they assist (White 2006). An individual may be consciously aware of this aspect of themselves or this aspect may be unconsciously present. It is an aspect of an individual that some prefer to keep private and may avoid discussing in a social context. Despite spirituality usually being unconscious, it is often when an individual feels vulnerable that this aspect becomes conscious.

In the past 20 years there has been a growing interest in spirituality and religion among many of the health professions (Miller & Thorensen 1999). Despite the growing awareness of spirituality and the affect of this aspect on health and wellbeing (Miller & Thorensen 2003, Powell et al 2003, Seemen et al 2003), many health professionals fail to recognise the spiritual aspects of the 'other'. Failure of health professionals to recognise the importance of spiritual issues may be a major source of distress for particular 'others'. If spiritual issues are important to the 'other' they require recognition and attention (Hall et al 2004). Some cultures are constantly aware of a spiritual existence and thus a spiritual aspect for individuals from such cultures will be very significant. If the 'other' expresses needs with spiritual implications it is important that the health professional acknowledges and addresses those needs rather than ignoring them, regardless of the spiritual beliefs of the health professional.

CASE STUDY

You have been assisting an elderly Asian man for several weeks. He appears to benefit from seeing you and there is indication of rapport between you. He attends regularly but demonstrates limited progress. Through an interpreter, he indicates he is too tired to implement your suggestions except during your treatment sessions. Empathic questioning reveals that he cannot sleep because every night the spirits of his previous wives who died some years ago torment him.

Regardless of your spiritual beliefs, you know this man would improve quickly if he was able to implement your suggestions outside your treatment sessions.

GROUP ACTIVITY

List possible appropriate actions to assist this man.

There are many ways of addressing the spiritual needs and concerns of the 'other'. It is important to remember that no health professional has all the answers and it is acceptable to indicate this reality to the 'other'. Regardless of the personal beliefs of the health professional, it is important to identify whether the 'other' requires a person who understands their spiritual, religious or philosophical beliefs and connect them with such a person if necessary. Acknowledging the beliefs and values of the 'other' can motivate and sustain them in difficult situations.

When assisting someone for whom spirituality is significant it is important to

- Demonstrate respect for the person and their ideas of spirituality
- Recognise the source of spiritual support for the person and allow access to that form of support as required
- Understand when the person may be experiencing spiritual distress and behave in a manner that acknowledges and attempts to alleviate the distress.

Spiritual functioning affects the value the person assigns to their body, their spirit, their emotions, their thoughts and to those around them. It may affect the reaction to the suggestions and intervention of the health professional. It may limit or encourage the cooperation of the individual seeking assistance and that of their family. Ignoring the spiritual aspect, even when that aspect is obvious, is often detrimental to effective communication.

Spiritual issues may not appear relevant to the practising health professional; however, if the 'other' seeking their assistance considers them relevant they require specific attention. Such attention will contribute to positive outcomes and is therefore a necessary part of the intervention of the health professional.

Chapter summary

Health professionals relate to 'others' throughout a working day. Awareness of the holistic needs of the 'other' while demonstrating respect and empathy is essential for any health professional. Holistic care includes consideration of the physical, emotional, sexual, cognitive, social and spiritual needs that contribute to positive outcomes for the 'other'.

Complete the following:
1. What are the aspects that make up the whole person?

_____

_____

_____

2. What are the potential effects of failure to recognise each aspect of the whole person?

_____

_____

_____

3. List the 'others' who might seek assistance from a health professional.

_____

_____

_____

4. List the information a health professional requires in order to provide appropriate assistance.

_____

_____

_____

5. What three important elements does effective communication with the 'other' require?
    i.   _____
    ii. _____
    iii. _____

6. Physical aspects of the 'other' may appear obvious. Suggest reasons why they might not always be reliable.

_____

_____

_____

7. What might assist in meeting the needs of the emotional aspects of the 'other'?

_____

_____

_____

8. What are the components of the sexual aspects of an individual?

_____

_____

_____

9. How can a health professional communicate with an individual with limited cognitive skills?

_____

_____

_____

10. What can affect the social aspect of an individual?

_____

_____

_____

13. Why should a health professional acknowledge the spiritual aspect of an individual?

_____

_____

_____

References

American Psychiatric Association 2000 Diagnostic and Statistical Manual of Mental Disorders, 4th edn-TR. APA, Washington DC

Bergland C, Saltman D (eds) 2002 Communication for healthcare. Oxford University Press, Melbourne

Berk L 2006 Development through the lifespan, 4th edn. Allyn & Bacon, Boston

Beukelman D R, Mirenda P 2006 Augmentative and alternative communication: supporting children and adults with complex communication needs, 3rd edn. Brookes, Baltimore

Brill N I, Levine J 2005 Working with people: the helping process, 8th edn. Pearson, Boston

Burnard P 1992 Teaching interpersonal skills. Chapman & Hall, London

Davis C M 2006 Patient practitioner interaction. An experiential manual for developing the art of healthcare, 4th edn. Slack, Thorofare NJ

Devito J A 2007 The interpersonal communication book, 11th edn. Pearson, Boston

Egan G 2007 The skilled helper, 8th edn. Thomson, Belmont CA

Hall C R, Dixon W A, Mauzey E D 2004 Spirituality and religion: implications for counsellors. Journal of Counseling and Development 82:504–507

Higgs J, Sefton A, Street A et al 2005 Communicating in the health and social sciences. Oxford University Press, Melbourne

Holli B B, Calabrese R J, O'Sullivan Mailett J 2003 Communication and education skills for dietetics professionals, 4th edn. Lippincott, Williams & Wilkins, Philadelphia

Houghton A 2000 Using the Myers-Briggs type indicator for career development. British Medical Journal 320(2):366–367

Hymes D 1972 On communicative competence. In: Pride J B, Holmes J (eds) Sociolinguistics. Penguin Books, London, p 269–293

Long L 1978 Listening/responding: human-relations training for teachers. Brooks/Cole, Monterey CA

Miller W R, Thorensen C E 1999 Spirituality and health. In: Miller W R (ed) Integrating spirituality into treatment: resources for practitioners. American Psychological Association, Washington DC, p 3–18

Miller W R, Thorensen CE 2003 Spirituality, religion and health: an emerging research field. American Psychologist 58(1):24–35

Milliken M E, Honeycutt A 2004 Understanding human behavior: a guide for healthcare providers, 7th edn. Thomson Delmar, New York

Mohan T, McGregor H, Saunders S et al 2004 Communicating as professionals. Thomson, Melbourne

Northouse P G, Northouse L L 1992 Health communication: strategies for health professionals, 2nd edn. Prentice Hall, Englewood Cliffs NJ

Opt S, Loffredo D 2003 Communicator image and Myers-Briggs type indicator extraversion-introversion. The Journal of Psychology 137(6):560–568

Piaget J 1968 Six psychological studies. Vintage, New York

Powell L H, Shahabi L, Thorensen C E 2003 Religion and spirituality: linkages to physical health. American Psychologist 58(1):36–52

Purtilo R B, Haddad A 2002 Health professional and patient interaction, 6th edn. Saunders, Philadelphia

Rogers C 1967 On becoming a person. Constable, London

Rogers C 1975 Empathic: an unappreciated way of being. The Counselling Psychologist 5(2):2–10

Sander M R, Mitchell C, Byrne G J A (eds) 1997 Medical consultation skills: behavioural and interpersonal dimensions of healthcare. Addison Wesley, Melbourne

Schmid T 2005 Promoting health through creativity: for professionals in health, arts and education. Whurr, Philadelphia

Seemen T E, Dubin L F, Seemen M 2003 Religiosity/spirituality and health: a critical review of the evidence for biological pathways. American Psychologist 58(1):53–63

Stein-Parbury J 2006 Patient and person: interpersonal skills in nursing, 3rd edn. Elsevier, Sydney (Original work published 2005)

White G 2006 Talking about spirituality in healthcare practice: a resource for the multi-professional healthcare team. Jessica Kingsley, London

Awareness of different environments

8

CHAPTER OBJECTIVES

Upon completing this chapter, students should be able to

- Recognise the physical factors within the environment that influence the quality of the service and the outcomes of a health profession
- Understand the importance of the emotional environment for all individuals in a healthcare service
- Recognise the factors contributing to the creation of the emotional environment
- Identify the benefits of acknowledging and accommodating the emotional environments of all relevant people to ensure family/person-centred practice
- Justify the importance of considering the cultural environment of the individuals in a healthcare service
- Recognise some of the elements of a culture that vary across cultures
- Appreciate the possibility of varying sexual environments and understand that the sexual environment can influence health service delivery
- Demonstrate understanding of various social environments and their influence on the individuals in a healthcare service
- State the benefits of being aware of and understanding the spiritual environments of the individuals in a healthcare service
- Explain the importance of openness to all the environments that affect the outcomes of any health service.

Individuals develop in many types of environments. Such environments initially include the physical settings within the family home, the local community and the school. These physical environments provide the setting for other environments, particularly emotional, cultural, sexual, social and spiritual environments. These environments interact to form a dynamic system that determines the development and expectations of each individual. These expectations influence the expectations and outcomes of communicative interactions.

ACTIVITY

- Divide a page into two, top to bottom. On one side list the factors that have assisted your ability to understand in particular environments and on the other list those that have limited your comprehension (e.g. noisy, emotionally tense or spiritually unfamiliar environments). Consider the aspects of your whole person as well as cultural and financial aspects.
- Using this list construct the environment that best assists in establishing comprehension when providing or receiving information. Consider the perspectives of the health professional and the person receiving assistance.

There are unique factors that affect the responses within and the results of interactions. Some of these factors are age, gender, social expectations, economic status, cultural norms, sexual preferences, attitudes, experience, professional knowledge and associated expectations, problem-solving strategies, types of thinking, personality types and motivational forces (Blanche 2007, Chen 2006, Slahova et al 2007). Environmental factors also affect the outcomes of interactions. They are many and varied and each has its own effect on potential outcomes. Environmental factors are akin to the factors affecting the 'other', with some being obvious and others more obscure. Some are more immediate than others – directly affecting the individual in the present – while others have shaped them in their past. Some the health professional can manage within the routine of practice, while others require specific understanding and tolerance.

The physical environment

Physical appearance: Dress

The health professional has immediate control over their physical appearance, specifically clothing, jewellery and personal grooming. Certainly facial features and other inherited characteristics are uncontrollable, but consideration of personal codes of dress and grooming is essential for health professionals. While dress and grooming are components of body language (see Ch 12), from the perspective of the person seeking assistance the physical appearance of the health professional is part of the new and unfamiliar physical environment. Most healthcare services have specific codes of dress for some staff members, however, it is important to consider the effect of personal appearance upon the 'others' in the health service.

CASE STUDY

A health professional recently joined a health service. Upon arrival, the manager explained the personal appearance code along with many other behavioural expectations. The personal appearance code included smart conservative dress, removal of nose or lip rings, particular footwear and guidelines for jewellery and hair.

GROUP ACTIVITY

- Decide why health services have restrictive codes of personal appearance.
- List the reasons for and against such codes; consider healthcare interventions for individuals in various stages of the lifespan.

This new staff member chose to ignore many of the codes, arguing they wanted to maintain their individuality and that they were neat and clean. A nose ring, loose-fitting 'hippy' clothing, several large skull finger rings, sandals and unrestrained beautiful long hair were typical of the personal appearance of this health professional.

GROUP DISCUSSION

- If this were you, how would you respond to any attempt to change how you dress or groom yourself in a professional setting?
- How would your grandmother respond to a health professional with this physical appearance?
- Now think of a small child you know – how would they respond?
- Decide the best way to manage this behaviour to achieve a positive outcome for all.

When dressing as a health professional it is important to avoid expressions of economic status – either wealth or poverty – in clothing, footwear or jewellery (Holli et al 2003). Appearance of wealth or poverty might be intimidating and is sometimes misinterpreted by those seeking assistance.

REFLECTIVE GROUP ACTIVITY

- Discuss reasons for restrictive codes of personal appearance in health services – consider uniforms, hair restraint, jewellery and footwear.
  - Consider the importance of comfort and safety for all stakeholders.
  - List the benefits and disadvantages of wearing a uniform regularly.
- Decide whether restrictive codes of personal appearance are necessary and appropriate in every healthcare setting.

Familiarity with the physical environment and the usual procedures
Person seeking assistance

REFLECTION

- Have you ever sought assistance from a service about which you knew very little?
- How did you feel initially?
- What made you feel more comfortable?

Most people feel apprehensive when entering a new environment for the first time. New environments typically stimulate unsure and hesitant behaviours. If the new environment holds unknown procedures and perhaps pain there might even be feelings of fear and anger. Investing time to familiarise people to a new environment can avoid any negative emotions related to the novelty of the environment and the unknown procedures associated with the environment (Purtilo & Haddad 2002). In such situations it is helpful to imagine what the personal reaction of the health professional might be in a similar situation.

CASE STUDY

A person waking from a 10-day coma asks to get up to go to the toilet. A helpful nurse returns a few minutes later with a commode chair on wheels. This is a standard procedure where the person transfers onto the commode chair and the nurse wheels the person and commode to the toilet cubicle. This is appropriate for someone who is weak from lack of sustenance and exercise. Upon seeing the commode chair the person bursts into tears and states *I don't want to go that much!*

REFLECTION

- Can you explain this reaction? How would you react?
- Is there anything that could be done to avoid this reaction?
- If so, what? If not, why?
- Can you think of a regular procedure in your health profession that might illicit a similar reaction?

Knowing where to find toilets and other necessary facilities is reassuring, however, understanding what to expect during a procedure or intervention, or as a result of a particular need, is equally important. Assisting the person to become familiar with the environment – the facilities, people and procedures – is essential to ensure positive responses and outcomes (see Ch 3).

Health professional

There are times when health professionals may find themselves in unfamiliar environments when assisting a person. Some of these environments may feel cosy and relaxing, while others seem daunting, smelly or cluttered. (A visit to the home of a person who lives adjacent to a fertiliser factory does test the ability of the health professional to successfully complete their task in such an environment.) When visiting a person in their home or taking them to an unfamiliar environment as part of the intervention, it is important for health professionals to take the necessary measures to minimise their anxiety related to the novelty of the environment (e.g. outline every expectation and indicate the level of assistance available). In such circumstances it is imperative that the health professional continues to respond with respect and empathy.

Rooms

Furniture placement and physical comfort

Various factors require consideration when choosing the type of furniture and how to place the furniture within a room. Placement of furniture can encourage or discourage interaction. Chairs side-by-side facing the same direction do not encourage communication, nor do they demonstrate interest and care. A desk between the people communicating is not only a physical barrier, it is also an emotional barrier. Such a desk communicates a desire to keep others distant. It is important to avoid using furniture as a physical barrier when aiming at family/person-centred practice. Arranging the chairs around a desk, a comfortable distance apart, so they face each other or are adjacent to each other promotes communication that is more personal. This configuration facilitates eye contact, which is valued in most western cultures, although may not be in other cultures. It is important to ensure that all communicating individuals are physically comfortable before the commencement of the interaction. If a table is required for placement of written material, a round table allows a clear view for everyone seated at the table.

REFLECTIVE ACTIVITY

- Consider the effect of your physical comfort on your ability to concentrate, understand and remember specific details. Can you concentrate regardless of your comfort?
- Decide on the best way to establish whether a person is physically comfortable. Remember they are feeling vulnerable so may not tell you directly they are physically uncomfortable. How will you know they are comfortable or uncomfortable? What might you do to make them physically comfortable if you establish they are uncomfortable?

Waiting rooms

Waiting rooms are often crowded and noisy. Regardless of the busy nature of the room or the size of the room, there are basic principles that make a waiting room pleasant for those waiting. The colour of the room (paint and furniture), the texture and type of furniture, the lighting and the ventilation present either a warm, welcoming atmosphere or a cold, clinical feeling. The first encourages a feeling of comfort, relaxation and safety, while the other feels impersonal and unfriendly. The first encourages people to linger, while the other encourages people to leave as quickly as possible (Northouse & Northouse 1992). The more impersonal the waiting room, the greater the likelihood of expressions of frustration and hostility (Purtilo & Haddad 2002). Such behaviour can result from personal factors or having to wait too long, but may also result from the impersonal or clinical nature of the environment.

GROUP ACTIVITY

- For each member of the group list the colours and textures that create a feeling of comfort and emotional warmth. Have these changed with age?
- Consider the variations in personal taste.
- What does this mean for a health service and the health professional?

The feeling of comfort gained from sitting or lying on particular types of furniture varies from person to person according to size, height, physical condition, age and gender. Equipping waiting rooms with varying types of chairs and mattresses can assist to overcome these personal variations. Ventilation and natural light also contribute to the ambience of any room, but if these are not possible the colour and type of furniture can adequately compensate for their lack.

Treatment rooms and rooms with beds

The same principles outlined for creation of an appropriate waiting room atmosphere also apply to treatment areas. However, it is important to consider additional environmental factors when in such areas. Many treatment areas do not naturally facilitate confidential and private communication. It is important for health professionals working in such environments to consider individual needs for privacy.

REFLECTION

- How do you feel if you discover someone talking about something personal when they do not know you can hear the conversation?
- What do you do in such situations – do you keep listening or do you move? What does this reveal about you?
- What implications does this have for a health professional?
- How do you feel if you discover someone talking about you when they do not know you can hear? What do you do then?
- What does this mean for a health professional?

The need for privacy may vary according to personality type and the emotional state of the individual at any given time. Consistent consideration of these needs will promote personal disclosure when required and the development of rapport. It is important to consider the difference between visual privacy and auditory privacy. Drawing curtains around a treatment bed or a bed in a ward does not guarantee privacy. A private room will facilitate personal communication, while a public space will keep the communication at a superficial level in order to protect confidentiality.

Avoiding distractions and interruptions

The use of a private room for discussion of personal information is very important but may not achieve personal disclosure if there are constant distractions. Distractions come from the telephone, people, regular or loud noises, particular objects in the room and sometimes movement outside a window.

REFLECTION

Think of a time when someone or something distracted you during a conversation or lecture. What was the distraction? Was it important? How did you feel about the distraction? Were you able to return to the exact point after the distraction occurred? How long did it take to regain concentration and the 'flow' of the information?

GROUP ACTIVITY

- As a group find a movie only one member of the group has seen. Have that person tell another group member who wants to see the movie the story of the movie and describe the major characters in the movie.
- Every other member of the group takes turns to interrupt the retelling with an unrelated statement or noise – asking for the time or when the next bus is due, tapping on the floor, or pointing out an event outside the window etc.
- The person listening responds to each distraction, taking interest and where necessary answering or commenting.
- As a group, observe the effect of the distractions on the flow of the story and on the person attempting to tell the story.
- Have the listening person retell the story of the movie and check for accuracy.

Personal and emotional communication requires concentration and focus. Distractions make this focus difficult and disturb the flow of the communication. Restoring the concentration and information flow during exploration of emotion is often difficult. More importantly, responding to distractions communicates that the distraction is more important to the health professional than the communicating 'other'. Thus, avoidance of such distractions is very important (Bergland & Saltman 2002). This is achieved by not answering the telephone, leaving a message that indicates disturbances are not acceptable (e.g. a sign on the door indicating 'Do Not Disturb'), decreasing or removing distracting noises and/or objects where possible, and organising the seating to avoid distractions outside a window. If in a hospital ward, it is appropriate to arrange a time when there are no expectations from other health professionals or visitors.

Some sounds are so much a part of the environment that the health professional no longer notices them, such as sounds from equipment or machinery. These sounds are often necessary and unavoidable but may be distracting to a person unfamiliar with the environment. In such situations it may be necessary to recognise the distraction and encourage the individual to attempt to ignore it if possible. Sometimes the simple acknowledgement of the distraction may assist the individual to ignore it and focus on the communicative event.

Temperature

Different healthcare settings have different constraints relating to resources and type of service. This may affect the presence of temperature controls within the setting. The external climate may make temperature alterations desirable. Health services in very cold climates usually have heating; however, those in hot, humid climates may not always have air-conditioning. In such situations, the behaviour of those within the health service may reflect the temperature. If there is a pattern of irritability among people in those services – people seeking assistance and staff alike – consideration of the heat in the environment may explain the 'emotional temperature' (Purtilo & Haddad 2002).

Warm temperature and poor ventilation can encourage drowsiness, which will limit the quality of the communication. Feeling cold can be equally detrimental to communication, with the physical temperature of the person dominating their responses. Where possible, control of the temperature or compensatory measures when climate control is lacking are essential to ensure effective communication.

The physical ability of the person

Each individual has abilities and skills that facilitate their movement and comfort in particular environments. Children find stairs and large chairs and tables difficult to accommodate until they grow to a particular height and develop the abilities and skills to independently negotiate such objects in the environment. Extremely tall people can find the size of chairs and tables and the height of benches equally challenging – regardless of their abilities and skills. Individuals with physical limitations that restrict their ability to negotiate particular environments may find such objects to be barriers to participation and independent functioning. It is important for a health professional to consider the abilities and skills of the individuals seeking their assistance in order to adjust the environment to accommodate the needs of those individuals. Ramps with rails, height of chairs and tables, height of beds and toilets – in fact height of anything they must negotiate within the environment of the particular health profession – may be significant. Assistive devices that facilitate independent functioning for such individuals will reduce potentially negative emotions and increase the possibility of positive outcomes of communication and interventions.

Trust, empathy, good rapport and a therapeutic relationship will compensate for deficits in the physical environment. These develop over time, however, and an unfriendly clinical environment creates an initial impression that may be difficult to overcome.

The emotional environment

The emotional state and emotional response of individuals seeking assistance create a particular emotional environment that in many cases requires direct attention from the health professional. Direct and immediate attention to emotions can save time and effort for both the person seeking assistance and the health professional (see Ch 7). The emotional environment within an individual may be as simple as feeling a sense of inconvenience because they require assistance for something simple and relatively minor. The emotional environment of a person who has a life-limiting illness, however, is complex and requires management and collaboration to ensure positive outcomes for all stakeholders. Consideration of the emotional environments of those seeking the assistance of a health professional has numerous benefits that contribute to family/person-centred practice.

Formal versus informal environments

Different occasions and places demand different types of behaviour – some that is more formal than others. In formal situations individuals are expected to adhere carefully to particular norms. These norms might require the use of the family name when addressing an individual, they might require only speaking when asked a question, or they might perhaps require a controlled use of language. For example, the language and behaviour used in a courtroom is very different to the language and behaviour used with friends at a football game. The expected formality of a situation will affect the emotional response of the individual, their comfort when communicating and their willingness to communicate about personal matters.

GROUP ACTIVITY

- Divide a page into two halves, top to bottom. Label one column 'Formal' and the other 'Informal'.
- Consider the expectations of each type of environment and how that makes you feel. If you find it difficult to determine the expectations of each you might wish to consider a particular formal or informal occasion in your experience. For example, consider your emotional response to attending a formal dinner party or a barbeque where you are unsure about the expected level of formality. List the expectations of each environment.
- List the emotional responses group members might have to these types of situations.
- List the factors that might affect these responses (e.g. close friends present etc).

REFLECTIVE ACTIVITY

- How do the emotions associated with the formality of the situation affect your desire to communicate? Do they affect the superficiality of the conversation? Explain why they affect the type of communication and the topic of communication.
- On a separate piece of paper, list those things that facilitate your ability to talk about yourself at more than a superficial level.

GROUP ACTIVITY

Discuss the implications of the above factors for a health professional.

The various expectations and demands of the formality of the environment affect the individual. Situations that are more formal tend to create a more tentative and apprehensive emotional response in an individual. Less formal situations promote relaxation and generally encourage willingness to discuss personal matters at a deeper level.

Emotional responses to environmental demands

Emotional responses to the immediate environment

There is a continual and dynamic interaction between the individual and their immediate environment. This interaction creates a particular emotional environment that will vary according to the dominant need at any given time. If the personal emotional needs dominate an individual and the environment does not accommodate these needs, the stress level for that individual increases as they attempt to meet the demands of both self and the environment (Brill & Levine 2005). In such circumstances, it is beneficial for the health professional to note and where possible accommodate the emotional environment of the individual. Something as simple as the position of the health professional (e.g. standing over a person or standing too close or too far away) may evoke a negative response in particular individuals. Unfamiliarity with the surroundings, the individuals and the associated intervention or procedure in the environment can also create a particular emotional environment for the individual. This emotional environment may affect their responses and the quality of their interactions. It is possible to alleviate these particular emotional environments with direct attention, acknowledgement and action.

Emotional responses to an external environment

Individuals often exhibit emotions because of an emotional environment established from a source external to the immediate environment of the health service. Potential contributing causes of negative emotional environments include financial stress, social stress, physical discomfort or anxiety about an unknown future. It is not the role of every health professional to treat the causes of the dominating emotional environment. However, validation of the associated emotions, empathic responses and referral to a relevant professional will reduce the consequences of the particular emotional environment.

CASE STUDY

Mrs Gilles is a 78-year-old lady who lives alone with her cat. She is currently attending for weekly treatment. She generally appears happy and eagerly enters into collaborative goal-setting. Her level of improvement suggests she is implementing the particular regime suggested by you as her health professional.

One particular day you intend to introduce Mrs Gilles to a more demanding 'home program' during her treatment session. You have a good relationship with her and often talk about her past and present life when she attends. She appears to enjoy attending.

When Mrs Gilles arrives, she seems a little teary but smiles when she sees you.

- You have two choices – to investigate her apparent tendency to tears or ignore it.
- The treatment environment demands a happy and willing-to-participate Mrs Gilles. At this point, her emotional environment is not dominating her responses. She is able to respond to the demands of the treatment environment and continues in her happy, collaborative way of interacting.
- What will you do? You decide to ignore it – you have a full day and simply do not have the time to investigate.

The next time Mrs Gilles attends it is obvious she has not been implementing her home program; in fact, she seems to be back to her status of 3 weeks ago. She is teary and, although participating, does not smile or look at you.

- The emotional environment of Mrs Gilles is now beginning to dominate and she is no longer able to meet the demands of the treatment environment; she demonstrates being unable to continue her treatment regimen at home.
- You are busier this week with more appointments than normal because you are going on holidays at the end of the week. You decide to ignore the emotional environment surrounding Mrs Gilles and hope it will be better when you come back from holidays. You think to yourself that most emotional things improve with time and another person will see her while you are away.

You return from holidays 2 weeks later to find that Mrs Gilles has not attended since you went on holidays. You ring her and hear that she has been lying in bed since the last time you saw her – she says she cannot be bothered to get out of bed anymore.

- What will you do? You know Mrs Gilles was improving with your intervention.

You ask her a few questions but she is reluctant to talk to you. You finally ask her about her cat – she often talked lovingly about the cat, stating she had nothing else since the death of her husband. Mrs Gilles suddenly sobs uncontrollably – the cat had died the week when she was teary! This interaction took more than 10 minutes.

REFLECTION

- How long would it have taken to investigate the cause of the tears (the emotional environment affecting the person) the first time you saw the tears?
- Might it potentially have created a different scenario for Mrs Gilles?

ROLE PLAY

- Have one person play Mrs Gilles and another the health professional who validates the cause of the tendency to tears with empathic responses and questions.
- Time how long it takes to validate the emotions and demonstrate empathy.
- Discuss the possible direction of the conversation with Mrs Gilles.
- Should the health professional discuss the emotions related to grieving (see Ch 22) and strategies for dealing with the death of the cat?

Failure to note and accommodate the internal or external emotional environment of the individual can have negative results. Responding to the emotional environment does not usually take excessive amounts of time and has benefits for all involved. The ultimate benefit for the individual is improved outcomes, but it also saves time for the health professional if dealt with immediately.

The cultural environment

Individuals grow and develop in specific cultural environments. These cultural environments determine how individuals view themselves, how they view others and how others view them (Watson 2006). Examination and understanding of the cultural context of a person provides information about the rules and norms that govern their life, both individually and within groups. Cultural environments influence the values of societies and individuals. These values directly affect expectations and goals within the culture and outside the particular culture. Shared values and expectations (i.e. the cultural worldview) are inherent in cultural groups and thus individuals from those groups are often unable to verbalise the details of these values and expectations. An appreciation of the specific worldview of the individual seeking assistance promotes positive communication and family/person-centred practice.

Personal space

Different cultures have different norms that govern personal space, that is, the distance individuals stand or sit from each other during a communicative interaction. Recognising variations in ideas of personal space is important when relating to people from a different culture. If the person uses non-verbal cues that demonstrate emotional discomfort and moves away from standing a particular distance apart, the person has adjusted their emotional environment according to their cultural expectations. It is important to not move closer in response. Instead, the health professional should try to remain in their original spot, even if it feels impersonal and distant. If the health professional does move closer, they may 'chase the person around the room' throughout the discussion. Alternatively, if a person moves closer when interacting, demonstrating emotional distress unless they remain closer, this demonstrates a different cultural norm governing personal space. Variations in ideas of personal space when interacting, whether sitting or standing, require awareness in the health professional.

Colour

Colours can communicate different emotions to different individuals. Some of this communication is culturally determined and some results from individual preferences. Different cultures assign sometimes totally opposite meanings to different colours (Devito 2007).

REFLECTION

What is your favourite colour? Can you remember if there is a particular reason or experience that explains why it is your favourite colour? The colour of a favourite comfortable piece of clothing may become your favourite colour when that piece of clothing becomes a rag. Wearing the same colour every day may make that colour your least favourite.

GROUP ACTIVITY

- Consider each of the colours listed and together decide if the colour is symbolic of or relates to something particular.

  Black: Red:

  Blue: Green:

  White: Purple:

  Yellow:

- If there are various cultures represented in the group note the different meaning each colour has in each culture.
- Decide if the cultural meaning of colour is important to the practice of a health professional.

Time

Different cultural environments have a different awareness of and place a different emphasis on time. Some cultures measure time by the movement of the earth around the sun, that is, a **seasonal calendar**. In these cultural environments the seasons regulate the lives and expectations of the people. If the winter is long and cold then that season determines the cultural expectations of interactions between people at that time. If there is little seasonal change then the cultural environment is unlikely to demand different ways of relating as the year changes. Some cultures regulate their interaction by the movement of the moon around the earth (phases of the moon) – the **lunar calendar**. In these cultural environments the movement of the moon determines the expectations and norms that govern interactions between people at particular times. This means that a New Year celebration may sometimes occur in late February and Easter may occur in mid-March. Other cultures regulate their interactions by the movement of the earth on its axis – a **24-hour schedule** based around the spinning of the earth. In these cultural environments the 24-hour clock regulates the events and expectations of the people. In other cultures, time has a different significance and is unrelated to schedules throughout the day.

The regard for time in different cultures delivers different messages. Some cultures value adherence to the time schedule above other cultural or social demands. In western cultures, punctuality communicates respect whereas being late communicates the opposite. Others consider the adherence to 'being on time' is not as relevant as other cultural or social demands – so much so that they may not attend a previously made appointment and not consider it necessary to notify the health professional that they are unable to attend. When differences in perceptions of the significance of time cause difficulties in the health professions, it may be important to sensitively communicate to some 'others' that the reality for the health professional of many appointments in one day makes it difficult to see someone after their allocated time.

In some cultures, inviting a person to have or do something requires a repeat of the request three times before the person answers in the affirmative. In other cultures, lack of an affirmative response after the first request might indicate that the person is ambivalent about accepting the invitation. For example, in China it is polite to ask a person three times if they would like a drink. If the request occurs once, the person will indicate a definite *no*, regardless of their desire for a drink. It is not until the occurrence of the third request that they might indicate their desire for a drink. In other cultures where one request is the expected norm, the first answer indicates the desire or lack of desire for a drink.

REFLECTION

- Is it important to you to be on time for social appointments?
- Is it important to you to be on time for professional appointments?
- Is there a difference? Why? Do you have friends who do not differentiate?
- Does it annoy you when others are late for an appointment?
- Consider the above points relating to different interpretations of the importance of time. What does that mean for a health professional?
- List the possible ways a health professional might accommodate cultural differences relating to time.

A cultural environment influences many components of human behaviour, too many to consider in this chapter. It is the responsibility of the health professional to acknowledge and accommodate the cultural variations in all interactions. Fulfilling this responsibility requires an awareness of the personal cultural expectations of the health professional and their emotional responses to variations in cultural expectations. It also requires an awareness of the cultural differences of the individuals the health professional assists. Such awareness potentially prepares health professionals to open themselves to exploring and understanding those differences. Understanding cultural differences empowers the health professional to accommodate variations in the diverse cultural environments potentially represented by both the individuals seeking their assistance and their colleagues in the particular health service.

The sexual environment

Different individuals may exist within different sexual and moral environments. These differences may affect the willingness of an individual to consider and discuss sexuality. They may also determine the expectations of individuals relating to sexual intimacy and the significance an individual places upon sexual experiences (Milliken & Honeycutt 2004). A person raised in an environment that practises regular casual sexual relationships will make particular assumptions about sexual practices and may either exhibit similar practices or carefully control any sexual activity. A sexually abused person may avoid any kind of physical touch or may have a fragile self-image that does not allow them to relate sexually or communicate about sexual matters.

It is important that health professionals understand that different individuals may have different sexual habits and preferences. Some individuals may practise sexual abstinence, others casual sexual relationships, and others may prefer sexual experiences with people of the same gender. Such sexual practices and preferences may or may not be the preference of the health professional; however, it is important to be aware of these various sexual environments to ensure a positive response to such individuals.

The social environment

Individuals usually mature in the context of other individuals. The social environment of an individual consists of all the social relationships they experience with people and animals. Such relationships can be encouraging and supportive, discouraging and unhelpful, or a combination of both. The social environment of the person seeking assistance can influence their responses and their ability to communicate effectively.

Family

A supportive family can assist the health professional (Holli et al 2003). When desired and if appropriate, supportive family members should be included in establishing and supporting the goals of the collaborative process between the person seeking assistance and the health professional. If the social environment of a family is a place of abuse and discouragement, this will shape the communication style of the individual. The behaviour associated with this type of social environment is not always interactive or easy. Understanding this behaviour might be difficult; however, it is important in such cases that the health professional relate to the individual with acceptance, consistency and definite boundaries. The creation of a safe, predictable environment for such a person within the context of the health service is the immediate goal of the health professional.

Pets

A relationship with a pet is often of great significance to a person (e.g. a dog to a child, a horse to a female adolescent, or a cat to an ageing person). Different cultures or geographical settings may mean that the animal is different (it may even be a whale), but, if a pet, the animal may serve to be the most significant comforting social relationship for a particular individual.

Friends, neighbours, interest groups and sporting teams

The social environment that includes groups outside a family is often significant to an individual. Friends, neighbours, special purpose groups or sporting teams may provide a social environment that reinforces the value of the individual, provides affection and affirms them in a unique way. Such friends or groups may become more significant if the individual lives alone. However, these social environments may also be the context for abuse (e.g. a 'helpful' neighbour may lock a person in a room thinking they are protecting them) and this may explain unreasonable behaviour in some circumstances.

Institutions

A health professional may assist an individual whose primary social environment is an institution. These individuals may have different styles of communication according to their experiences within the particular institution. In this situation, it is important for the health professional to demonstrate behaviour that reflects both the general (see Ch 2) and specific purposes (see Chs 3 & 4) of the health professions.

GROUP ACTIVITY

- Brainstorm and list possible strategies for managing an unsupportive social environment. Note these are not age-specific needs and occur throughout the lifespan.
- List strategies for managing an unsupportive family.
- List strategies for managing the loss of a special pet.
- List strategies for managing lost social environments through relocation of the family home, decrease in or loss of physical abilities, or the death of someone significant.
- List strategies for managing experiences from institutional social environments – whether pleasant or unpleasant.

The social environment of each health service team may vary. It is important that health professionals resolve any personal responses to their colleagues in that environment to avoid negatively affecting those seeking their assistance.

The spiritual environment

Individuals adopt particular elements of spirituality that create their own spiritual environment for many reasons. Some simply adopt the dominant spiritual environment of their native culture while others may choose a particular spiritual environment. The spiritual environment of an individual may be more relevant to particular health professions than others and thus some health professionals may appropriately choose not to relate to this environment. Regardless of the relevance of spiritual issues to the particular health profession, it is important that health professionals demonstrate respect and sensitivity to the way in which the spiritual environment may assist in the management of the health issue and healing of the individual seeking assistance (Purtilo & Haddad 2002). Health professionals can choose to relate to or to ignore the spiritual environment of the people they are assisting (Egan 2007). Many western health professionals prefer to avoid consideration of spiritual environments. However, growing interest in spirituality is producing an increasing body of knowledge that provides guidance for the use of spiritual understanding in the practice of health professionals (Miller 1999, Miller & Thorensen 2003, Powell et al 2003, Richards & Bergin 1997, White 2006.) Acknowledging and accommodating the spiritual environment of the 'other' can create deeper understanding of that environment as well as encourage the individual in the use of images, medicine and rituals typical of that environment. The use of these elements of a particular spiritual environment may promote participation, healing and function.

Chapter summary

Health professionals may experience multiple environmental demands while fulfilling their role. These demands may arise from the physical, emotional, cultural, sexual, social and spiritual environments of the health professional, the particular health service or the person seeking assistance. It is the responsibility of health professionals to overcome any personal and negative responses to the specific environmental demands experienced as part of their role. Successfully meeting the demands of particular environments while practising as a health professional will ensure positive outcomes and family/person-centred practice.

Complete the following:

1. Various environments form a dynamic system that affects each individual. These environments include:

    i. _____

    ii. _____

    iii. _____

    iv. _____

    v. _____

    vi. _____

2. List seven elements of the physical environment that affect the individual seeking assistance.

    i. _____

    ii. _____

    iii. _____

    iv. _____

    v. _____

    vi. _____

    vii. _____

3. Name three ways the health professional can accommodate the emotional environment.

    i. _____

    ii. _____

    iii. _____

4. Cultural environments vary and the heath professional must be open to differences between their own cultural environment and those of the individuals seeking assistance. Health professionals must respond with willingness to understand and accommodate such differences. Name three culturally specific elements that require understanding.

    i. _____

    ii. _____

    iii. _____

5. What do social environments include?

    i. _____

    ii. _____

iii. _____

iv. _____

6. What is important to remember about social environments?

_____

_____

_____

7. Why is the spiritual environment of each individual important?

_____

_____

_____

References

Bergland C, Saltman D (eds) 2002 Communication for healthcare. Oxford University Press, Melbourne

Blanche E I 2007 The expression of creativity through occupation. Journal of Occupational Science 14(1):21–29

Brill N I, Levine J 2005 Working with people: the helping process, 8th edn. Pearson, Boston

Chen M 2006 Understanding the benefits and detriments of conflict on team creativity process. Creativity and Innovation Management 15(1):105–116

Devito J A 2007 The interpersonal communication book, 11th edn. Pearson, Boston

Egan G 2007 The skilled helper, 8th edn. Thomson, Belmont CA

Holli B B, Calabrese R J, O'Sullivan Mailett J 2003 Communication and education skills for dietetics professionals, 4th edn. Lippincott, Williams & Wilkins, Philadelphia

Miller W R (ed) 1999 Integrating spirituality into treatment: resources for practitioners. American Psychological Association, Washington DC

Miller W R, Thorensen C E 2003 Spirituality, religion and health: an emerging research field. American Psychologist 58(1):24–35

Milliken M E, Honeycutt A 2004 Understanding human behavior: a guide for healthcare providers, 7th edn. Thomson Delmar, New York

Northouse P G, Northouse L L 1992 Health communication: strategies for health professionals, 2nd edn. Prentice Hall, Englewood Cliffs NJ

Powell L H, Shahabi L, Thorensen C E 2003 Religion and spirituality: linkages to physical health. American Psychologist 58(1):36–52

Purtilo R B, Haddad A 2002 Health professional and patient interaction, 6th edn. Saunders, Philadelphia

Richards P S, Bergin A E 1997 The need for a spiritual strategy. American Psychological Association, Washington DC

Slahova A, Savvina J, Cack M et al 2007 Creative activity in conception of sustainable development education. International Journal of Sustainability in Higher Education 8(2):142–145

Watson R M 2006 Being before doing: the cultural identity of occupational therapy. Australian Occupational Therapy Journal 53(3):151–158

White G 2006 Talking about spirituality in healthcare practice: a resource for the multi-professional healthcare team. Jessica Kingsley, London

THREE

DEVELOPING CORE SKILLS IN COMMUNICATION

Communication with the whole person

9

CHAPTER OBJECTIVES

Upon completing this chapter, students should be able to

- Demonstrate understanding of the concept of and components of the whole person
- Synthesise all aspects of the whole person in order to achieve effective communication with the 'other'
- Consider and develop strategies to overcome the difficulties associated with assisting the whole person
- List the various meanings of the concept of holistic care
- Understand the importance of holistic communication
- List some characteristics of holistic communication.

Defining the whole person

The concept of the whole person is important to many health professions. Those professions require inclusion, understanding and care for the whole person. There is detailed discussion about the components of the whole person in Chapters 7–8 of this book. In summary, there are five basic aspects of the whole person (Brill & Levine 2005). Four of these aspects are the physical, cognitive, emotional/psychological and spiritual functioning of the person. The physical functioning is the most obvious and includes the body of the person, the functioning of their internal organs and their external body parts. While there is some debate about the components of the mind, cognitive functioning definitely includes thoughts and memory processes. Some believe that emotional or psychological functioning is part of the mind, others believe it originates in the heart while others believe it originates in the liver. Regardless of origin, psychological and emotional functioning is an aspect of every person and a component of the dynamic system of the whole person. Spiritual functioning refers to that aspect of the person that gives meaning to self, life and the universe. It involves moral values and relating to the world at a spiritual level. Whole people exist in a social context and thus, while the person may consist of the four above-mentioned aspects, past and present social experiences create the fifth aspect of the whole person – the social aspect. The social aspect influences and often determines responses in the other four aspects. These five components of the person interrelate to exist as a dynamic whole. It is impossible to separate the individual aspects from the whole because they are mutually dependent on each other and mutually affect each other.

GROUP ACTIVITY

- Do the five aspects of the whole person ever operate separately? Explain.
- List ways in which each aspect may affect the functioning of the person.
- Consider how the health professional might recognise the influence of each aspect of the whole person.

While it is possible to focus upon one aspect of the whole person, dividing the whole into parts for analysis can be problematic (Dossey et al 2003, Harms 2007, Reed & Sanderson 1999) because each aspect exists in an intricate and sometimes delicate relationship with the other parts. Analysis of one aspect is often useful and transformative. Such analysis, however, should always consider the effects of the other aspects.

There are times during life when one particular aspect may dominate the dynamic system of the whole individual. The demands of life at that time or the particular choices made by the individual result in the person giving greater priority to a particular aspect of their whole more often than the other aspects. For example, the physical aspect of an elite athlete may dominate their focus and functioning because of the requirement for physical training. A student is required to use the cognitive aspect regularly and thus the cognitive aspect may prescribe their focus and functioning. A grieving person may experience extreme emotional stress and thus the psychological aspect of a grieving person may dominate their functioning. A person who chooses to be a monk or nun usually makes choices based upon the spiritual aspect. The need for social acceptance during adolescence may mean that the social aspect of the adolescent drives/dominates their existence at that stage in life.

REFLECTION

- Consider the five aspects of the person. Do you agree that these aspects create the whole person? Do you feel there are any more internal aspects of the person? If so, ensure your answers do not belong in one of the other five aspects.
- Consider times in your life when one of the aspects may have dominated your functioning (e.g. when playing competitive sport or when studying). Were the other aspects dormant at that time? How did the focus affect your overall functioning? Did other aspects become less predictable or more sensitive? How did you manage this? What facilitated a sense of wellbeing despite the focus upon one aspect?

Holistic care

The principle of holism always considers the person to be a whole, regardless of the specific demands upon that person at a particular time. The concept of holism is not a new idea for many health professions (Brill & Levine 2005, Dossey et al 2005, Milliken & Honeycutt 2004, Reed & Sanderson 1999, White 2006); in fact, a variety of health professions have developed because of a holistic philosophy of care (Punwar & Peloquin 2000). There are various ways of understanding holistic care. It can mean inclusive care that accommodates diverse cultural and spiritual systems (Taylor 2000), in particular the medicine of traditional indigenous healers and the traditional interventions of eastern cultures. Holistic care can also mean complementary and alternative medicine (CAM; Dossey et al 2003) as opposed to traditional medical care. A holistic concept of healthcare is the basis of CAM (Milliken & Honeycutt 2004) and thus some consider holistic care as synonymous with CAM. Some health professions perceive holistic care as the consideration of the whole person – every aspect of the unique individual – using a variety of interventions depending on the needs of the individual. In these professions, holistic care means avoidance of focusing upon one aspect of the individual over another aspect. It requires recognition that healthcare is more than a focus upon the physical needs of the individual (White 2006). Holistic care fulfils more than the immediate needs relevant to the particular health profession; it recognises there are many causes contributing to those needs. It recognises that the immediate needs may arise from more than the physical aspect of the person, even though the need initially may appear to be physical. Holistic care understands there is more than one way to fulfil a need and to achieve healing. It considers the less obvious and often forgotten aspects of the cultural, psychological, social and spiritual functioning of the individual.

REFLECTION

- Consider the aspect of the person to which you feel most comfortable relating. Why?

GROUP ACTIVITY

- Have each group member explain which aspect of a person they would feel most comfortable addressing in their health profession.
- As a group decide which aspect of the person is the easiest to relate to or address. Discuss why.
- As a group decide which aspect is the most difficult to address. Discuss why. Suggest strategies that might assist in overcoming this difficulty.

Holistic care does not merely treat symptoms but also searches for causes, understanding there are often multiple causes that arise from and relate to every aspect of the whole person. Mutual respect is the foundation of holistic care and it assumes equality (see Chs 2 & 12) within the therapeutic relationship. Mutual respect seeks involvement from the person seeking assistance in the collaborative goal-setting and decision-making associated with their care and future (Dossey et al 2005). In holistic care, the responsibility for change and healing lies within the person. The role of the health professional is to facilitate and empower the person to achieve their set goals (Milliken & Honeycutt 2004).

Unless specifically taught to provide holistic care, a developing health professional may require experience to provide holistic care consistently (Liu et al 2000). It is possible for a health professional who practises within a particular specialty area to provide holistic care, despite a focus upon their specialty area. Regardless of the situation, it is possible to consider the whole person while practising as a health professional. Holistic care is fundamental in achieving family/person-centred practice in any healthcare service and thus should be an aim of every health professional.

Holistic care includes consideration of context

To provide holistic care it is important that health professionals consider the interrelating aspects of the whole person regardless of the presence of an obviously dominating aspect at any one time. It is also important to consider that individuals with whom health professionals communicate develop within diverse and multiple contexts. Recognition of these contexts is essential when communicating (Harms 2007, Milliken & Honeycutt 2004, Purtilo & Haddad 2002, White 2006; see Chs 6 & 7). Some consider these contexts to be physical, financial, cultural and social (family or kinship groups, friends, colleagues or acquaintances), while others consider them to also include a spiritual element (Colbert 2003, Taylor 2000). Regardless of their composition, these contexts provide experiences that promote positive or negative responses within the cognitive, spiritual and psychological functioning of the individual. Such responses ultimately affect the physical and social aspects of the individual (Colbert 2003, Golman 2006) and, therefore, all of these contexts require the attention of health professionals.

The requirements of holistic care

There are currently many health professions, each with their particular expertise and focus. An awareness and understanding of the various health professions is important to ensure holistic care and positive outcomes. Openness to the involvement of multiple health professionals when assisting individuals, regardless of the presence of an inter/multidisciplinary team, increases the potential for holistic and positive outcomes (White 2006).

ACTIVITY

- State the aspect(s) upon which your particular health profession focuses.
- How can you ensure holistic care for those seeking your assistance?
- Divide a page into two, top to bottom.
    - On one side, make a list of every health profession you know.
    - On the other side, list the aspect(s) upon which that health profession focuses. If you are not sure, do some research and then list the aspects.

GROUP ACTIVITY

- Compare your list with two others and adjust it according to the contents of the other lists, requesting clarification where necessary.
- How can you use this list to ensure holistic care that empowers the individual to achieve their goals and transform their functioning?

CASE STUDIES

Each of the individuals below is awaiting a diagnosis relating to physical symptoms, however, this is what they express.
- A 43-year-old regularly expresses anxiety about his/her diagnosis.
- A 17-year-old expresses stress because of matriculation assessments.
- A 7-year-old just wants to continue playing weekend sport.
- A 54-year-old male with an intellectual disability wants to marry his 22-year-old girlfriend who also has an intellectual disability.
- A 28-year-old overeats constantly because of fear.   ↳

↳ •   A 45-year-old expresses disappointment that his/her same-gender partner of 20 years has been unfaithful recently.
   •   A 76-year-old expresses distress over his/her lost cat.
   •   A 52-year-old expresses confusion because of his/her dementing parent.
   •   A 39-year-old expresses despair because of his/her dying child.
   •   A 60-year-old is depressed because he/she cannot attend his/her religious group.
   •   A 32-year-old is devastated because she has just given birth to her first (much-awaited) child only to be told the child has Down Syndrome.

GROUP ACTIVITY

   •   Decide how to best acknowledge and fulfil each person's need.
   •   What would your health profession do to assist each person?
   •   Decide whether it is appropriate for one health professional to meet all the needs of every person they see.
   •   How can you ensure holistic care for these people?

Holistic care requires consideration of the whole person, however, it also requires care of self. It requires health professionals to assume responsibility for themselves – for their thoughts, words, actions and related outcomes. This of course requires health professionals to balance their personal and professional needs (Dossey et al 2003, Dossey et al 2005). Holistic care requires health professionals to acknowledge the effects of their professional encounters and seek assistance as necessary. It requires reflection about, and self-awareness within, the practice of the health professional that guides and promotes change as appropriate – change that will develop and strengthen holistic communication.

GROUP ACTIVITY

Using the information contained in this chapter and the beliefs held within the group, list ways of achieving holistic healthcare.
   Consider the following questions when compiling this list:
   •   Can an individual health professional achieve holistic care alone?
   •   Can traditional medical intervention alone achieve holistic care?
   •   Can CAM alone achieve holistic care?
   •   How can a health professional from a profession typical of either the medical model or CAM achieve holistic care?
   •   How important are traditional indigenous treatments for an indigenous person? Why?
   •   How important are traditional eastern treatments for a person with an Asian background? Why?
   •   Do all aspects of the whole person require attention to achieve holistic care? Why?

Holistic communication

Holistic communication requires health professionals to apply the principles of effective communication to every individual within the context of their practice. These individuals include other health professionals (some in the same team and others not), support staff and people seeking assistance. Holistic communication requires a willingness to communicate about contexts, experiences, thoughts, emotions, needs and desires, because in so doing the health professional will relate to all aspects of the whole person (Brill & Levine 2005, Milliken & Honeycutt 2004, White 2006; see Ch 7). When communicating holistically it is important to understand that the individual perspectives of each person (Gordon et al 2006, Harms 2007), as well as previous and present events, affect the choice of topics of communication, the interpretation of events and messages during communication, and the results of communication. Holistic communication requires health professionals to consider elements of the particular context of the interaction because these will affect the quality and success of the communication. The immediate context involves the resources associated with the service (both people and objects) and the various aspects of the individual at the time. It is necessary for health professionals to consider and care for these aspects within themselves as well as within those with whom they communicate (Devito 2007, Purtilo & Haddad 2002, Stein-Parbury 2006; see Ch 6).

Purtilo & Haddad (2002) note that it is essential to understand that the person seeking assistance will attribute a different significance, most often a greater significance, to their need than the health professional. They will generally be aware of their need from a physical perspective and this may be the reason they are seeking assistance. The person will also perceive the emotions, thoughts and social experiences associated with their need. In addition, many will also perceive a spiritual element depending on their background and beliefs. Awareness of variations in the level of significance and influence of the aspects, perspective and context of the individual will assist the health professional to communicate holistically.

REFLECTION

What is your emotional and physical response to the following questions?
- Can you tell me where I can perform my daily prayers while I am here?
- Can you talk with me about my religious beliefs?
- Can I ask my family to bring me a copy of the writings of my faith?
- May I keep my placenta please?
- I must go back to where I was born to 'finish off' (die). When can I go?
- Can I use the medicine made by my Elder (Aboriginal or Torres Strait Islander) or *tohonga* (Maori)?
- Can I use herbal remedies as well?
- Can you tell me where I can have an abortion? My husband and I are not ready to have children.
- Can I also have acupuncture while having your treatment?
- Can I also have physiotherapy while having acupuncture?
- You won't tell my father he is dying, will you? It is not our way.

GROUP DISCUSSION

- How should health professionals respond to these requests?
- Is there anything they should do in response to these requests?

Dossey et al (2005) state that holistic communication requires genuine and sincere care that acknowledges the uniqueness of each individual. It requires a flow of expression and interchange between people and significant beings – pets, nature, God/life force and others around them. Dossey et al (2005) admit the importance for individuals of recognising and understanding that humans share their humanity. Humans, regardless of race, culture, gender, age, status, intelligence, material possessions or any other factor, share the same needs and concerns. Recognition of this fact assists health professionals to accept diversity and communicate holistically, thereby creating collaborative relationships in practice (Milliken & Honeycutt 2004).

Effective and holistic communication with any individuals relating to the health professions requires understanding of those individuals, that is, both the self and the 'other'. It requires a holistic understanding of the constituent aspects of the person (Brill & Levine 2005) and knowledge of the roles of the various health professions. Holistic communication requires an investment of time but is essential for effective communication.

Chapter summary

The whole person comprises physical, cognitive, emotional, spiritual and social aspects. It is important for health professionals to synthesise all five aspects to achieve effective communication with the 'other'. Holistic care recognises that the needs of a person seeking assistance may arise from more than the physical aspect. Holistic communication requires that health professionals remember the principles of effective communication when relating to every person involved in their practice.

Complete the following:
1. What are the five aspects of the whole person?
   i. _____
   ii. _____
   iii. _____
   iv. _____
   v. _____
2. What are the three meanings of holistic care?
   i. _____
   ii. _____
   iii. _____
3. What does holistic care seek to achieve?
   _____
   _____
   _____
4. What does holistic care require?
   i. _____
   ii. _____
   iii. _____

5. Why is it important to have knowledge of the role of other health professions?

6. With whom do health professionals communicate?

    i.

    ii.

    iii.

7. What does holistic communication require?

    i.

    ii.

    iii.

    iv.

8. What should health professionals be willing to communicate about?

    i.

    ii.

    iii.

    iv.

    v.

    vi.

References

Brill N I, Levine J 2005 Working with people: the helping process, 8th edn. Pearson, Boston

Colbert D 2003 Deadly emotions: understand the mind body spirit connection that can heal or destroy you. Thomas Nelson, Nashville TN

Devito J A 2007 The interpersonal communication book, 11th edn. Pearson, Boston

Dossey B M, Keegan L, Gussetta C 2003 Holistic nursing: a handbook for practice, 4th edn. Jones & Bartlett, Sudbury MA

Dossey B M, Keegan L, Gussetta C 2005 A pocket guide for holistic nursing. Jones & Bartlett, Sudbury MA

Golman C 2006 Social intelligence: the new science of human relationships. Hutchinson, London

Gordon R, Druckman D, Rozelle R et al 2006 Non-verbal communication a behaviour: approaches, issues and research. In: Hargie O (ed) The handbook of communication skills, 3rd edn. Routledge, New York, p 73–120

Harms D 2007 Working with people: communication skills for reflective practice. Oxford University Press, Melbourne

Liu K P Y, Chan C H, Hui C W Y 2000 Clinical reasoning and the occupational therapy curriculum. Occupational Therapy International 7:173–183

Milliken M A, Honeycutt A 2004 Understanding human behavior: a guide for healthcare providers, 7th edn. Thomson Delmar, New York

Punwar A J, Peloquin S M 2000 Occupational therapy: principles and practice, 3rd edn. Lippincott, Williams & Wilkins, Baltimore

Purtilo R B, Haddad A 2002 Health professional and patient interaction, 6th edn. Saunders, Philadelphia

Reed K L, Sanderson S N 1999 Concepts of occupational therapy. Lippincottt, Williams & Wilkins, Philadelphia

Stein-Parbury J 2006 Patient and person: interpersonal skills in nursing, 3rd edn. Elsevier, Sydney (Original work published 2005)

Taylor B J 2000 Reflective practice: a guide for nurses and midwives. Allen & Unwin, Crows Nest, Sydney

White G 2006 Talking about spirituality in healthcare practice: a resource for the multi-professional healthcare team. Jessica Kingsley, London

'Other'-centred communication

10

CHAPTER OBJECTIVES

Upon completing this chapter, students should be able to
- Explain the importance of listening in 'other'-centred communication
- Identify and accommodate the benefits of active listening
- Describe the barriers to listening
- Explain the importance of preparing to listen
- Discuss the characteristics of effective listening
- Explore and examine cultural variations that affect listening
- Understand the importance of appropriate disengagement.

The fundamental nature of the health professions as helping professions mandates 'other'-centred communication. The skill of placing the 'other' at the centre of communicative interactions is one that is also beneficial in everyday relationships (Adler et al 2005, Devito 2007, Lauer 2003). Although achieving 'other'-centred communication is often challenging, it is essential in the health professions and requires effective listening. Listening is the most widely used communication skill in life. Individuals listen every day – some more actively than others. Studies indicate that individuals who listen effectively tend to assume various roles, some of which are in the health professions. Considering the amount of time people spend listening each day it is amazing that effective listening requires practice and conscious effort.

GROUP DISCUSSION

- What is listening? List the necessary abilities to achieve effective listening.
- How do you know someone is listening to you? What non-verbal and verbal behaviours indicate they are listening? How can you establish whether the listener has understood you?

Effective listening as well as skills in speaking, reading and writing are useful for any person to facilitate communication in general life, but are essential for a health professional (Egan 2007, Giroux et al 2002, Harms 2007, Holli et al 2003, Milliken & Honeycutt 2004, Parker 2006, Stein-Parbury 2006).

Benefits of active listening

Effective listening benefits the health professional, the people they assist, and ultimately the outcomes of intervention. The health professional who listens effectively is able to make appropriate decisions that influence the quality of care (Brown et al 2003). When a health professional is committed to effective listening the person seeking assistance feels valued and is more confident in the health professional because of their demonstrated listening skills (Nyström et al 2003). Thus, the therapeutic relationship develops appropriately because of effective listening skills (Egan 2007, Stein-Parbury 2006). In addition, effective listening increases the probability of the fulfilment of mutually established goals (Lauer 2003, Mohan et al 2004).

Specifically, active listening enables the health professional to Assist, Enjoy, Influence, Observe and Understand (AEIOU; Devito 2007; see Table 10.1).

AEIOU: Benefits of active listening for the health professional	
Assist	Listening allows the health professional to gather information that promotes collaboration. The information gathered increases the ability of the health professional to assist the 'other' in collaborative problem-solving.
Enjoy	Listening enables the health professional to enjoy (if appropriate) the thoughts and feelings of the 'other'. Listening encourages connection and enhances collaborative and trusting relationships with the person seeking assistance and with colleagues.
Influence	Listening indicates the interest and concern of the health professional. This encourages the 'other' to impart information that produces insights. These insights, once communicated, can positively influence the ideas and responses of the health professional and the 'other'.
Observe	When effective listening occurs the health professional is able to observe the non-verbal messages of the 'other'. It is the non-verbal messages that often encapsulate the less-obvious needs of the 'other'. These observations offer the opportunity to validate and sometimes diffuse emotions that may dominate the observed messages.
Understand	It is undeniable that listening in combination with validation unravels the complex needs of the 'other'. The effective listener uses the information gathered to reduce unnecessary events and the likelihood of difficulties while ultimately increasing the possibility of appropriate outcomes.

TABLE 10.1 Adapted from Devito 2007.

Barriers to listening

Awareness of the **barriers** to effective listening prepares health professionals so they can avoid potential hazards that might negatively affect the listening process. There are various external and internal factors that hinder effective listening (see Chs 6 & 8). The **external** (environmental) factors are important and not always obvious. Consideration of external interferences (Stein-Parbury 2006) – including noise levels, distractions and unrelated activity in the space allocated for the interaction – and adjustments where possible will contribute to the understanding of the listener and enhance their confidence. A health professional who continues listening instead of answering a telephone or pager indicates commitment to the needs of the 'other' and encourages the development of a therapeutic relationship.

An effective listener attends to the **internal** 'noise' of their emotions before listening, thereby ensuring they can listen unhindered by their needs (Bergland & Saltman 2002). A listener who is not psychologically prepared to listen because they are preoccupied with their own thoughts may misunderstand messages. Alternatively, a listener who is focused on their own ideas and assumptions may also fail to listen carefully if they attempt to predict what they will hear (Purtilo & Haddad 2002).

Individuals may have habitual internal barriers that affect their ability to listen (Gordon 2004; see Ch 5). These barriers fall into three major categories: i) judging; ii) ignoring the needs; and iii) stipulating the solution. Overcoming these barriers is essential for a health professional because they significantly limit the effectiveness of listening.

The **language** of the listener may hinder the effectiveness of the communication if their ability in the language of the 'other' is poor. Mutual understanding requires both communicators to have some level of competence in a common language. Effective listening is impossible without a common language.

Preparing to listen

Effective listening requires preparation and awareness of the factors that contribute to interested and efficient listening. Systematic preparation of the necessary external and internal factors guarantees positive outcomes for the listening process.

Cultural expectations change the requirements for effective listening

Some skills associated with active listening may not be appropriate in some cultures, for example, eye contact (Higgs et al 2005). In some cultures the age and gender of the speaker will affect the expectations of the listener. A factor considered important for effective communication in one cultural context is often inappropriate or unimportant in another culture. For example, the use of direct questions facilitates sharing of information in many western middle-class contexts, while in some indigenous cultures direct questions are offensive. In such indigenous cultures information may be shared through story-telling while performing activities together.

The principle of SAAFETY (see Table 10.2) reminds the health professional of the necessary factors and stresses the importance of a feeling of safety for the 'other' when communicating in the health professions.

SAAFETY: Principles of preparing to listen for the health professional	
S	Schedule an interpreter if required to ensure effective communication.
A	Arrange your mind to enable complete focus and concentration on the 'other'.
A	Arrange the seating in a culturally appropriate way and remove physical barriers.
F	Familiarise yourself with the history and/or culture of the 'other'.
E	Environmental factors affect effective listening. Remove all distractions and reduce noise or activity.
T	Time alone with the 'other(s)' is important to ensure privacy.
Y	Y – Why listen? Clarify and understand the purpose of the interaction.

TABLE 10.2

- Find someone you do not know well. Ask them to tell you about their fondest memory about school.
- Before preparing to listen consider the principle of SAAFETY (see Table 10.2).
- Listen carefully – ensure that they
  - Describe the environment at the time of the event
  - State who was present during the event
  - Describe every action during the event
  - Describe *and* explain the reactions of each person during the event
  - Explain why it is their fondest memory.
- If the person does not include these five factors, ask questions that will encourage them to provide this information.
- Make a verbal summary of the content of the description and have the 'other' verify the accuracy of your listening.

Characteristics of effective listening

Effective listeners use all of their knowledge and skills to understand and respond appropriately to the 'other'. They use active listening in preference to passive listening. Passive listening does not encourage continued interaction because the listener fails to engage with the speaker or the verbal or non-verbal content of their message. Active listening facilitates comprehension of all the messages of the 'other' and is a core skill in effective listening.

REFLECTION

- Consider your usual style of listening. Are you naturally an active or passive listener? What conditions encourage you to listen actively?
- List the situations in which you adopt passive listening.
- How could you change your listening to active listening in these situations?

Table 10.3 describes the essential elements of effective listening for health professionals.

For more than 20 years the SOLER model (see Table 10.4) has highlighted the major non-verbal methods for communicating solidarity with the 'other' (Egan 2007). This model is an excellent guide for the use of non-verbal communication while listening in some sectors of western society. However, the SOLER model gives little weight to cultural variations in expectations while listening.

Disengagement

Disengagement is the process that leads to the disconnection of the individuals communicating. It consists of the actions required to satisfactorily close the interaction. Disengaging is as important as introducing. It leaves the 'other' with a definite impression of the level of interest and care on the part of the health professional. Disengagement is essential to ensure the conversation is finished and that everyone understands the content of

How to listen effectively as a health professional	
Always:	**Avoid:**
• Prepare yourself to listen (Stein-Parbury 2006) • Adjust to all contexts and needs (Devito 2007) • 'Tune in' visibly to the 'other' (Egan 2007) • Listen with your whole self (Davis 2006) • Focus attention fully on the 'other' (Holli et al 2003) • Carefully observe all non-verbal messages of the 'other' • Use appropriate non-verbal cues • Communicate interest and commitment to the 'other' • Search for the meaning of all verbal and non-verbal messages (Devito 2007) • Predict and clarify their meaning • Seek areas of interest to assist focus (Mohan et al 2004) • Communicate the importance of the contribution of the 'other' in the process (Stein-Parbury 2006) • Consider cultural variations in listening (Harms 2007).	• Stereotyping the 'other', regardless of their appearance or skill in communicating (Purtilo & Haddad 2002) • Judging – this imposes personal values and beliefs onto the 'other' • Advising the 'other', even if they request it • Taking extensive notes while listening • Losing concentration because of thoughts about external matters (e.g. the next appointment or dinner) • Interrupting with thoughts or ideas; instead allow the 'other' to finish • A closed mind when listening (Holli et al 2003) • Double-guessing the meaning by making assumptions (Devito 2007) • Over-identification – this interrupts the ability to remember and problem solve • Changing the focus to yourself, regardless of the similarity of experiences • Negative and non-supportive non-verbal behaviours • Passive disengagement while listening, regardless of your interest in the subject.

TABLE 10.3

SOLER: A model of active listening for the health professional	
Sit	Sit to facilitate ease of sight and interaction between yourself and the 'other'. The orientation in space indicates an interest in and a commitment to the 'other' that communicates *I am here for you.*
Open posture	Assume a posture and facial expressions that communicate alert interest and openness to the 'other'. Avoid crossed arms because this may not indicate involvement and availability.
Lean towards the 'other'	Lean towards the 'other' slightly when listening to them. This will occur naturally if you are interested in the 'other'.
Eye contact	Use eye contact to indicate interest in the 'other'. When listening to a person with a visual impairment, communicate interest by facing the person as though they can see you. In cultures that consider eye contact rude there are other methods of communicating interest. Investigate these methods to assist you to communicate interest and concern to such 'others'.
Relax	Relax in order to assist development of trust and to encourage the 'other' to relax. Avoid loss of concentration through thoughts about unrelated things while listening – this is interpreted as lack of interest and is easily communicated to the speaker.

TABLE 10.4 Adapted from Egan 2007.

the interaction and the implications for the future. If each person engaging in the interaction has a different understanding of the interaction, there was neither effective listening nor speaking and certainly no effective communication.

There are definite non-verbal cues that signal the impending end of an interaction. These cues vary across cultures. In the health professions it is sometimes necessary to explicitly state that the interaction is near completion. With the younger 'other', a signal that indicates the amount of time left or the number of games remaining before the conclusion of the conversation/intervention often makes the difference between uproar and an easy departure. With the 'other' from another culture and indeed any 'other', a direct statement indicating the end of an interaction, along with a question to ensure satisfaction, is beneficial; for example, *We have finished now – do you have anything else you want to say?* Disengagement is the polite method of concluding an interaction.

Chapter summary

'Other'-centred communication cannot occur without effective listening, which requires active listening skills. Effective listening is beneficial for the health professional, the 'other', the therapeutic relationship and the possible outcomes. It is important that health professionals are aware of the barriers to effective listening, the preparations for listening effectively and the characteristics of effective listening. Health professionals must consider the cultural variations that govern expectations for effective listening, as well as the need for appropriate disengagement.

Complete the following:
1. What is a basic characteristic of effective listening?

_____

_____

_____

2. What abilities are required to listen effectively?

_____

_____

_____

3. What are the benefits of active listening?

_____

_____

_____

4. Active listening allows the health professional to A, E, I, O and U. What do the letters in AEIOU mean?

A: _____

E: _____

I: _____

O: _____

U: _____

5. List the barriers to effective listening.

_____

_____

_____

6. What do the letters in SAAFETY mean?

S:_____

A: _____

A: _____

F:_____

E: _____

T: _____

Y:_____

7. List six characteristics of effective listening and give examples of each.

i.   _____

ii. _____

iii. _____

iv. _____

v.   _____

vi. _____

8. List six behaviours a health professional should avoid when listening.

i.   _____

ii. _____

iii. _____

iv. _____

v.   _____

vi. _____

9. Suggest ways that cultural expectations might change the requirements for effective listening.

_____

_____

_____

10. Explain SOLER. What does each letter stand for?

S: _____

O: _____

L: _____

E: _____

R: _____

11. Explain the limitation of the non-verbal SOLER model of active listening.

_____

_____

_____

12. How does effective disengagement contribute to 'other'-centred communication?

_____

_____

_____

References

Adler R B, Proctor R F, Towne N 2005 Looking out, looking in, 11th edn. Wadsworth, Belmont CA

Bergland C, Saltman D (eds) 2002 Communication for healthcare. Oxford University Press, Melbourne

Brown G, Esdaile S A, Ryan S 2003 Becoming an advanced healthcare professional. Butterworth-Heineman, London

Davis C M 2006 Patient practitioner interaction: an experiential manual for developing the art of healthcare, 4th edn. Slack, Thorofare NJ

Devito J A 2007 The interpersonal communication book, 11th edn. Pearson, Boston

Egan G 2007 The skilled helper, 8th edn. Thomson, Belmont CA

Giroux Bruce M A, Borg B 2002 Psychosocial frames of reference: core for occupation-based practice, 3rd edn. Slack, Thorofare NJ

Gordon J (ed) 2004 Pfeiffer's classic activities for interpersonal communication. Wiley & Sons, San Francisco CA

Harms D 2007 Working with people: communication skills for reflective practice. Oxford University Press, Melbourne

Higgs J, Sefton A, Street A et al 2005 Communicating in the health and social sciences. Oxford University Press, Melbourne

Holli B B, Calabrese R J, O'Sullivan Mailett J 2003 Communication and education skills for dietetics professionals, 4th edn. Lippincott, Williams & Wilkins, Philadelphia

Lauer C S 2003 Listen to this. Modern Healthcare 33:34–37

Milliken M A, Honeycutt A 2004 Understanding human behavior: a guide for healthcare providers, 7th edn. Thomson Delmar, New York

Mohan T, McGregor H, Saunders S et al 2004 Communicating as professionals. Thomson, Melbourne

Nyström M, Dahlberg K, Carlson G 2003 Non-caring encounters at an emergency care unit – a life-world hermeneutic analysis of an efficiency driven organization. International Journal of Nursing Studies 40:760–769

Parker D 2006 The client-centred frame of reference. In: Duncan E A S (ed) Foundations for practice in occupational therapy, 4th edn. Elsevier, London, p 193–215

Purtilo R B, Haddad A 2002 Health professional and patient interaction, 6th edn. Saunders, Philadelphia

Stein-Parbury J 2006 Patient and person: interpersonal skills in nursing, 3rd edn. Elsevier, Sydney (Original work published 2005)

Ethical communication

CHAPTER OBJECTIVES

Upon completing this chapter, students should be able to

- Explain the importance of ethical communication
- List and understand the characteristics of ethical communication
- Appreciate the ethical responsibility of health professionals when communicating about their professional life
- Consider and develop strategies that ensure ethical communication and practice.

Ethical communication is essential in any health profession. Ethical communication relates to appropriate behaviour when communicating and is necessary for the maintenance of harmonious, productive and beneficial therapeutic relationships. The ability to communicate ethically requires motivation, character and self-awareness (Dossey et al 2003, Dossey et al 2005, Tyler et al 2005). Awareness of and commitment to ethical communication may depend on the familial, social and cultural background of the health professional (Egan 2007, Harms 2007). Violation of ethical responsibilities when communicating has serious consequences for both the person seeking assistance and the health professional (Egan 2007). Thus, it is important for the health professional to know the rules or codes of behaviour expected by the government, their profession and their particular health service (Higgs et al 2005, Purtilo & Haddad 2002). This chapter examines some of these expectations and rules.

GROUP ACTIVITY

- Discuss what is right and what is wrong when communicating. Consider possibly inappropriate topics, places of communicating, styles of communicating and reasons for communicating. Your answers here should look beyond personal preference.
- Use the ideas raised in this discussion to list the possible fundamental elements of ethical communication in the health professions.

Mohan et al (2004) state that most health professionals, while being aware of ethical requirements at a theoretical level, rarely consider them during everyday practice. However, it is not awareness or consideration of ethical requirements alone that produces ethical communication. It is the knowledge of, commitment to and application of these requirements into communicative behaviours that creates an ethical communicator. Devito (2007) considers every communicative act to have the potential to be constructive or destructive. This reality indicates that every communicative interaction in the health professions, if ethically sound, has the potential to create and sustain constructive therapeutic relationships (Rider & Keefer 2006).

The main purpose of this chapter is to outline the characteristics of, and strategies to achieve, ethical communication.

Respect regardless of differences

An overall characteristic and value of the health professions is respect of all people, whether those seeking assistance or those working alongside the health professional (see Ch 2). Every health professional must respect the rights of all individuals. These rights include equal opportunities, equal consideration and equal treatment regardless of status or condition (Harms 2007). Ethical communication requires health professionals to express unconditional positive regard for all human beings (Purtilo & Haddad 2002, Rogers 1967; see Ch 7). These are fundamental steps in achieving the ultimate purpose of the health professions – family/person-centred practice (see Ch 2). Expression of unconditional positive regard for all human beings is ethical and is in accordance with the *Universal Declaration of Human Rights* (United Nations 1948), the *Human Rights Council* (United Nations 2006) and the *Convention on the Rights of Persons with Disabilities* (United Nations 2006). The challenge for the health professional is not usually in respecting rights, however, but in respecting the actual person.

REFLECTIVE ACTIVITY

- How do you demonstrate respect for someone who is quite different from you? For example, someone who
  - Lives on the street
  - Works the streets
  - Will only wear/not wear designer clothes
  - Hates/loves football
  - Has a different religious code than you
  - Believes terrorism is/is not appropriate
  - Has a different political allegiance?
- List the values or beliefs a person may have that make it difficult for you to demonstrate respect.
- What can you do to ensure you demonstrate respect regardless of such differences?

Demonstration of respect for others requires health professionals to first respect themselves. Respecting and valuing self begins with an awareness of the thoughts about self that affect self-image and self-esteem; some of these thoughts may have their origin in comments made by others. Regardless of their origin, these thoughts require reflective consideration and adjustment (Backus & Chapian 2000). If health professionals find it difficult to value and respect themselves it is imperative they seek expert assistance to maximise their potential to be effective communicators.

Health professionals demonstrate respect through verbal and non-verbal communicative behaviours. Such behaviours automatically reflect the underlying values and beliefs of an individual (Brill & Levine 2005, Tyler et al 2005). Thus, critical awareness of personal values and beliefs is essential for establishing and practising ethical communication (Harms 2007).

Honesty

The truthful statement of thoughts, feelings and desires is the common understanding of honesty. *The New Shorter Oxford English Dictionary on Historical Principles* (1993) suggests that honesty is a characteristic, not merely a linguistic or social occurrence. Words such as 'honourable character' and 'uprightness of disposition and conduct' imply that honesty is about more than truthful statements; it is an underlying characteristic of an individual. The dictionary presents the opposites of honesty as being cheating, stealing and lying. These definitions provide 'food for thought' that may assist the health professional when considering honesty. They suggest that honesty is a characteristic that generates honest statements and produces consideration of the needs of all interacting individuals.

CASE STUDY

You are very busy today, with more than the usual number of people to assist. The young person seeking assistance is the same age as you and has similar interests. They are usually optimistic and relaxed when they attend, but today they suddenly begin to tell you all the things that are going wrong in their life and how depressed they are feeling.

A holistic communicative approach alone, without consideration of the therapeutic relationship that is essential for positive outcomes, dictates that you should stop, actively listen, empathise and seek permission to refer the person to another professional if appropriate.

However, you are extremely busy and not interested in hearing any more because you have problems in your life too! You do not want a reminder of those things while at work, nor do you want to fall behind today because you have a personal appointment immediately after work. Besides, there are other people waiting to see you.

GROUP DISCUSSION

- Consider the possible ways of responding. Discuss the potential outcomes of each response.
- What is an ethically appropriate response?
- Which needs are the appropriate ones in this situation – the needs of the person or those of the health professional?

Honest responses from a health professional are important. Many people seeking assistance are able to recognise a verbal or non-verbal response that does not reflect honesty. Such responses affect the level of trust in the relationship and if detected potentially create anxiety in the person seeking assistance concerning reasons for the lack of honesty. It is important to consider particular situations and questions that could cause difficulty for the health professional and prepare possible responses (Higgs et al 2005). This consideration will assist in the development of a therapeutic relationship and contribute to family/person-centred practice.

DISCUSSION

- What do you need to consider before responding to the following?
  - Someone is reluctant to follow a treatment regimen.
  - Someone is unhelpful when you have asked for their assistance.
  - Someone is dismissive when you have asked them a question.
  - Someone relates differently from their previous interactions.
  - Someone shares that they are lonely and depressed but asks that you tell no-one.
  - Someone requests your assistance and what they are asking is inappropriate.
  - Someone waiting for results asks *Do I have cancer?* You know they do.
- Consider other possible situations that require honest responses.

If the health professional genuinely seeks the wellbeing of those with whom they interact, honest responses will develop trust and safety for all communicating individuals.

Clarification of expectations

When entering a new situation or environment, most individuals strive to understand that situation or environment. They may feel tentative or insecure and thus appreciate a friendly health professional who demonstrates genuine interest and concern. In such situations it is reassuring for the person to know what to expect and how to gain answers or assistance through either verbal or written information. Asking the person seeking assistance to voice their expectations of the service allows the health professional to clarify any uncertainties and will also serve to reassure the person.

REFLECTION AND DISCUSSION

- As a health professional, what do you feel a person seeking your assistance should know about your expectations and their rights before they receive your assistance?
- What do you feel such a person would like to know about their rights and the services available as they seek your assistance?
- What would you like to know about their expectations of your service?

There are various ways of communicating about the available services and the rights of the individual seeking assistance. Verbal and written explanations of rights and procedures with opportunity for clarification are usually successful and potentially improve the outcomes of both the communication and the service.

Consent

Agreement about information

In an attempt to achieve ethical behaviour from staff, particular health services use signed agreements that outline privacy and related issues. All people seeking assistance are asked to sign such agreements. These agreements are explicit statements of the usually implied rules that guide the relationship between the health professional and the person seeking assistance. Such rules assume that health professionals will never seek to harm the person seeking assistance and that they will always seek to assist and fulfil appropriate goals for that person (Purtilo & Haddad 2002). Signed agreements may provide information about the service, what to expect when receiving assistance, the responsibilities of all stakeholders and guidelines for lodging a complaint. They usually make statements about responsible use of gathered information based upon the assumption that every individual has a right to privacy (Mohan et al 2004). For more information relating to privacy in Australia, see Australian Government policies and acts such as the *Privacy Act 1988*, *Disability Services Act 1986* and *Commonwealth Disability Strategy 2003*. For a similar policy in New Zealand see the New Zealand Government *Privacy Act 1993*. These acts may state that the health service agrees to protect privacy. They may indicate that health professionals might share revealed information with other health professionals but only for the benefit of the person seeking assistance, never for illegal or inappropriate reasons.

REFLECTION AND DISCUSSION

- If you sign an agreement to protect your privacy, what would you expect that to mean regarding the information you provide to different health professionals about your needs or condition?
- Would you feel it was appropriate for a particular health professional to discuss your information with another person? If so, with whom and why?
- Would you like to have access to and explanation of any notes or reports the health professional(s) wrote about you?
- What are the implications of your answers for a health professional?

It is important to remember that the person seeking assistance will be more willing to provide information if the health professional has explained how the information will be used and why it is necessary for the health professional to have this information (Harms 2007, Stein-Parbury 2006). To encourage sharing of information, health professionals must act to indicate they are worthy of trust (Brill & Levine 2005).

Informed consent

Although the 'informed consent' type of agreement often refers to research involving humans (Malone 2003), within the health professions it usually refers to procedures associated with a particular health profession. This type of agreement requires the health professional to provide clear information about the procedure, the associated risks and the expected outcome of the procedure (Purtilo & Haddad 2002). Informed consent is an attempt to give the vulnerable individual a sense of control in a situation where they often feel they have little power, control or autonomy. In many places there is a legal requirement to provide such information at an appropriate level of complexity for the person seeking assistance.

Confidentiality

Protecting shared information

The person seeking assistance requires a safe 'space' in which to express their feelings, thoughts and concerns. The basis for that safe place and the expression of concerns is a trusting therapeutic relationship (Brill & Levine 2005, Stein-Parbury 2006). It requires the health professional to state explicitly what they intend to do with the shared information.

Some of the information given by the person is required for the development of appropriate interventions and should be available for all involved health professionals. However, there will also be information shared that does not contribute to their overall treatment. It is not essential to share this information. Sometimes it is not obvious whether the information is necessary for the success of the overall goals. Awareness of the necessity of information increases with experience. A relatively inexperienced health professional who is unsure about why someone is sharing particular information might be advised to ask the person two questions. First, *Are you telling me this for a reason?* meaning *Is there any action required because of this disclosure or do you simply trust me?* Second, the health professional might ask whether it is acceptable to pass the information on to a more senior health professional, for example, *Do you mind if I tell X what you have told me?* These questions will promote awareness in the person about the type of information they are sharing and the reason for sharing it. This may be particularly important when a young person shares information with a young health professional of the opposite gender. The possibility for attachment, whether romantic or not, is real and is best avoided because it can be destructive for both the person and the health professional. A guiding principle for deciding what information to share with other health professionals should be whether the information affects the health and wellbeing of the person seeking assistance.

Protecting ethical responsibility

Health professionals have ethical responsibility to protect information about the people they assist. This refers to information both read and heard. Such information belongs exclusively in the professional context – records, files, experiences, feelings and memories of shared information all belong at work.

Protecting the health professional

There are many times when health professionals simply need to 'unload' the thoughts and feelings associated with the information gathered from a particular person or from an entire day. The emotions and thoughts associated with a particular interaction or several interactions over a day require some form of resolution. Accumulation of these emotions can produce cynicism and burnout (Rupert & Morgan 2005). Discussing the emotions with someone provides an opportunity for resolution and dissipation of the intensity of the emotions. Sometimes a particular person makes a deep impression in the mind of the health professional and thus the health professional may require time and discussion to process the depth of and the implications of this impression.

Protecting the 'other' from gossip

Words once said are very difficult to retract, regardless of the intention of the words. Words cause an immediate emotional or cognitive reaction and it is often impossible to change those emotions even with an explanation of the intended meaning. This means that the health professional must take care when they say anything about any of the people with whom they are working – colleagues or otherwise.

REFLECTION

Think honestly about the following questions.
- How easy do you find it to talk about others when they are not present?
- How easy do you find it to tell someone directly what you think of them – either positive or negative thoughts?
- How easy do you find it to believe things said about other people, whether you know them or not?
- Is what you say about other people usually positive or negative?
- If negative, can you isolate the reason why you often say negative things about people? Are you jealous? Are you naturally judgemental? Have you been hurt by these people? Are you responding to something that someone else has said about these people?
- How do you feel when you discover someone has been talking about you – saying things, whether true or not, without you knowing?

Boundaries

Roles

Ethical communication requires definite understanding of the limits of the role of each health profession and the relationship between the person and the health professional. Each health profession has a particular role. Regardless of the level of knowledge of the health professional about the interventions of other health professions (Milliken & Honeycutt 2004), it is important that they practise within the limitations of their particular profession-related knowledge and skills. This is important for ethical, safety and insurance reasons.

Relationships

The limitations of the therapeutic relationship relate to the whole person. There are physical, emotional, social, cognitive and spiritual reasons for health professionals to practise within particular boundaries or limits. These limits include **time**, **friendship** and **dependency** boundaries (Brill & Levine 2005, Harms 2007, Purtilo & Haddad 2002). Each encounter with a person seeking assistance should have time limits. These limits allow the person to rest and the health professional to assist others and complete the requirements of their role.

Practising within the boundaries of the health professional role means understanding the role to be that of a 'therapist' not an intimate friend. If the health professional needs to have a real 'friendship' with people they assist this is an abuse of the role and can potentially damage the vulnerable individual (Heron 2001). That health professional must ask themself whether the relationship is fulfilling their needs rather than those of the person. Being friendly within the role is essential but is different to connecting in a personal and intimate manner.

Many of the people health professionals encounter will share personal and intimate information. This self-disclosure from the person seeking assistance assists them and assumes a particular understanding of confidentiality. If self-disclosure occurs between people of opposite genders, the health professional may misinterpret the meaning of this disclosure. They may assume it is simply an expression of emotions at the time and not understand that there are expectations of a deeper relationship that the health professional is unable to reciprocate. Dependence may develop and an expectation of exclusion of all others in the relationship that removes any therapeutic benefits (Egan 2007, Purtilo & Haddad 2002).

DISCUSSION

Egan (2007) and Harms (2007) suggest that to be therapeutic you have to 'come close'.
- How do you achieve this while maintaining boundaries?
- How do you achieve this without developing reliance and dependence?

Self-disclosure

It is sometimes appropriate for health professionals to share their own experiences, but only in particular circumstances. Self-disclosure on the part of the health professional should only occur to promote a connection with a person or to demonstrate understanding and particular strategies (Harms 2007). Self-disclosure should never occur to move the focus to the health professional or to make the health professional appear connected and knowledgeable. It should only take place to encourage and maintain the relationship (Devito 2007) – in this case, the therapeutic relationship.

DISCUSSION

- If someone asks you personal questions, what should you do? For example, *Do you do drugs? Do you have children? Do you have a girlfriend/boyfriend?*
- How do you decide whether or not to answer? What criteria should you use?

Sharing information about self can develop rapport. In New Zealand, a normal process that develops rapport for the Maori is disclosure about their iwi (tribe). In other cultures, disclosure about birthplace or immediate family is the norm. People from certain cultures may benefit from the health professional disclosing particular kinds of personal information. This information might be about family, country or town of origin, events or experiences, but is not usually about deep emotional experiences or emotional reasons for their demeanour. Some individuals are more comfortable than others with sharing personal details (Vogel et al 2006) and thus the comfort level of the health professional may assist in deciding the appropriate level of self-disclosure.

Over-identification

Over-identification can cause difficulties in the therapeutic nature of a relationship (Purtilo & Haddad 2002). Over-identification may occur when a health professional has experienced a very similar situation to the person seeking assistance, for example, when assisting someone who has a child, sibling or parent with a disorder the same as that of the health professional.

When a health professional over-identifies they can be anxious to share their experiences to indicate a connection, thereby focusing on themself. Emotional competence (Heron 2001) becomes important when the health professional experiences over-identification. Emotional competence means that the health professional will not allow their own experiences or emotions to affect the assistance offered to the vulnerable person. If the health professional is not able to function with emotional competence, the resultant self-focus is detrimental to the therapeutic relationship because it fulfils the needs of the health professional rather than the person seeking assistance (Heron 2001, Purtilo & Haddad 2002).

Ethical codes of behaviour/conduct

There are principles and in some cases legislation that guide and direct the behaviour of all health professionals (Collins 2004). These principles are usually the basis for the specific code of ethics adopted by individual health professions. If a particular health profession does not have a code specific to their practice, the government policy exists to guide their practice in ethical conduct. For example, in Australia, see the Queensland Government *Public Sector Ethics Act 1994*, the Queensland Health *Code of Conduct 2006* and the NSW Health Department *Code of Conduct, Appendix 27 2007*. In New Zealand, see *The Health and Disability Commissioner Act 1994* and the *Health Practitioners Competence Assurance Act 2003*.

The legislation, principles and ethical codes do not define the word 'ethical', nor do they necessarily provide exact answers to all ethical dilemmas experienced during practice (Banks 2006). They do provide guidelines that assist a practising health professional. It is important to understand that a code of ethics can produce rigid doctrinarian attitudes that are insensitive to the rights of others (Taylor 2000). This is never the intention of such a code and health professionals should use their code of ethics to encourage and empower individuals, not to paralyse them.

ACTIVITY

- Using the code of ethics specific to your profession, list behaviours that reflect this code.
- List characteristics of communication that conform to this code.

Chapter summary

Ethical issues that relate to communication are important because they ensure positive outcomes for all people involved in a health service.

Complete the following:
1. What does ethical communication achieve in a health service?

_____

_____

_____

2. Explain why some health professionals might not consciously apply ethical requirements in their practice?

_____

_____

_____

3. Why must a health professional fulfil ethical requirements?

_____

_____

_____

4. A health professional must provide certain information to fulfil ethical requirements.
   • What information must a health professional provide?

   _____

   _____

   _____

   • What forms can this information take?

   _____

   _____

   _____

   • What characteristic must this information have?

   _____

   _____

   _____

5. What must a health professional ensure when communicating ethically?

_____

_____

_____

6. What must a health professional remember to achieve ethical communication?

_____

_____

_____

7. Define emotional competence and explain how it assists a health professional to achieve ethical communication.

_____

_____

_____

8. What are the requirements of the code of conduct relevant to your health profession?

_____

_____

_____

References

Australian Government 1986 Disability Services Act. Available: www.austlii.edu.au/au/legis/cth/consol_act/dsa1986213 27 Mar 2008

Australian Government 1988 Privacy Act. Available: www.comlaw.gov.au 27 Mar 2008

Australian Government. Commonwealth Disability Strategy 2003 Available: www.facs.gov.au/internet/facsinternet.nsf/disabilities/cds_introduction.htm 27 Mar 2008

Backus W, Chapian M 2000 Telling yourself the truth. Bethany House, Bloomington MN

Banks S 2006 Ethics and values in social work, 3rd edn. Palgrave Macmillan, Basingstoke UK

Brill N I, Levine J 2005 Working with people: the helping process, 8th edn. Pearson Education, Boston

Collins D 2004 The balancing act: self determination versus duty of care. In: Brown R (ed) Living, striving, achieving: an Australian perspective on disability. Life Activities, Newcastle, Australia

Devito J A 2007 The interpersonal communication book, 11th edn. Pearson, Boston

Dossey B M, Keegan L, Gussetta C 2003 Holistic nursing: a handbook for practice, 4th edn. Jones & Bartlett, Sudbury MA

Dossey B M, Keegan L, Gussetta C 2005 A pocket guide for holistic nursing. Jones & Bartlett, Sudbury MA

Egan G 2007 The skilled helper, 8th edn. Thomson, Belmont CA

Harms D 2007 Working with people: communication skills for reflective practice. Oxford University Press, Melbourne

Heron J 2001 Helping the client: a creative, practical guide, 5th edn. Sage, London

Higgs J, Sefton A, Street A et al 2005 Communicating in the health and social sciences. Oxford University Press, Melbourne

Malone S 2003 Ethics at home: informed consent in your own backyard. International Journal of Qualitative Studies in Education 16:797–815

Milliken M A, Honeycutt A 2004 Understanding human behavior: a guide for healthcare providers, 7th edn. Thomson Delmar, New York

Mohan T, McGregor H, Saunders S et al 2004 Communicating as professionals. Thomson, Melbourne

New South Wales Health Department 2007 Code of Conduct. Available: www.health.nsw.gov.au/pubs/a/ar9697/a2700.html 27 Mar 2008

New Zealand Government 1993 Privacy Act. Available: www.legislation.govt.nz 27 Mar 2008

New Zealand Health and Disability Commissioner. The Health and Disability Commissioner Act 1994 (Amended 2003). Available: www.hdc.org.nz 27 Mar 2008

New Zealand Ministry of Health 2003 Health Practitioners Competence Assurance Act. Available: www.moh.govt.nz/hpca 27 Mar 2008

Purtilo R B, Haddad A 2002 Health professional and patient interaction, 6th edn. Saunders, Philadelphia

Queensland Government 1994 Public Sector Ethics Act. Available: www.legislation.qld.gov.au/LEGISLTN/CURRENT/P/PublicSecEthA94.pdf 27 Mar 2008

Queensland Health 2006 Code of Conduct. Available: www.health.qld.gov.au/about_qhealth/cc.asp 27 Mar 2008

Rider E, Keefer C 2006 Communication skills competencies: definitions and a teaching toolbox. Medical Education 40:624–629

Rogers C 1967 On becoming a person. Constable, London

Rupert P A, Morgan D J 2005 Work setting and burnout among professional psychologists. Professional Psychology: Research and Practice 36:544–550

Stein-Parbury J 2006 Patient and person: interpersonal skills in nursing, 3rd edn. Elsevier, Sydney (Original work published 2005)

Taylor B J 2000 Reflective practice: a guide for nurses and midwives. Allen & Unwin, Crows Nest, Sydney

The new shorter Oxford English dictionary on historical principles, 1993. Oxford University Press, Oxford

Tyler S, Kossen C, Ryan C 2005 Communication: a foundation course, 2nd edn. Pearson, Prentice Hall, Frenchs Forest, Sydney

United Nations 1948 Universal declaration of human rights. Available: www.un.org/Overview/rights. html 24 Feb 2008

United Nations 2006 Convention on the rights of persons with disabilities. Available: www.un.org/ disabilities/default.asp?id=150 24 Feb 2008

United Nations 2006 Human Rights Council. Available: www2.ohchr.org/english/bodies/hrcouncil 27 Mar 2008

Vogel D, Wester S, Heesacker M et al 2006 Gender differences in emotional responses: do mental health trainees overestimate the magnitude? Journal of Social and Clinical Psychology 25:305–332

Further reading

Australian Government 1999 National standards on ethical conduct in research involving humans. Commonwealth of Australia, Canberra

Human Rights and Equal Opportunity Commission 2006 Disability standards and guidelines. Available: www.humanrights.gov.au/disability_rights/standards/standards.html

New South Wales Department of Ageing, Disability and Home Care 2006 Stronger together: a new direction for disability services in NSW 2006–2016. NSW Government, Sydney

The New Zealand Ministry of Health 2000 The New Zealand health strategy, Chapter 5. Available: www.moh.govt.nz/moh.nsf

United Nations Enable. About us: secretariat for the convention on the rights of persons with disabilities. Available: www.un.org/disabilities

United Nations Enable. Standard rules on the equalization of opportunities for persons with disabilities. Available: www.un.org/disabilities

Websites: Codes of conduct for some health professions (mainly Australian)

Ambulance: Ambulance Service of NSW 2007 Code of conduct. Available: www.ambulance.nsw. gov.au

Dental Hygiene: International Federation of Dental Hygienists 2003 Code of ethics. Available: www. ifdh.org

Dietetics: Dietitians Association of Australia 2006 Statement of ethical practice. Available: www.daa. asn.au

Nursing and Midwifery: Australian Nursing and Midwifery Council 2005 Code of professional conduct for nurses in Australia. Available: www.anmc.org.au

Occupational Health and Safety: Safety Institute of Australia. Occupational health and safety professionals code of conduct. Available: www.sia.org.au

Occupational Therapy: Occupational Therapy Australia 2001 National code of ethics. Available: www.ausot.com.au

Osteopathy: New South Wales Osteopaths Registration Board 2001 Code of conduct for board members. Available: www.osteoreg.health.nsw.gov.au

Physiotherapy: Australian Physiotherapy Association 2001 Code of conduct. Available: apa.adusol.com.au

Podiatry: Podiatrists Registration Board 2005 Code of professional conduct. Available: www.podreg. health.nsw.gov.au; Podiatrists Board of Queensland 2007 Code of conduct. Available: www. podiatryboard.qld.gov.au

Radiography/Radiation Therapy: Australian Institute of Radiography 2003 Guidelines for professional conduct for radiographers, radiation therapists and sonographers. Available: www.a-i-r.com.au

Social Work: Australian Association of Social Workers 1999 Code of ethics. Available: www.aasw. asn.au

Speech Pathology: Speech Pathology Australia 2000 Code of ethics. Available: www.speechpathology australia.org.au

Traditional Medicine: Australian Traditional-Medicine Society Ltd 2006 Code of conduct. Available: www.atms.com.au

Informed consent

This extract from an original article by Malone (2003) relates to a research study involving postgraduate students as subjects. While many health professionals do not partake in research projects, the principles of informed consent are the same. Health services require any person receiving assistance to sign a form indicating their responsibilities and the responsibilities of the health service. Many require signing of an 'informed consent' form. This means that the person has been informed about and understands the implications of any interventions or procedures. There are many assumptions behind such letters, as the following extracts indicate. It is important to consider the ethical implications of such assumptions when requesting a signature from a vulnerable person seeking assistance.

Note: The repeated dots indicate removed text. The words in italics were not included in the original letter but have been added to highlight the difficulties associated with such letters. They indicate the potential meaning of the words in the letter – a meaning that was not evident until the project had been completed.

Ethics at home: Informed consent in your own backyard
Reproduced from Malone S 2003 Ethics at home: informed consent in your own backyard. International Journal of Qualitative Studies in Education 16:797–815 by permission of the publisher (Taylor & Francis Ltd, www.tandf.co.uk/journals).

A fully informed consent letter

Dear Graduate Student:

I am a doctoral candidate from ……….. doing dissertation research. The purpose of my proposed study is to develop an understanding of how doctoral students learn to write the accepted language, or discourse, of their discipline. ……………… I am interested in looking specifically at doctoral students in mathematics education.

The study will last for one semester (approximately 15 weeks). As a part of the project I would like permission to collect data from you in three ways.

Observations: I would also like an opportunity to observe your involvement in activities related to writing. ……….. I am also interested in observing such activities as collaborative writing with a group on a class project, a peer review of some of your writing as part of the composing process, or a discussion between you and a professor about a piece of writing; you might be able to direct me to other relevant activities as well. [*My presence in your class and continuing requests to be present in these other situations will initially make you very uncomfortable…………. In the class, you will never really know how to think of me – but you will not dare to bring up this issue because the professor has agreed to let me in and you will believe that expressing concern or discomfort will put you in the position of resisting him. You and he will say and do and think about things that you never would have except for my presence in your lives – it will change the nature of the class, perhaps in some negative ways.*]

After our initial interview, we will decide together which of your semester's writing projects I will examine in depth………………. I might also ask for samples of writing you produced before the semester in which the study takes place, in order to determine a baseline by which to judge your writing development. [*My assurance that this is something we will decide together might mislead you to think that you will have more power in this situation than you will actually have; it is highly unlikely that either of us will have time for you to be very involved in many of the decisions, especially those regarding the interpretation and rendering of the data.*]

Other than the possible inconvenience posed by the extra printing, I do not believe your participation in this study will pose any risks for you. [*Except for putting you into a position of extreme vulnerability in your relationships with your professor and your fellow graduate students. You also might learn things about yourself that will be painful; you will almost certainly share with me or discover things that you will not want anyone else to know about you and you will have to trust me to not do things that will hurt you. It is probable that I will not always know what might hurt you.*] .... You will have the opportunity to read the report before it is made public and to see how any data from your case study are used. [*The potential for 'harm' will continue even beyond the data collection phase and into the reporting phase; that harm could include your discomfort with things the study – and my interpretations – reveal about you. Even your feedback on the report and on how I have represented you will end up being 'data', to be interpreted along with the rest of it.*] ....

If you agree to participate, please sign the form below. Participation in this project is completely voluntary and you may withdraw at any time. [*In reality, you are very unlikely to feel free to withdraw from this study once you've begun – you would be too concerned with what others, particularly your professor, would think and the repercussions of such a decision. You probably are not even free to volunteer – you have been drafted, coerced by your professor's decision to work with me and, possibly, to some extent, by your own position as a graduate student/novice researcher. In short, you will not have a great deal of personal autonomy, given the political realities of the situation.*] If you would like additional information, please feel free to contact me at…. Thank you for responding to this request.

Sincerely, ...

Non-verbal communication

12

CHAPTER OBJECTIVES

Upon completing this chapter, students should be able to

- Explain and give examples of non-verbal communication
- Discuss the significance of non-verbal communication
- Examine the benefits of non-verbal communication
- List and explain the results of non-verbal communication
- Recognise and synthesise the components of non-verbal communication.

Non-verbal communication is, as the name implies, communication without words. It encompasses the environment, manner and style of communicating and the internal values of the person communicating (Holli et al 2003). Non-verbal communication includes the behaviours that accompany words (Burgoon & Hoobler 2002). Crystal (2007) states that even though non-verbal messages carry meaning, they are less flexible and adaptable than verbal modes of expression. While this may be true, non-verbal cues significantly influence the meaning of a sent message and as such are often more important than the spoken words (Egan 2007).

Body language is the general name given to non-verbal cues. Body language includes gesture, facial expression, posture, eye contact, gait and clothing. However, some elements of our speech are also non-verbal. The technical name for non-verbal characteristics of the voice is suprasegmentals. There are two types of suprasegmentals: prosodic and paralinguistic. The prosodic features of the voice include volume, pitch and rate of speech, which combine to create the unique 'rhythm' of a language. The paralinguistic features (also called paralanguage) of the voice use other vocal effects to convey meaning; they include emphasis (see Ch 1), timely pauses and tone, as well as laughing, whining, moaning and other non-verbal sounds (Crystal 1997). Suprasegmental vocal characteristics along with body language can change meaning, and thus are worthy of recognition and examination when considering non-verbal communication.

The significance of non-verbal communication

Researchers have investigated the significance of non-verbal cues in communicating meaning. Mehrabian (1981) suggests that the words only carry 7–10% of the meaning of a message. The suprasegmentals of a message carry 38% of the meaning and body language delivers 55% of the meaning. While such statistical reduction of messages is interesting, it does not change the reality that health professionals must use both verbal and non-verbal forms of communication consciously and with care, regardless of the relative significance of either in delivering the meaning.

The benefits of non-verbal communication

Burgoon & Hoobler (2002) indicate that skill in interpreting and using non-verbal behaviour increases the attraction, popularity and psychosocial wellbeing of an individual. However, they also state that the ability to use non-verbal behaviours increases the likelihood of manipulating others. Thus, individuals who are skilful in using non-verbal communication can be influential in assisting and supporting as well as deceiving others.

The effects of non-verbal communication

Non-verbal behaviour regulates or adjusts verbal communication (Egan 2007). It can

- Substantiate or reiterate the meaning of the words (e.g. yelling *Yeah!* at a football game is often reiterated by throwing arms up in the air or jumping up and down)
- Contradict or complicate the meaning of the words (e.g. stating *I am OK* with a faltering voice and quivering lip may indicate the opposite meaning to the words)
- Reinforce or accentuate the meaning of the words (e.g. saying *No thanks* along with specific non-verbal gestures and body positions, such as covering a cup with a hand, makes the message very clear)
- Influence the response of the 'other' regardless of words (e.g. avoiding eye contact may indicate a desire to evade interaction, or holding up a hand may indicate a need to stop an interaction).

ACTIVITY

Non-verbal communication can achieve positive and negative results.
List the positive and negative results of the non-verbal behaviours listed above. Consider the results from the perspectives of both parties – the sender and the receiver.

The components of non-verbal communication

Environment

The environment communicates clearly the level of interest in, and care for, the 'other' (Brill & Levine 2005; see Ch 8). Seating arrangements in a cosy room that promote appropriate levels of connection communicate careful attention to the needs of those using the room. Health professionals who focus, rather than being distracted by responding to every other event in the service, deliver specific messages that develop trust and positive outcomes.

Body language

Body language is a worldwide component of communication. There are particular rules for the use of body language that vary from culture to culture. The interpretation of body language must take into consideration the context and the particular circumstances of the person communicating.

DISCUSSION

- Discuss the different meanings of standing while waving both arms frantically above the head. When have you done this or seen others do it?
- How does context assist the interpretation of body language?

The physical appearance of a health professional communicates particular messages. Conscious consideration of those messages assists the health professional to communicate equality and acceptance.

Facial expression

Facial expressions can be powerful additions to words and generally express emotions. Facial expressions can also convey messages without the use of words (Purtilo & Haddad 2002). Some individuals have expressive faces while others rarely use their face to express their emotions. Some comedians are excellent examples of people who, when performing, rarely use facial expressions to communicate their emotions (i.e. the classic 'deadpan' delivery). Individuals with expressive faces must take care when communicating with others not to demonstrate emotions they regret. Health professionals should consciously use and control facial expressions to express respect, empathy and attention.

REFLECTION

- Do you use your face to express your emotions regularly?
- How successfully do you express your emotions with your face?

GROUP ACTIVITY

- Each member of the group chooses an emotion (e.g. happy, sad, embarrassed, tired, angry, frustrated, disgusted, anxious, confused, peaceful, lonely, bored, sleepy, interested). Do not tell anyone in the group your chosen emotion.
- Each person uses their face to express their chosen emotion.
- The other group members write down the name of the person and the emotion they are expressing on a piece of paper.
- When everyone has expressed their emotion, check the interpretations of the emotion. How many were incorrect? How could you vary your facial expression to more accurately express the emotion? How many variations of the same emotion were there?
- What are the implications for a health professional if different people assume different emotions from similar facial expressions?

There are cultural variations in the use of facial expression to convey messages. These variations include both how the face is used and the meaning of particular facial expressions.

Eye contact

Eye contact in some cultures signals interest and attention, while avoiding eye contact can indicate the opposite (i.e. disinterest). Eye contact can regulate turn-taking in an interaction and indicate the nature of the relationship between the people communicating. Using eye contact can assist the health professional to assess the feelings or functioning of the 'other' while communicating.

There are cultural variations in the use of eye contact. Some Aboriginal and Torres Strait Islander Peoples may communicate discomfort or pain by turning their heads to avoid any possibility of eye contact. Some cultures have different rules or beliefs about eye contact relating to gender, age and status.

ACTIVITY

- In pairs, look each other in the eye. How long can you continue this until you feel uncomfortable? Continue beyond the point of discomfort. What was the result?
- Discuss the variations in comfort with eye contact. What does this mean for a health professional?

Gesture

Gestures vary from individual to individual and convey attitudes, feelings and ideas. They do not necessarily require words. Gestures can use the entire upper limb or one finger; using an arm to wave or a finger to wave conveys very different meanings. Folded arms can communicate lack of openness or unhappiness, a tapping foot along with folded arms communicates impatience, and looking at a watch while tapping a foot with folded arms has a different meaning again (i.e. anger). In these cases the action clearly communicates the meaning without words.

Understanding subtle as well as obvious gestures is essential for effective communication (Purtilo & Haddad 2002). When working with people from different cultures it is appropriate for a health professional to state the conventions of gesture in their own culture and ask for the convention in the culture of the person seeking assistance. For example, the health professional might say *When we do this it means this; what does it mean to you?* Asking such a question of the person will assist understanding and build rapport.

ACTIVITY

Think of five common gestures (e.g. waving). Do they have the same meaning every time they are used? If not, what changes the meaning?

If gestures can change meaning within a single culture due to context, it is inappropriate to assume that the gestures of one culture have the same meaning in another culture.

Specifically asking about the meaning of particular gestures in the relevant culture is often conducive to the development of the therapeutic relationship.

Space

The use of space or proximity while interacting is important because it communicates interest (Mohan et al 2004) and, in some cultures, the nature of the relationship. In some South Pacific cultures, the authority figure must always be at a higher level than others. Generally, however, it is important to attempt to communicate on the same level with people seeking assistance. That is, if they are sitting it is beneficial to attempt to sit as well.

REFLECTIVE ACTIVITY

- Converse in pairs while one person is sitting and the other standing. Then swap positions.
- Discuss how each person felt in the different positions.
- What are the implications of these feelings for the health professional?

The distance between two interacting people communicates interest in the interaction and can indicate the intimacy of the relationship. The comfortable distance between standing individuals while relating varies from country to country. Cultural differences can result in individuals from a country with a small acceptable space 'chasing' individuals from a country with a larger acceptable space around a room, as the first steps into the personal space of the second and the second moves away. Until they realise what is causing the constant movement they will both experience discomfort during the interaction, one because they are standing too far apart and the other because they are too close.

Suprasegmentals: Prosodic features of the voice

Volume

The volume of a voice refers to whether the voice is loud or soft. Some individuals have voices that seem loud even when the person thinks they are speaking softly. Such voices are distinctive and can often be heard clearly from a distance or among other noises. Different situations require changes in volume depending on the context and the environmental noise conditions. Some individuals lower their volume when they are nervous, while others will raise their volume when nervous. Using appropriate volume is very important when speaking with people seeking assistance because this demonstrates the characteristics of a caring health professional. Many Aboriginal and Torres Strait Islander Peoples speak with a low volume when discussing personal or important information and may find a loud volume in such situations uncomfortable (Australian Government Department of Health and Ageing 2004).

REFLECTION

- Are you ever asked to change your volume when speaking?
- Are there particular circumstances that make you speak more quietly or more loudly?

Pitch

Pitch refers to the frequency of the voice, which makes the voice sound low or high. Pitch changes the style of expression and communicates feelings. Variations in pitch change meaning and may give greater force or intensity of feeling to spoken words (Crystal 1997, Crystal 2007). In some cultures variations in pitch can also indicate the opinion of the speaker. Pitch falls or rises depending on the starting point of the voice. Various languages use falling or rising pitch to indicate meaning. For example, changes in pitch can mean the difference between a statement and a question. In some South Pacific groups, however, raising the pitch at the end of a sentence is a common feature of the language and does not indicate a question.

Rate

The speed or rate of speaking also affects comprehension. Different communities and cultures use particular rates of speaking and most people within those communities adopt the rate that represents the norm. Some cultures value rapid speech while others consider slow speakers to be competent speakers (Devito 2007). Within a particular culture, however, some people naturally speak more quickly or slowly than the majority. Speaking in public or in situations that are anxiety-provoking may affect the speed of speaking; in turn, this may limit the ability of the listener to concentrate, which will decrease their understanding.

It is important for health professionals to be aware of situations that potentially affect the rate of their speech, and to consciously adjust their rate in these situations to ensure adequate comprehension. Another situation that might require an adjustment in speech rate is when the health professional is communicating with someone who has limited skills in the language of the interaction. In this situation using a slower than usual speech rate may facilitate understanding for the listener.

Suprasegmentals: Paralinguistic features of the voice

Volume, pitch and rate combine to create rhythm while speaking. However, there are other important non-verbal characteristics of speech.

Emphasis

Emphasis is a characteristic of the voice that can be used to change meaning. Emphasis refers to the stress placed on words within phrases or sentences. When used skilfully it is a powerful communicating tool. Care must be taken when using emphasis to communicate meaning, however, because it can easily produce negative effects in addition to positive effects. *You did* **what?** stresses the action and can have a positive or negative meaning. **You** *did what?* stresses the person and again may indicate disbelief that has a positive or a negative meaning.

Pauses

Pauses when speaking occur within sentences as well as in conversations. They provide opportunities for taking a breath or for looking up from papers if referring to notes. They provide opportunities for thinking in both the speaker and the listener. Pauses allow the speaker to compose their next sentence and the listener to process, understand and perhaps consider any questions they might want to ask of the speaker. A speaker may pause in response to non-verbal cues given or not given by the listener. Such a pause allows the speaker to decide whether to clarify the words or ask if the listener requires clarification, or, in some cases, to ask whether they are listening.

Different cultures view pauses or silence differently (Vainiomaki 2004). Some interpret them negatively while others consider them essential when attempting to become familiar with an unknown individual. In general it is best to avoid pauses over 10–15 seconds in length, because long pauses can feel uncomfortable (Cormier et al 1986). However, in some Aboriginal and Torres Strait Islander cultures, pauses and silence facilitate communication and information-processing (Harms 2007); in these cultures, pauses of less than several minutes can feel uncomfortable.

Pauses associated with vocalisation (e.g. *ah* or *um*) may communicate uncertainty (Devito 2007) or a level of incompetence. It is best for health professionals to avoid such vocalised pauses. It is important for health professionals to communicate confidence when speaking, whether through words, non-verbal cues or silence, because this assists the listener to trust and feel confident in the accuracy of the message.

DISCUSSION

- Is a pause an appropriate response when you do not know what to say or how to respond?
- What might be an appropriate response in this circumstance?
- Is a pause or silence appropriate when someone has asked a question and is waiting for a response?
- What might be appropriate if you need time to consider your answer?

REFLECTION

- How do you respond to pauses in conversations?
- How do you feel if you have verbally shared something personal and there is a pause with no response?
- What do you do in such situations?
- How do you feel if someone has shared something personal with you and you simply have to stop, process and consider while they are waiting for a response?
- What would you say in this situation?

GROUP DISCUSSION

- Suggest situations when a pause might occur or be required for a health professional.
- Suggest possible responses to these situations.

Tone

Emphasis and tone may occur together. Tone is associated with quality of voice and is the manner of expressing words that indicates feelings, attitudes or thoughts about a particular topic. Tone is usually expressed through changes in pitch, volume or duration of a word. Tone of voice can be used to change meaning in particular circumstances. The tone of the voice usually affects the entire utterance, unlike emphasis, which usually affects a few words.

- Say each of the following statements. Then change your tone to indicate a change in meaning.
    - *Do you really want that?*
    - *What do you think you're doing?*
    - *Have you finished yet?*
    - *Why is this here?*
- Decide how tone of voice changes the meaning of these statements.
- If something is important for the safety of the person seeking assistance, is it appropriate for the health professional to use a particular tone of voice to indicate that importance? For example, when talking about using a device, taking medication, doing exercises, keeping to a diet or cleaning a device.
- Can you think of a situation in which a health professional might appropriately use tone to enhance meaning?

Non-verbal behaviours, while powerful communicators of various emotions and ideas, can be easily misunderstood. It is essential to validate perceptions of non-verbal messages because these vary from individual to individual and from culture to culture. Requests for validation allow the person to either state or deny the emotions and ideas they are experiencing at that moment. They sometimes remind the person of the power of their non-verbal messages and encourage them to take responsibility for their non-verbal behaviours and the associated emotions or ideas.

Different individuals use non-verbal communication in different ways. Some use it consciously while others use it unconsciously. Many individuals have been surprised while watching themselves on video to see their non-verbal use of their body or voice. Unconscious hair-twirling, arm-crossing, upper-lip-stroking or nail-biting while concentrating may be a habit so unconscious that the person is surprised when they see themselves doing it. Health professionals must learn to observe and interpret non-verbal messages, but must also be aware of their own non-verbal behaviours. Health professionals should use non-verbal messages to communicate exactly what they mean.

Chapter summary

Non-verbal communication refers to communication without words, and is often more important than spoken words in influencing the meaning of a message. There are two main elements of non-verbal communication. Body language includes facial expression, eye contact, gesture and proximity. Suprasegmentals refer to the non-verbal characteristics of the voice; they include volume, pitch, rate, emphasis, pauses, tone and non-verbal sounds such as laughing. Non-verbal communication can have negative and positive results, and thus it is important that health professionals are aware of their own non-verbal messages.

Complete the following:
1. What does non-verbal communication encompass?

_____

_____

_____

2. What are the four major components of non-verbal communication?

    i.   _____

    ii.   _____

    iii. _____

    iv.   _____

3. How much of the meaning of a message do the words carry?

    _____

    _____

    _____

4. What are the benefits of using non-verbal behaviour skilfully?

    _____

    _____

    _____

5. What are the effects of non-verbal communication?

    _____

    _____

    _____

6. Give three examples of three of the four components of non-verbal communication.
    *   Component 1:_____
        i.   _____
        ii.   _____
        iii. _____
    *   Component 2:_____
        i.   _____
        ii.   _____
        iii. _____
    *   Component 3:_____
        i.   _____
        ii.   _____
        iii. _____

7. Explore the four components of non-verbal communication.
    *   Choose one aspect of the environment and explain how a health professional might use that aspect to achieve positive results when communicating.

    _____

    _____

    _____

    *   Choose two forms of body language and explain how a health professional might use those forms to achieve positive results when communicating.

    _____

    _____

    _____

- Choose two forms of prosodic features and explain how a health professional might use those forms to achieve positive results when communicating.

  _____

  _____

  _____

- Choose two forms of paralinguistic features and explain how a health professional might use those forms to achieve positive results when communicating.

  _____

  _____

  _____

8. Context can affect the meaning of non-verbal behaviour. Give an example of how context might affect the interpretation of non-verbal behaviour.

   _____

   _____

   _____

9. Culture can affect the use of non-verbal communication. Give two examples of ways of using non-verbal behaviour to communicate messages in different cultures.
   i. _____
   ii. _____

10. Consider your own non-verbal behaviour. Do you have friends or family members who tell you that you express yourself non-verbally without realising you are doing it? For example, do you play with your hair, use a strong tone of voice when you are not angry, fidget/fiddle when listening, or sit in a disinterested manner when you are actually listening and interested? If so, is this something that could be detrimental to your role as a health professional? How could you learn to control the behaviour? If you have never had someone tell you about your non-verbal messages, ask a friend if there are particular times when you send non-verbal messages that may deliver a different message to the intended one.

References

Australian Government Department of Health and Ageing 2004 Providing culturally appropriate palliative care to Aboriginal and Torres Strait Islanders: resource kit. Commonwealth of Australia, Canberra. (The Mungabareena Aboriginal Corporation assisted in the preparation of this resource kit.)

Brill N I, Levine J 2005 Working with people: the helping process, 8th edn. Pearson Education, Boston

Burgoon J K, Hoobler D 2002 Nonverbal signals. In: Knapp M L, Daly J A (eds) Handbook of interpersonal communication, 3rd edn. Sage, Thousand Oaks CA, p 240–299

Cormier L S, Cormier W H, Weisser R J 1986 Interviewing and helping skills for health professionals. Jones and Bartlett, Boston

Crystal D 2007 How language works. Penguin Books, London

Crystal D 1997 The Cambridge encyclopedia of language, 2nd edn. Cambridge University Press, New York

Devito J A 2007 The interpersonal communication book, 11th edn. Pearson, Boston

Egan G 2007 The skilled helper, 8th edn. Thomson, Belmont CA

Harms L 2007 Working with people: communication skills for reflective practice. Oxford University Press, Melbourne

Holli B B, Calabrese R J, O'Sullivan Mailett J 2003 Communication and education skills for dietetics professionals, 4th edn. Lippincott, Williams & Wilkins, Philadelphia

Mehrabian A 1981 Silent messages. Wadsworth Thomson, Belmont CA

Mohan T, McGregor H, Saunders S et al 2004 Communicating as professionals. Thomson, Melbourne

Purtilo R B, Haddad A 2002 Health professional and patient interaction, 6th edn. Saunders, Philadelphia

Vainiomaki T 2004 Silence as a cultural sign. Semiotica 150:347–361

Stereotypes, judgement and communication

13

CHAPTER OBJECTIVES

Upon completing this chapter, students should be able to

- Understand and recognise stereotypical judgement
- Account for the effect of stereotypical judgement upon communication
- Examine some of their personal stereotypical prejudices and expectations
- Demonstrate the importance of communicating without stereotypical judgement
- Describe the characteristics of a health professional who communicates without stereotypical judgement
- Explain how to overcome tendencies to stereotype and judge
- Develop strategies that promote non-judgemental communication.

Communicating without judgement occurs when the individual *avoids* making a judgement about a person based on personal values and beliefs. Value-laden judgements often occur because of appearance or some observable behaviour or characteristic that creates stereotypical expectations (Purtilo & Haddad 2002). The values and beliefs of an individual, although not always observable (Ellis et al 2004), provide the foundation for biases that create stereotypical judgements. These often-irrational biases develop over time from significant others or parental models (Milliken & Honeycutt 2004). They can create prejudice towards particular types of people or groups (Brill & Levine 2005). Stereotypical judgements may be positive or negative. For example, a judgement stating that all surfers are able-bodied and fit is positive, if being able-bodied and fit are considered positive attributes. However, this statement may not always be true. Similarly, a judgement stating that all Muslims condone violence and terrorism is negative, if violence and terrorism are considered negative attributes, but this statement is definitely not always true. A stereotype is a fixed impression about a person or group (Devito 2007) that may have some connection with reality because there may appear to be some similarities within the people or group. A stereotype in itself may initially be beneficial because it provides a framework from which to commence communication. However, if the stereotype produces judgements that dominate all communication with an individual it can be detrimental, because it limits the possibility of relating to more than the stereotype (Holliday et al 2006).

Reasons to avoid stereotypical judgement when communicating

Biases, prejudice and resultant judgements can greatly affect communication – they may result in conflict (see Ch 14), misunderstandings (see Ch 17) and communication breakdown (Mohan et al 2004). These are good reasons why health professionals should avoid stereotypical judgements based on prejudice (Egan 2007). However, there are additional reasons to avoid stereotypical judgement. Stereotypical attitudes often develop from limited information (ignorance) or misinformed assumptions (Brill & Levine 2005, Holliday et al 2006) and thus the resultant judgement may be incorrect. This potentially means that if a health professional is relating to someone through a stereotype, they have reduced the person to something that is less than who they are and therefore the health professional is not allowing the person to have thoughts and opinions that do not conform to the stereotype. It is also possible that the stereotype is based on an unconscious belief about an 'in' group and a subordinate 'out' group (Bowe & Martin 2007). This suggests the beliefs or culture of the person making the stereotypical judgement are the standard for evaluating the 'other' person or culture (Tyler et al 2005). Stereotypical judgement usually occurs unconsciously and thus has serious implications for the health professional (Lyons & Kashima 2003). If unconscious, prejudice and possible resultant stereotypical judgements will unknowingly influence the communication of the health professional, with potentially unpleasant results.

REFLECTION

Explore your prejudice (Adapted from Devito 2007)
- What are your honest answers to the following questions?
    - Are you willing to have a close friend from any other culture or religious group?
    - Are you willing to have a long-term romantic relationship with someone from another culture, political party or religious group?
    - Are you willing to choose to talk to someone who 'lives on the street' (is homeless) when you are out shopping?
    - Are you willing to allow people who are obviously different to you to have value and credibility?
- Are you able to answer with a definite yes? If not, are you able to determine the source of your biases?
- What can a health professional do to overcome any unconscious tendency to stereotypical judgements?

Although a stereotypical judgement may benefit the person holding the stereotype because it justifies their own characteristics or value, it produces lenses that negatively affect communication. Devito (2007) states that a stereotypical judgement creates two major barriers when communicating. The first barrier occurs if there exists a set idea about the person or their group. This idea will limit the ability to hear or experience anything that is different to the constructs of the stereotype. The second barrier limits the possibility of relating to particular qualities or abilities within the person if those qualities contradict the stereotype. In such cases, the stereotypical judgement may not allow the person to be unique or different to the stereotype. For example, a young health professional can be as competent as an older one, but a stereotypical judgement may not allow them to be competent. Alternatively, an elderly person may lead a very active life despite the stereotypical judgement that states elderly people are frail and dependent. If such stereotypical judgements occur, all communicators experience limited mutual understanding, and negotiation of meaning – if it does occur – is likely to fail. More importantly, while these barriers limit the possibility of effective communication, they also limit the potential to achieve family/person-centred practice.

Stereotypical judgement that relates to roles

Stereotypical judgements often lead to expectations of particular behaviour within particular roles. This is potentially as detrimental as applying a stereotype to the characteristics of a person or group. Expectations of particular behaviour from a person in the role of an administration assistant, for example, are beneficial whenever that person behaves according to those expectations. If an individual expects an administration assistant to make their favourite hot drink every morning but the administration assistant does not consider that activity part of their role, there will be disappointment in one person and anger in the other. Understanding stereotyping facilitates consideration of what behaviour a health professional expects from the 'other' (Thompson 2006) and what the 'other' might expect from a person in the role of a health professional.

> **REFLECTION AND DISCUSSION**
> - What behaviour represents an 'ideal' person seeking assistance? Answer this question alone, making a list of behaviours. Use your expectations not those of other health professionals.
> - Discuss the individual lists within a group and together agree upon a list.
> - How would these expectations affect the reactions to, and communication with, someone who does not behave according to these expectations?
> - How can a health professional ensure they allow the 'other' to be unique and thus fulfil their unique needs regardless of the particular role of the health professional?

Expectations of a health professional

Many individuals have stereotypical attitudes that affect their expectations of people and situations. While parental influences contribute to the creation of these attitudes, experience will also influence them. A person who has a negative experience with one health service or health professional may generalise this experience to expect similar experiences from all health professionals (Holliday et al 2006). It may take only one negative experience with a particular health professional to create the expectation that all individuals from that health profession will be the same (Harms 2007). It is the responsibility of the health professional to communicate without stereotypical judgement or expectations, because it is important to avoid reinforcing any existing negative stereotypes.

CASE STUDY

A young mother brings her 3-year-old child who has Down Syndrome to a speech pathologist for assistance with oral communication. At home, the child verbalises and communicates. However, in the clinic the child is nervous and overwhelmed by the situation so does not communicate or respond in any way. The health professional assumes the child cannot verbalise and, not listening to the mother, provides strategies to manage a non-verbal child.

GROUP DISCUSSION

- How would you respond?

The mother, upset and infuriated, never returned to that speech pathologist and took some time to seek the assistance of another.

   This health professional demonstrated stereotypical judgements that negatively affected the vulnerable mother for some time. This response was not conducive to fulfilment of family-centred practice and certainly limited communication.

An 'ideal' health professional demonstrates differing behaviours and communicative qualities according to the needs of the individual and the requirements of the particular situation (Green et al 2006). The following list highlights the characteristics and behaviours of an ideal health professional that will affect the quality of their communication.

An ideal health professional should be

- Knowledgeable about and skilled in their health profession (Stein-Parbury 2006)
- Respectful and caring (Brill & Levine 2005)
- Warm and genuine (Ellis et al 2004, Harms 2007)
- Open and humble (Devito 2007)
- Willing to be human and supportive, often emotionally and sometimes through touch (Dossey et al 2003, Egan 2007, Harms 2007)
- Concerned about others and open to differences (Tyler et al 2005)
- Honest and sensitive (Devito 2007, Higgs et al 2005)
- Reflective and self-aware (Dossey et al 2005, Harms 2007, Purtilo & Haddad 2002).

REFLECTION AND DISCUSSION

- If you have sought assistance from a health professional, what were your expectations? Is there anything else to add to the above list?
- Do the characteristics in the above list assist in the creation of a health professional who communicates without stereotypical judgement? Explain how and why.

People sometimes expect specific physical characteristics of an individual in a particular role. For example, some people seeking assistance refuse to see a young health professional. They believe a young health professional cannot possibly have enough experience to be competent and therefore will only see a health professional over a particular age. Some young health professionals take special care to appear older in order to combat this stereotypical expectation. Some people apply gender stereotypes to particular health professional roles. In such cases, a person may insist on receiving assistance from a health professional of a particular gender if they believe that only a female/male should fulfil that role. For example, some people believe that nurses or massage therapists should be female and medical specialists or physiotherapists should be male.

If a person seeking the assistance of a health professional holds any stereotypical expectations, this can affect the development of rapport and any subsequent communication. Overcoming the stereotypical expectations of others requires perseverance and sound professional practice. Similarly, if a health professional holds stereotypical expectations of the person seeking assistance there are usually comparable consequences. Overcoming personal stereotypical judgement in the health professional requires careful, self-aware vigilance and tolerance to maintain non-judgemental attitudes and communication that avoids stereotypical judgement (Mohan et al 2004).

Developing attitudes that avoid stereotypical judgement

Most individuals have unconscious values and beliefs that create unconscious biases and stereotypical judgements. Many biases develop when a parent expresses a particular sentiment that the child then adopts (Milliken & Honeycutt 2004), often with more conviction than the parent. Such convictions create stereotypical judgements which, when superimposed upon information and behaviour, increase the complexity of any interaction and certainly create barriers to effective communication. Honest evaluation of current values and beliefs that cause bias and prejudice is essential to produce communication in health professionals that avoids stereotypical judgement (Brill & Levine 2005, Devito 2007, Egan 2007).

REFLECTIVE ACTIVITY

Honest evaluation of values and prejudice
- Read the following points and write down your immediate and honest response to each of these groupings. Avoid trying to explain or change your thoughts – simply write down the thoughts that immediately come into your mind. What are your attitudes or bias towards
  - A person who is obese
  - A person with an intellectual disability
  - A person who smokes
  - A person who has a hearing impairment
  - A person who is homeless or lives on the street
  - A person who is Muslim (Did you know there are various types of groupings within the Muslim faith?)
  - A person with a different sexual orientation to you?
- Are there any other 'groups' of people that elicit a negative stereotypical response in you? Explain why.
- Consider how your reactions will affect your ability to communicate without stereotypical judgement if assisting anyone from these groups.

It is essential to overcome the biases that create stereotypical judgements that negatively influence responses to people who are different (Milliken & Honeycutt 2004). Self-awareness is essential to overcome these biases (see Chs 5 & 6). Seeking exposure to particular groups or people who are different with an open and accepting attitude is also beneficial in this process (Purtilo & Haddad 2002). Such exposure will allow development of perceptions based upon experiences; it will provide information about similarities as well as differences. Exposure to particular groups or people will reveal that there are many variations within any grouping and reinforce the uniqueness of every individual regardless of their ethnicity or their departure from societal norms. An example of a common stereotypical judgement from many westerners is that Asians are all the same. In reality, there are many different countries in Asia and within those countries there are a multitudinous number of ethnic groups. It takes exposure and willingness to perceive and accept the differences to understand that Asians are definitely not all the same. If the health professional finds it difficult to expose themself to and accept differences, it can be beneficial to explore the basis of the attitudes of other health professionals who regularly communicate without judgement (Mohan et al 2004). Discussion about how the non-judgemental individual achieves this may assist a health professional who is struggling to overcome stereotypical judgements that negatively affect communication.

It is important that health professionals understand and accept those around them despite the differences. In order to avoid judgemental communication health professionals will benefit from being aware of their personal stereotypical attitudes and seeking experiences that will change those attitudes. It is beneficial for health professionals to be flexible and willing to regularly evaluate their personal opinions and attitudes (Devito 2007). When reacting with a negative attitude based upon a stereotypical prejudice, it is important that health professionals strive to overcome that judgement. An awareness of the bias that produces the judgement facilitates change in that bias and ultimately acceptance of the 'different' individual or group.

Stereotypical judgement will limit any perception of the worth or value of the person or their opinions. The judging person will find reasons why that particular individual does not have value or worth. For example, thoughts such as *They will be lazy because they are overweight* or *They will be unreliable because they smoke – they'll always be off smoking* limit the ability to acknowledge any hard-working or reliable behaviour from that individual. Alternatively, thinking *Oh here is another extremist – looks like recycling will be more important than the quality of the work they do* limits the possibility of acknowledging the benefits of recycling or the value of the 'extremist'. Stereotypes and biases prompt judgement of the person on outward appearances or behaviour (e.g. age, gender, skin colour, clothing, jewellery, religious grouping, nationality, political party or particular behaviours), rather than perceptions of their personal attributes and value. In the health professions, this tendency results in the labelling of people. The overweight person is 'lazy', the person who smokes is 'unreliable' and the person who values recycling is an 'extremist' or fanatic. While labels may reflect something, in reality they are unhelpful and dehumanise the person, removing them from emotions and value. It is common to hear statements such as *The knee in Room 407* within some health professions and, while understandable from many perspectives, such statements are unhelpful and unnecessary.

REFLECTION

- What labels did you or another student have at school?
- How did these labels make you or the other student feel?
- What are the implications of these feelings for health professionals?

A bias restricts the ability to understand a person, their thoughts and actions. The presence of bias and stereotypical judgement in a health professional does not allow the health professional to view the person as they actually are and, therefore, seriously restricts their ability to demonstrate empathy, acceptance and a sense of equality.

Overcoming the power imbalance: Ways to demonstrate equality in a relationship

Non-judgemental thoughts and behaviours promote equality and acceptance. The understanding that each person is vital and important (Milliken & Honeycutt 2004) assists in achieving equality when communicating. It is important to remember that health professionals are in a position of power because of their knowledge and familiarity with their role and the particular health service. This understanding emphasises the need to express acceptance and avoid communicating a sense of superiority. Flexibility and humility are key characteristics (Devito 2007) that contribute to the construction of equality in relationships in all health services. In addition – if differences stimulate stereotypical judgements – there are particular responses that promote equality when communicating (see Table 13.1).

Promoting equality when communicating as a health professional	
Do:	Do not:
• Acknowledge the person • Acknowledge what they say, regardless of agreement with the statements • Acknowledge cultural differences and learn about those differences • Adjust practice to accommodate cultural differences • Be tolerant of differences.	• Make demands (e.g. *Get that done now*) – instead make polite requests • Make 'should' or 'must' statements (e.g. *You must do these exercises or keep to that diet*) – they imply judgement • Interrupt – this suggests your ideas are more important than those of others.

TABLE 13.1 Adapted from Devito 2007.

Non-judgemental communication requires conscious awareness of consistent thoughts and repeated responses to avoid stereotypical judgements in communication. It requires self-awareness and tolerance that promotes acceptance and respect for the 'other' regardless of the challenges. Non-judgemental communication has many rewards.

Chapter summary

Stereotyping refers to biases that develop over time and create prejudice towards certain people or groups. Communication based upon stereotypical judgements limits the possibility of relating to the whole person and can result in misunderstandings. It is important for health professionals to develop attitudes of unconditional positive regard for all people who seek their assistance. Non-judgemental communication is the key to overcoming the inherent power imbalance in the relationship between the health professional and the 'other'.

Complete the following:
1. How can a health professional avoid communicating a stereotypical judgement?

_____

_____

_____

2. What is a value-laden judgement?

_____

_____

_____

3. What can value-laden judgements often create?

_____

_____

_____

4. Where do values and beliefs originate?

_____

_____

_____

5. What can values and beliefs create?

_____

_____

_____

6. Focus upon stereotypes:
   • Define 'stereotype' and give an example of a positive and a negative stereotype.

   _____

   _____

   _____

   • Are the stereotypes you isolated representative of the social norms within your health profession?

   _____

   • If not, are they important?

   _____

   • What should you do to adjust your ideas?

   _____

   _____

   _____

7. Give three reasons why it is important for health professionals to avoid communicating stereotypical judgement.
   i. _____
   ii. _____
   iii. _____

8. What communication barriers can stereotypical judgement produce?
   i. _____
   ii. _____

9. Give original examples of stereotypical expectations of behaviour that accompany particular roles.

_____

_____

_____

10. Give original examples of stereotypical expectations of characteristics that accompany a particular role.

_____

_____

_____

11. Identity the characteristics of a health professional that are most closely related to effective communication skills. Explain why and how.

_____

_____

_____

12. Suggest three ways a health professional can avoid stereotypical judgement.

   i. _____

   ii. _____

   iii. _____

13. List five behaviours (some of which are communicative) to overcome the power imbalance in the relationship between the health professional and the person seeking assistance. Give original examples of each behaviour.

   i. _____

   ii. _____

   iii. _____

   iv. _____

   v. _____

References

Bowe H, Martin K 2007 Communication across cultures: mutual understanding in a global world. Cambridge University Press, Melbourne

Brill N I, Levine J 2005 Working with people: the helping process, 8th edn. Pearson, Boston

Devito J A 2007 The interpersonal communication book, 11th edn. Pearson, Boston

Dossey B M, Keegan L, Gussetta C 2003 Holistic nursing: a handbook for practice, 4th edn. Jones & Bartlett, Sudbury MA

Dossey B M, Keegan L, Gussetta C 2005 A pocket guide for holistic nursing. Jones & Bartlett, Sudbury MA

Egan G 2007 The skilled helper, 8th edn. Thomson, Belmont CA

Ellis R, Gates B, Kenworthy N 2004 Interpersonal communication in nursing: theory and practice, 2nd edn. Churchill Livingstone, London (Original work published 2003)

Green R, Gregory R, Mason R 2006 Professional distance and social work: stretching the elastic? Australian Social Work 59:449–461

Harms L 2007 Working with people: communication skills for reflective practice. Oxford University Press, Melbourne

Holliday A, Hyde M, Kullman J 2006 Intercultural communication: an advanced resource book. Routledge, New York (Original work published 2004)

Higgs J, Sefton A, Street A et al 2005 Communicating in the health and social sciences. Oxford University Press, Melbourne

Lyons A, Kashima Y 2003 How are stereotypes maintained through communication: the influence of stereotype sharedness. Journal of Personality and Social Psychology 85:989–1005

Milliken M E, Honeycutt A 2004 Understanding human behavior: a guide for healthcare providers, 7th edn. Thomson Delmar, New York

Mohan T, McGregor H, Saunders S et al 2004 Communicating as professionals. Thomson, Melbourne

Purtilo R B, Haddad A 2002 Health professional and patient interaction, 6th edn. Saunders, Philadelphia

Stein-Parbury J 2006 Patient and person: interpersonal skills in nursing, 3rd edn. Elsevier, Sydney (Original work published 2005)

Thompson N 2006 Antidiscriminatory practice. Palgrave Macmillan, Basingstoke

Tyler S, Kossen C, Ryan C 2005 Communication: a foundation course, 2nd edn. Pearson, Prentice Hall, Frenchs Forest, Sydney

Conflict and communication

14

CHAPTER OBJECTIVES

Upon completing this chapter, students should be able to

- Recognise the mutual benefits of communicating appropriately during conflict
- Identify the typical causes of conflict
- Understand the importance of evaluating severity of emotions during conflict
- Demonstrate some awareness of their own patterns of dealing with conflict
- Discuss the different responses to conflict
- Outline the characteristics of assertive communication
- Demonstrate ways of communicating assertively in difficult situations.

Most communicative interactions are relatively straightforward and, although they may require concentration and energy, do not present major difficulties. However, wherever people interact difficult communicative interactions involving conflict are inevitable (Bowe & Martin 2007, Brill & Levine 2005, Devito 2007). Conflict involves a disagreement or clash between people; such communicative interactions are not only difficult, they are also potentially unpleasant. It is beneficial for health professionals to develop understanding of and skills in managing conflict – both to achieve effective communication and to develop skills and confidence when communicating. It is advantageous if health professionals feel confident to resolve situations of conflict calmly and appropriately for the mutual benefit of themselves and the vulnerable individual(s).

Conflict during communication

REFLECTION

- How do you feel about
  - Disagreeing with someone
  - Presenting a point of view that is different to a popular view
  - Saying *no* to a request
  - Discussing an emotionally charged topic?
- Consider your answers to these questions. Your answers indicate the reality of how you face potentially difficult situations involving conflict.

Causes of conflict

Conflict while communicating can involve

- Disagreement about supply of information, reasons for decisions, supervisory feedback (Higgs et al 2005)
- Differences in ideas, principles or even in people
- Differences in ideas about the way things should be organised (Stein-Parbury 2006)
- Different understanding of the same words (Purtilo & Haddad 2002)
- The relative value of certain procedures (Holli et al 2003)
- The order of priority for particular tasks
- Not understanding expectations (Mohan et al 2004).

These are some of the differences that may result in conflict and thus potentially a difficult communicative interaction. Conflict may occur between the health professional and the person seeking assistance, but it may also occur between the health professional and their colleagues. Conflict in itself does not cause difficulty; it is the management of conflict that produces negative or positive results (Rakos 2006). Gaining positive results from situations of conflict requires self-awareness and self-control (Devito 2007).

REFLECTION AND DISCUSSION

- How could an understanding of your blocks to listening and barriers to emotions assist communication during conflict? How could this understanding contribute to changing the way you communicate during conflict?
- How could the need to always be right affect communication during conflict?
- How could the need to appear knowledgeable affect communication during conflict?
- How could being judgemental affect communication during conflict?
- How could feelings of insecurity affect communication during conflict?
- Will explicitly noting these tendencies in yourself or in others assist you to respond appropriately when communicating in difficult situations in the future? If you have these tendencies, will you need to do more than recognise them? That is, will you need to act to overcome these tendencies when communicating?

Identifying emotions during conflict

In order to understand how to communicate appropriately during conflict it is important to identify the severity of the emotions in all communicating parties during the conflict. This recognition will assist in deciding how to control or resolve the conflict. The severity of the emotions associated with the conflict may also indicate the effort and action required to resolve the conflict. If the emotion is simply one of uneasiness or awkwardness, it is probably not too serious. The uneasiness may indicate totally unrelated causes (e.g. tiredness, hunger or lateness). A simple question to clarify the reason for the lack of ease can quickly resolve the awkwardness (e.g. *Are you feeling all right today?*). Alternatively, a statement to explain the uneasiness (e.g. *I am sorry, I have just been to the funeral of a close friend*) will assist in clarifying the situation.

Another emotion associated with conflict when communicating is irritation. Irritation or annoyance can occur during an interaction when the potential outcome of the interaction appears unsatisfactory to at least one of the people communicating. In this situation the use of questions (e.g. *You seem irritated today – is there something upsetting you?*) or an 'I' statement or question (e.g. *I feel irritated because you said you would be on time today and you were half an hour late again* or *Are you upset because of something I have done?*) can be powerful in highlighting and potentially resolving a difficult communicative event. Despite the use of 'I', these responses focus on the problem. They can clarify the cause of the emotion and potentially resolve the situation for the person who feels irritated.

Another result of difficult communicative interactions can be misunderstandings (see Ch 17). A misunderstanding occurs when there is a failure to understand or correctly interpret the meaning of thoughts, intentions, words, associated feelings, non-verbal behaviours or actions. This situation can cause confusion, dissatisfaction and discouragement in all communicating parties. The failure in understanding is not always easy to resolve if there were associated emotional responses. However, if one party feels misunderstood it is possible the other communicating individuals will also feel misunderstood. Honestly acknowledging the misunderstanding, admitting any mistake and apologising is a powerful course of action that can resolve the conflict. This action often allows the other person to apologise and say that it is all right. Remembering that each individual is in control of their emotional responses and can choose what they will feel is important for the health professional in such circumstances.

Choosing to ignore

In some situations it is important to identify the purpose of expressing the emotions. Recognising the reason for the passionate expression of any negative emotion may assist the health professional to determine their response. Such expressions of emotion may cause discomfort for those present in the room. In these situations it is important to assess whether ignoring the expression is the appropriate course of action. Sometimes a person simply needs to express their emotions with minimal response from another person. It may be difficult to evaluate and respond with the correct action. The action might be to quietly leave the room and close the door or perhaps remain quietly in the room until the completion of the expression of the emotion. Whether or not the health professional chooses to ignore, in situations similar to these it is best for health professionals to avoid responding emotionally, nor should they absorb blame if they are not responsible. Dealing appropriately with expressions of emotion will assist the person and the resolution of the situation.

Resolving negative attitudes and emotions towards another

Sometimes negative attitudes and prejudice towards a person can cause constant stress when thinking about or communicating with that person. Such responses may occur between the health professional and the person seeking assistance, and in the health professions they can also occur among colleagues. The opinion that creates this stress may seem justified because of the attitudes or actions of the other person. It will, however, be a source of constant strain. This strain could negatively affect every working relationship connected with that person and would certainly affect the thoughts and ultimately attitudes of the stressed health professional. In order to avoid habitual unproductive ways of relating to that person it is important to resolve such emotions quickly.

Unresolved stress in a relationship can result in a breakdown in both communication and the relationship. This suggests that resolving the attitude and associated emotions creating the stress is important. Recognition of the source of the attitude of the health professional can assist in resolving the emotions associated with the other person. Investment of time to understand the person and the factors that stimulate a negative response in the health professional can promote a positive attitude and assist the health professional to relate in a positive manner. A focus on the positive attributes of the person as well as similarities shared in experiences or values can also assist in changing a negative attitude. Appropriate management of conflict situations is essential in the health professions. It requires awareness, preparation and commitment to resolution of unresolved emotions on the part of the health professional.

Patterns of relating during conflict

There are always underlying requirements that must guide communicative interactions in the health professions, whether or not the interactions involve conflict. During any type of communication, but particularly during conflict, it is important to focus on the needs of the person. Remember that they have a right to feel and to express their differences of opinion or their emotions. They do not have a right to 'abuse' another person, however, regardless of the strength of their emotions. Communicative practice during conflict must be guided by respect for and protection of the rights of self and others (Tyler et al 2005) as well as the need for family/person-centred goals (Unsworth 2004). Understanding the difference between aggressive, passive and assertive responses assists health professionals to protect their own rights and the rights of others while achieving positive results from conflict. Awareness of these differences empowers health professionals to develop the skill of asserting rather than reacting with a fight or flight response. Assertiveness skills assist in the confident and constructive management of conflict situations.

Aggressive

The individual with an aggressive pattern of relating during conflict expresses their perceptions, opinions and feelings in a manner that intimidates or attacks the other communicating individuals. Their manner expresses the desire to be right and make everyone else agree with them, thus indicating they are right, or it expresses a desire to achieve what they want regardless of the feelings of others. Aggression expresses the desire to 'win'. This manner precipitates two major reactions in listeners: fight (aggression – *I will win this*) or flight (escape from the uncomfortable situation and emotions).

Passive

The individual who relates passively during conflict does not express their perceptions, ideas or opinions. The belief that the individual does not have the right to express or feel anything is the basis of this response. Limited confidence, self-esteem and self-respect produce passive responses. In turn, encountering regular and repeated passive responses from an individual may negatively affect and ultimately destroy the confidence, self-esteem or self-respect of their communicative partner. This person too may eventually relate passively in every communicative event due to limited confidence, self-esteem and self-respect.

Assertive

The assertive individual expresses their perceptions, ideas or opinions in a manner that respects the worth and rights of others to have and express perceptions, ideas or opinions. Assertion affirms the interests and rights of the self and the other. It facilitates positive communication outcomes and strengthens relationships (Devito 2007, Rakos 2006), and thus is the preferred manner of responding during difficult communicative interactions (Alberti & Emmons 2001).

ACTIVITY

Label the following responses as aggressive, passive or assertive.

Tom and Jenny are deciding which people they will each assist of those just referred to them.
- *I am familiar with people who have that difficulty, but all right, you can see them.* (Thinking: *I'll struggle with these people – I have no idea what I will do with them, but hey, what does it matter.*)
- *I am experienced with people with those difficulties so I am assisting them.*
- *I would prefer to assist these people and you prefer them as well, so why not divide them and help each other with ideas for assisting the people with difficulties we are unsure about?*

Jean and Fred are choosing which piece of equipment to buy.
- *I am familiar with X and it has the best results. We are buying X.*
- *Mmm, X is good, but I was reading about Y (that latest development) – research seems to indicate it has great results. Why don't we look at the budget to see if we can afford both? If not, perhaps we can do some research and see if we can buy one now and one later.*
- *Oh, all right, we can buy X.* (Thinking: *Who cares what is the best or what I want anyway!*)

Create assertive ways of responding to the following.
- You are angry because a colleague promised to assist you with something and instead they read research articles all day.
- You are struggling with a task and a colleague is watching you struggle without attempting to assist you.
- You have a day's leave promised and now, without explanation, the decision has been reversed and you have heard that someone else has leave that day instead of you.
- A person is yelling and swearing at you and you have no idea why they are yelling or what the problem is.
- A person seeking your assistance appears not to be listening to you.

REFLECTION

Think of a situation in which you regularly communicate passivity or aggression. How could you respond in a more mutually satisfying manner that reflects awareness of the rights and dignity of everyone communicating?

How to communicate assertively

The following points are suggestions of how to use assertive behaviour when communicating.

- Establish and focus on the problem, not the emotions (Higgs et al 2005).
- Remain calm and avoid responding in an emotional manner (Harms 2007).
- Avoid placating with *Calm down, you're OK.*
- State the facts about the situation; do not evaluate or judge (Devito 2007).
- Listen carefully, allowing the person to finish each sentence (McLean 2005).
- Use 'I' statements (Mohan et al 2004).
- Take responsibility for your feelings and actions (Holli et al 2003).
- Be aware of your non-verbal behaviours; use a relaxed body position (McLean 2005).
- Use normal speed and tone of voice (Devito 2007).
- Avoid talking slowly because this may appear patronising.
- Observe carefully the non-verbal behaviours of the upset person.
- State how the problem affects you, not how you feel about the situation.
- If appropriate gently and calmly repeat a question or statement until the person hears and responds (e.g. *Shall we talk about how to solve this now?*). The timing of such questions is significant and may negatively or positively affect the situation (Higgs et al 2005, Rakos 2006).
- Emphasise collaboration, asking for an indication of their thoughts throughout the discussion.
- Seek achievable solutions that require specific action within a particular timeframe.

ACTIVITY

- Use the points on the previous page – 'How to communicate assertively' – while role-playing the following cases. It may assist if the players choose names for their roles.
- During each role play, have observers classify every statement or question according to the behaviours listed in 'How to communicate assertively'.

Role play 1

Person 1: You are the supervisor of Person 2. You feel angry because Person 2 is always late in completing their work and it reflects badly on you.

Person 2: You do your best every day with limited assistance and do not really understand the problem. The work will be done, just maybe not on time.

Role play 2

Person 1: You are a young health professional seeing Person 2 for the first time. They have previously received assistance from your health service, but the health professional who saw them is no longer available. You sense they are disappointed and do not really want to see you.

Person 2: You are disappointed that you have to see Person 1 because you had a good relationship with the previous health professional. You really do not want to see Person 1 because they seem too young, but you do not want to hurt their feelings.

Role play 3

Person 1: You are the supervisor of Person 2, a student who has been discussing confidential matters in the dining hall. During their orientation you outlined confidentiality, ethical practice and legislation. You indicated what these meant in practice and asked questions to clarify their meaning.

Person 2: The needs of some of the people assigned to you are overwhelming and there has been no time to talk about this except during lunch.

Role play 4

Person 1: You are a health professional who feels Mrs Stathos can continue living in her home. You have consulted all the health professionals assisting Mrs Stathos and intend to organise various supports (weekly home care and shopping, daily nurses for showering, meals on wheels) and attendance at a weekly program to maintain her in her home. Person 2 has requested an appointment with you and you feel he disagrees with you. You intend to show him how Mrs Stathos can stay safely and independently at home.

Person 2: You are married to Mrs Stathos' daughter. You know how forgetful and dependent Mrs Stathos has become because your wife has been caring for her, often staying with her overnight. You are really angry that this young health professional (Person 1) thinks they know what is best for *your* family; you think they have no idea. You intend to make sure Mrs Stathos is placed in residential care – not in a nursing home but in a 'village' with her own unit.

Role play 5

Person 1: You are a health professional who has been assisting Terry, a young man with paraplegia. You have been working consistently with him and his motivation to walk again is maintaining his mood. You are furious with a new colleague (Person 2) because they have just told him it is unlikely he will walk again. You have experience with people like Terry and in the past you have seen young men with worse damage than Terry walk (with assistive equipment, but walking independently of another person) against all the medical odds. You feel this colleague is ignorant and should not have spoken to Terry.

Person 2: You are new to the Spinal Injuries Department and heard the doctor say that Terry would probably not walk again. You feel it is important to be honest so you tell Terry he will probably not walk again. You cannot see why Person 1 is upset.

Chapter summary

It is important that the health professional develops strategies and skills to manage conflict situations in an effective and resolute manner. Recognition of the emotions causing the conflict begins the process of resolution (Milliken & Honeycutt 2004). Perceptions of the emotions behind the conflict require validation through honest statements or questions relating to these perceptions. Validation of perceptions promotes a clearer understanding of the cause of the conflict in the person expressing the emotion (Egan 2007). It allows disengagement from the argument and a focus on possible resolution of the emotions and the problem. Questions asked with an appropriate tone of voice (see Ch 12) can diffuse the expression of strong emotions, for example, *You are obviously upset; can you tell me about the problem?* or *Do you want to tell me why you are shouting?* Such questions allow focus on solving the problem rather than focus on the emotions that are creating the argument or emotional behaviour.

Resolution of conflict in difficult situations is facilitated by acceptance of differences, compromise and assertive collaboration with a calm focus on problem-solving (Devito 2007). It is important for the health professional to develop confidence in managing interactions involving conflict. Such confidence develops with self-awareness, self-control, appropriate supervision, specific instruction in conflict management, understanding of possible management strategies and, ultimately, experience.

Complete the following:
1. Define conflict.

_____

_____

_____

2. State the major cause of conflict.

_____

_____

_____

3. What is your natural tendency when communicating during conflict? Suggest at least two ways of overcoming this tendency if it is unproductive.

  i. _____

  ii. _____

4. Describe the effects of the severity of emotions resulting from conflict.

_____

_____

_____

5. Describe ways of resolving each emotion during conflict.

_____

_____

_____

6. Describe ways of resolving your negative attitudes towards particular people.

   _____

   _____

   _____

7. In your own words, describe one of the ways of responding during conflict.

   _____

   _____

   _____

8. In your own words, list five ways of communicating assertively and provide examples of each.

   i. _____

   ii. _____

   iii. _____

   iv. _____

   v. _____

References

Alberti R, Emmons M 2001 Your perfect right: assertiveness and equality in your life and relationships, 8th edn. Impact, Atascadero CA

Bowe H, Martin K 2007 Communication across cultures: mutual understanding in a global world. Cambridge University Press, Melbourne

Brill N I, Levine J 2005 Working with people: the helping process, 8th edn. Pearson, Boston

Devito J A 2007 The interpersonal communication book, 11th edn. Pearson, Boston

Egan G 2007 The skilled helper, 8th edn. Thomson, Belmont CA

Harms L 2007 Working with people: communication skills for reflective practice. Oxford University Press, Melbourne

Higgs J, Sefton A, Street A et al 2005 Communicating in the health and social sciences. Oxford University Press, Melbourne

Holli B B, Calabrese R J, O'Sullivan Mailett J 2003 Communication and education skills for dietetics professionals, 4th edn. Lippincott, Williams & Wilkins, Philadelphia

McLean S 2005 The basics of interpersonal communication. Pearson, Boston

Milliken M E, Honeycutt A 2004 Understanding human behavior: a guide for healthcare providers, 7th edn. Thomson Delmar, New York

Mohan T, McGregor H, Saunders S et al 2004 Communicating as professionals. Thomson, Melbourne

Purtilo R B, Haddad A 2002 Health professional and patient interaction, 6th edn. Saunders, Philadelphia

Rakos R 2006 Asserting and confronting. In: Hargie O (ed) The handbook of communication skills, 3rd edn. Routledge, New York, p 345–381

Stein-Parbury J 2006 Patient and person: interpersonal skills in nursing, 3rd edn. Elsevier, Sydney (Original work published 2005)

Tyler S, Kossen C, Ryan C 2005 Communication: a foundation course, 2nd edn. Pearson, Prentice Hall, Frenchs Forest, Sydney

Unsworth C A 2004 Clinical reasoning: how do pragmatic reasoning, worldview and client-centredness fit? British Journal of Occupational Therapy 67:10–19

Culturally appropriate communication

15

CHAPTER OBJECTIVES

Upon completing this chapter, students should be able to

- Define culture and culturally appropriate communication
- Clarify the importance of culturally appropriate communication
- Describe factors affecting culturally appropriate communication
- Explain the impact of cultural difference upon communication
- Develop useful strategies to achieve culturally appropriate communication
- State some of their personal cultural assumptions and expectations
- List the necessary steps required for the use of an interpreter
- Give a basic description of the culture of their particular health profession
- Recognise and understand the culture of disease or disability.

Effective communication requires the health professional to understand that there are *different ways of 'doing and being'* (Wilcock 2006). These ways of 'doing and being' result in many different patterns of everyday life (Brill & Levine 2005). The values and beliefs of the group generate these patterns or traditions (Purtilo & Haddad 2002). **Culture** is the word commonly used to describe the patterns that develop from within the context of a group or community. Thus, 'culture' influences every person and every activity, every day (Devito 2007). This chapter may begin the journey of exploring cultural difference. It cannot provide an exhaustive understanding of work practices with people from all cultural groups, but it can provide awareness of the cultural diversity in the world and ways to embrace, understand and accept this diversity.

It is important for health professionals to realise that they will relate to individuals from both 'large' and 'small' cultures (Holliday et al 2006). A 'large' culture is one that has extensive membership and considerable impact upon that membership in all aspects of life. The culture of a nation is an example of a 'large' culture. A 'small' culture is one that has a smaller membership and usually affects the lives of the members only when fulfilling roles expected by that culture. Thus, 'small' cultures have a limited impact on the lives of the members. An example of a 'small' culture is a particular health profession or a sports group. Therefore, health professionals will experience cultural differences with many people they assist, whether they are people from other countries, other socioeconomic groups or other 'small' cultures. They will also experience cultural differences with other health professionals. These differences develop within particular group settings and affect the outcomes of communication.

Defining culturally appropriate communication

In order to achieve culturally appropriate communication it is important for health professionals to understand that cultures differ (Tyler et al 2005). It is also important for health professionals to understand that each person has diverse experiences, worldviews and values that affect their understanding of power and privilege (Miller et al 2004). This understanding is especially important for health professionals because the relationship between the health professional and the person seeking assistance has an inbuilt power imbalance that can affect communication. This reality is especially relevant in communicative interactions with individuals from various indigenous cultures because many have experiences that negatively affect their expectations of the relationship with a health professional. Their perceptions of power and privilege in combination with their experiences of this relationship (with its inbuilt power imbalance) suggest they should not trust a health professional.

It is important for the health professional to behave with tactful and compassionate acceptance of the different cultures represented by the individuals relating to the health professional, and to demonstrate understanding of these cultures. It seems then that a consideration of culture is required to assist the health professional to achieve culturally appropriate communication. The understanding of the word culture has changed over time (Goddard 2005) and there are currently many ways of understanding the concept of culture. Purtilo & Haddad (2002) present culture as a broad concept that embraces all aspects of life, including customs, beliefs, technological achievements, language and the history of a group of similar people. Devito (2007) states culture relates to the 'specialised lifestyle of a group of people'. Tyler et al (2005) suggest culture to be the 'shared and systematic ways of living' within a particular society. Similarly, culture can be described as a system of beliefs, values and behaviours that characterise a particular group (Egan 2007, Purtilo & Haddad 2002, Stein-Parbury 2006, Verderber & Verderber 2004).

None of these descriptions of culture are contradictory; they all suggest that culture relates to a group and is an expression of similarities of some kind within that group. Groups might express their culture through their particular beliefs, spirituality, language, family roles, ways of living and working, expectations, dress, artefacts, artistic expression, attitudes, food, remedies, identity and non-verbal behaviours, as well as through the value they place on their land (Mohan et al 2004, Parbury 1986). Each generation shares these patterns of behaviours and understanding with each new generation.

Dean (2001) states it is impossible to be 'completely culturally competent' in every culture. In fact it is impossible to be completely culturally competent in any particular culture unless born into that culture. However, the health professional must be open to and accepting of the different cultures encountered during practice. Culturally appropriate communication involves being aware of, sensitive to and appreciative of the cultural variations common among individuals/groups and mandates tolerance of these variations (Egan 2007, Mohan et al 2004). It invites the health professional to acknowledge the validity of the other culture (Bowe & Martin 2007) rather than ridiculing or trivialising it. Culturally appropriate communication requires knowledge, mutual respect and negotiation (Purtilo & Haddad 2002) to achieve effective communication and thus outcomes specific to the needs of the person and the skills of the health professional.

Why consider cultural differences?

Cultural differences produce a diversity of behaviours, but they also produce the health beliefs and behaviours of individuals. These health beliefs and behaviours can profoundly affect expectations and ultimate outcomes of any health service (Purtilo & Haddad 2002).

REFLECTION

What are your health beliefs and behaviours?
- What would you do if you had
  - A cold for more than a week?
  - Prolonged nausea?
  - Neck or back pain?
  - Anxiety attacks?
  - A toothache?
  - Feelings of euphoria and highly irregular behaviour?
- Who would you go to if you had a health concern?

Individuals vary in their responses to physical and psychological distress; these variations affect the responses of both the health professional and the person seeking assistance. It is often particular health beliefs that regulate these responses. It is initially surprising to realise that different people have different beliefs and behaviours associated with their health. It is important to resist the application of particular health beliefs to those relating to the health professional because this will negatively affect communication.

Factors affecting culturally appropriate communication

Language

Words, non-verbal behaviours and intention can have different meanings among people from the same culture and cause difficulties in communication. For example, asking someone for dinner for some means a meal at midday, for others a meal around 5.30 p.m. and still others a formal meal after 8 p.m. It is not surprising then that individuals from different cultures experience communication difficulties because of variations in meanings of words and non-verbal behaviours. For example, directional nods and shakes of the head have different meanings in different cultures and, therefore, this can cause miscommunication (see Ch 17).

Context

Understanding a particular context can promote effective communication (Bowe & Martin 2007). The context of the person seeking assistance can affect communication and mutual understanding. Similarly, the context of a health service is confusing and unfamiliar for many individuals within their own culture, but for someone from a different culture it is often frightening. Understanding the particular contexts affects the expectations of each communicating individual – both the person seeking assistance and the health professional – and thus the effectiveness of communication.

Ethnocentricity

When an individual believes their particular method or way of approaching a situation is superior and indeed the best way then they are ethnocentric. Purtilo & Haddad (2002) state that ethnocentricity is a common phenomenon in health professionals and can negatively affect communication.

CASE STUDY

A man from a different culture is admitted to hospital with a stroke (cerebrovascular accident). His family are absent. The health professionals are curious as they settle the man into the ward. His language skills seem adequate because he asks appropriate questions and responds appropriately when asked to do something. However, he sits by the bed quietly and passively; he does not look around or relate to anyone.

Around 4.30 p.m. people of varying ages from the same culture arrive and the health professionals assume they are family. The man suddenly seems happy and takes an interest in what is happening. These people have brought woven mats, food, plates and utensils with them. In an out-of-the-way corner in the ward, they place the mats on the floor and serve the food onto plates. One person – an older lady – sits by the man and assists him with his meal. The rest of the family sit on the mats on the floor and eat together, including the man in all the interactions while talking quietly in their own language. They are obviously all enjoying themselves.

ACTIVITY

- What are the possible explanations for the behaviour of this family? Do you think it strange?
- How would you respond to this behaviour? (After asking if I could join them I sat with them on the floor! This caused reactions of mirth, horror and bemusement among my colleagues.)
- List the possible ways of responding. What are the possible consequences of these responses?
- What is a culturally appropriate response?

The behaviour in the case study outlined above was 'strange' in a western culture and there were various responses from the health professionals present. Some were direct expressions of personal attitudes and others were personal attitudes expressed through health service regulations. In most situations it is important, but in such situations it is essential, to consider more than the behaviours by looking below the surface to the multifaceted and complex reasons for the behaviours (Krepp cited in Purtilo & Haddad 2002, p 39). Different situations and countries have different services available. This family came from a country where hospitals do not provide many services and thus the family were expecting to do everything for the person in hospital, including supplying meals, providing clothes and assisting with showering and toileting. In addition, their culture values mealtimes as social occasions and therefore they could not imagine their relative having a meal alone. In this culture, a person is alone when they are among strangers. Understanding cultural differences in this situation provided explanations for the 'strange' behaviour and facilitated a compromise that met the needs of all involved in the care of this culturally different man and his family.

- Consider the previous case study and outline the
  - Needs and expectations of the person/family
  - Needs and expectations of the health professionals
  - Expectations of the health service.
- Brainstorm ways of compromising to be culturally appropriate while still completing the required routines of health professionals and meeting the occupational health and safety requirements of the health service.

In situations presenting cultural differences it is important to accept and appreciate diversity (Egan 2007). If the health professional merely recognises the differences this may separate and distance. Perception and appreciation of the similarities, however, will promote connection and development of rapport. In such situations it is important that culturally different individuals experience acceptance and understanding, not fear and misunderstanding.

CASE STUDY

A southern European family lives with several generations in four adjacent houses. The retired father, Mick, is recovering from surgery that established he has inoperable brain tumours. He currently requires assistance to complete simple self-care tasks. The health professionals involved are reluctant to suggest how long he might live.

Each health professional (HP) has different thoughts about what should happen.
- HP1 suggests he should go to a hospice to die.
- HP2 suggests he needs more time to recover from surgery.
- HP3 suggests placing him in a high-dependency unit.
- HP4 says that Mick's daughter cannot see her mother managing if he goes home.
- HP5 suggests that with the right assistance he could die at home.
- HP6 suggests that talking to the family is important.
- HP7 suggests that asking Mick might be a good idea.
- HP8 says that Mick should not be told that he will die soon (his prognosis).

GROUP DISCUSSION

- Consider each response and decide what that person believes, values and fears.
- Which of the responses do you consider is the one that suits the family?

The family conference includes health professionals 1, 4 and 5 as well as several members of the family, including Mick's wife, Roma, his eldest son, his youngest daughter and his youngest son's wife.

The aim of the conference is to establish where Mick will go upon discharge. Each health professional explains the options. The first discusses hospice care and states they feel that would suit them all. The second indicates they understand that certain members of the family are concerned about managing if Mick goes home and supports this view. While both these health professionals are explaining the options, Mick's wife is crying uncontrollably. The third health professional outlines the possible assistance that is available if Mick goes home, carefully explaining the possible difficulties but stating that Mick may be more independent when he recovers from the surgery. As the third health professional explains, Roma begins

↳

to listen and stares at this health professional. When this health professional finishes, Roma stands and says in broken English *That is what we want – Mick to come home*. She states this emphatically and says it will mean that he will not know he is going to die soon. A family argument ensues with some family members supporting Roma and others supporting the idea of Mick being told what is happening and going where he can receive expert care.

GROUP DISCUSSION

Discuss how to manage this situation so that Mick receives family-centred care.

Managing personal cultural assumptions and expectations

It is relevant to remember that cultural differences do not only occur between people from different countries, but also between people from different socioeconomic backgrounds; states or provinces; indigenous groups; religious groups; occupations; societies; and families. Cultural differences can even occur between different health professionals. Such variations are limitless.

Cultural differences occur in everyday life in practices relating to hand shakes; greetings; what to talk about; what to avoid talking about; the meaning and use of colours; personal space; eye contact; humour; music and songs; ways to wash and dry clothing; food (including its value, ways to prepare it, timing of meals and how to arrange the place of eating); habits of personal hygiene/personal cleaning rituals; bed linen and ways of arranging a bed; spirituality and religious practices; expression of beliefs and values; understanding and meaning of the land; and artistic expression.

The list is extensive and could fill many pages. In the health professions it is important to understand for particular individuals that there are differences that might affect the outcome of the health service. Wosket (2006) states consideration of cultural difference is essential when planning outcomes for individuals and groups. When setting goals it is easy to apply the cultural values, assumptions and expectations of the health professional, but this does not produce family/person-centred practice.

CASE STUDY

At a local health service, an older man holds the door open for a mother with a baby in a stroller and a toddler. The young mother is thankful but hurries past him mumbling something about being late. He walks slowly behind this mother to the desk to register his arrival.

The person at the desk is polite but their non-verbal communication indicates they are unhappy with the mother. The elderly man smiles and states his name and appointment time.

The receptionist looks up and says politely *You are very late Sir – could you ring if you are going to be this late. We assumed you were not coming.*

GROUP DISCUSSION

- Discuss the possible reasons why the health service staff would assume someone late was not coming.
- What reasons do they have to assume the man has access to a phone when in transit?
- What are their cultural expectations?

The older man sits down next to the mother. They both watch the receptionist ring the health professional who was scheduled to see the mother and hear her say *Yes she is here, but she was late last time she came and she was told to ring if she was going to be late. I just don't think she really cares about your schedule.*

GROUP DISCUSSION

- What is a culturally appropriate way to respond to individuals such as this man and young mother?
- What is it about the cultural assumptions and expectations of the health service staff that make it difficult for culturally appropriate communication?
- Suggest possible explanations for the lateness of these individuals.

The mother looks at her children, one asleep in the stroller and the other curled up on the floor. She quietly says *She has no idea how hard it is to organise two littlies, rely on a bus service that is always late and is 10 minutes walk from my unit, change buses twice and then walk 10 more minutes to actually reach the front door of this place.*

The older man smiles and looks at both children. He looks at his watch. *How late are you?* he enquires.

The mother says quietly *What is the time?* She looks to see it is 9.30 a.m. *Oh I left home in plenty of time, but the first bus was 20 minutes late and they were digging up the path from the bus stop closest to here, so it took longer to get here. I am 45 minutes late. I couldn't help it, I don't have a mobile phone, we can only afford one between the two of us, and so my husband takes it so he can ring during the day to see how we are. He's out on the road a lot. How late are you?*

The older man smiles and says *I don't like to be late, but this morning I found it hard to get going, there is a bit more pain than usual, and I stopped to help a little boy who I have not seen before, whose cat had run up a tree. I knew the cat would be fine, but the boy was worried about his cat so I retrieved it for him. Both cat and boy seemed happy, but obviously our friend here isn't! I don't have a mobile phone either. My children bought me one, but I found someone who needed it more than me – her family could pay for the calls but not buy the phone – so I asked my kids if it was all right for me to give it to that person. They said it was OK. They weren't surprised at all, they said.*

Both people in the case study above have good explanations for their tardiness. When a health professional considers more than the superficial characteristics of an individual they can explain behaviour that seems strange or unacceptable at the time. Health professionals often originate from particular socioeconomic backgrounds and thus they may apply particular cultural assumptions and expectations to those they assist. It is important that health professionals attempt to avoid applying these assumptions and expectations to the individuals seeking their assistance.

Strategies for demonstrating culturally appropriate communication

It is important for health professionals to expand, maintain their understanding of and accept cultural differences across the myriad of cultures they experience everyday (Harms 2007), including the cultures within different health professions. Many strategies contribute to positive experiences in cross-cultural communication.

Self-awareness

The first step in achieving culturally appropriate communication is to consider individual and personal cultural values, beliefs and traditions (Holli et al 2003, Purtilo & Haddad 2002). It is difficult to be a culturally appropriate health professional if unaware of personal biases. If unaware of personal cultural biases it is impossible to confront any tendency to stereotype (see Ch 13), and this limits the potential to understand and accept different cultures.

REFLECTIVE ACTIVITY

Consider your beliefs and attitudes
Write your honest answers to the following questions (adapted from Devito 2007).
- Equality of genders: Do women and men really have equal opportunities?
- Family: Are your personal priorities more significant than family or kinship priorities?
- Religion: Does it provide the ultimate guide for living and the concepts of right and wrong? Alternatively, is it simply a social construct?
- Group versus individual performance: Do you prefer to perform with a team or are you too competitive and prefer to perform alone?
- Money: Is it an important component of any major decision you make or is it something you do not consider when making major decisions?
- Relationship permanency: Do you feel relationships are forever or do you feel as long as there is more good than bad in them then they are sustainable?
- Expression of negative emotions: Do you feel it should occur freely or that this should never occur in public?
- Work habits: Do you prefer to work as much as possible or do you prefer to take every opportunity to enjoy yourself?
- Time orientation: Do you consider time and attempt to be prompt or do you live in the moment and are not concerned about time?
- A just world: Do you believe that good behaviour leads to good events in life or do you believe good and bad happen to everyone?

These questions highlight some of the differences in culture that might cause difficulties when communicating. Honest answers to these questions will assist you to understand your own beliefs about some aspects of culture. Consider and write down how your beliefs in these areas can affect your communication.

Personal commitment to understanding differences

The requirements of effective communication are the basis of culturally appropriate communication (Purtilo & Haddad 2002). Commitment to these requirements will assist health professionals to adopt appropriate strategies when communicating with people from cultures different to their own. Such commitment will assist the health professional in predicting the requirements of communicating with individuals from different cultures.

Exposure and learning

The best way to communicate across cultures is to become familiar with the relevant culture(s) (Devito 2007). There are many ways to achieve this familiarity, including reading books and articles written by individuals from the culture about the culture, watching relevant movies (beware of bias), reading information on the internet and socialising with friends from the culture. Another way to achieve familiarity with a culture is to approach the culturally different person with an open, accepting attitude and express interest within the context of the practice. Asking questions about traditions as well as styles of communication can increase understanding. As the health professional conducts their interventions, discussion about the cultural differences can be reassuring for both the individual and the health professional. Purtilo & Haddad (2002) suggest that the health professional should recognise the differences and consider the interaction an opportunity to learn about the other culture. It is important when considering cultural differences to also account for the individual because often there are individual variations that limit the application of a general understanding of any cultural norm.

Investment of time to negotiate meaning and ensure understanding

There is a certain amount of insecurity about communicating with someone who is from a different culture, speaks a different language, or has differing values, beliefs and traditions, even when it is only a different health language and belief. Investment of time and energy to understand the individual is imperative. There is no reason to be afraid because while it is important for the health professional to restructure their worldview to accommodate and understand the differences, they do not necessarily need to profess, internalise or assimilate these differences in their everyday life. Cultural understanding simply allows the health professional to demonstrate respect of the worldview, which will assist in developing rapport and fulfilling the needs of the person seeking assistance.

Anticipation of difficulties

There are a variety of possible difficulties within any communicative interaction. Anticipation of these difficulties may assist the health professional to respond appropriately (Verderber & Verderber 2004). The health professional can overcome some of the difficulties associated with achieving culturally appropriate communication by being aware of personal cultural attitudes, the aspects of that culture and the factors that affect culturally appropriate communication.

CASE STUDY

Marianna is a 5-year-old Fijian girl with no English. The interpreter informs the health professional that Marianna appears to understand only ten words of Fijian. Marianna appears friendly but unsure about the strange place, people and behaviours. An interpreter taught the health professional a few Fijian words this child understands: hello, goodbye, thank you, please, toilet, wee, sorry, help.

REFLECTION

- How might the health professional form a connection with this unsure 5-year-old?
- What are the immediate aims of the health professional in such a situation?

A major difficulty in intercultural communication can be the lack of a common language. This creates apprehension for both the health professional and the individual seeking assistance. An open and relaxed demeanour will assist any attempt to connect with the individual despite the lack of a shared language. When communicating without a common language, anticipating the need for an interpreter is paramount.

Using an interpreter

ACTIVITY

- What difficulties might arise when using an interpreter?
- When using an interpreter, who do you predict will most easily develop rapport with the person seeking assistance?
- How could the health professional use the interaction to build rapport?

When considering use of an interpreter to achieve culturally appropriate communication it is important to first note that there are different types of interpretation (Bowe & Martin 2007). **Simultaneous interpretation** requires the interpreter to translate information while it is being presented. This type of interpretation does not usually occur when translating for one person, but often occurs when there is a group of listeners. Simultaneous interpretation is common when interpreting for groups of people who have a hearing impairment. This type of interpretation is demanding because the interpreter speaks at the same time as the speaker and must concentrate and listen carefully to interpret. **Sequential interpretation** allows the speaker to present a small portion of the information and then the interpreter translates this portion. During this type of interpretation, only one person speaks at any one time. Sequential or consecutive interpretation is the usual form of interpretation for interactions in the health professions (Higgs et al 2005).

There are also two styles of interpretation. **Transliteration** is the exact translation of each word or sound spoken, regardless of meaning; such utterances often have limited meaning. **Interpretation** is the translation of the meaning of the utterance regardless of the spoken sound or word.

There are particular steps required to use an interpreter effectively. This process requires skill, concentration and careful planning, just as the act of interpreting itself requires skill, concentration and specific knowledge of both languages. Many interpreters, unless particularly trained in the use of medical terminology (Stein-Parbury 2006), may find medical or technical words unfamiliar and thus it is best to avoid using such terms.

It is important to understand that professionally trained interpreters are not always available. In remote areas interpreters may not be available at all while in other areas there are interpreters of only a limited number of languages available. In some areas telephone interpreters are available; they usually require an appointment made in advance. It is possible to use colleagues as interpreters if available, but remember that colleagues are rarely trained for interpreting and thus may require additional allowances while interpreting. In some situations health professionals might use family members to interpret. This practice is not always appropriate and can cause family tension. The use of an *adult* family or community member might be appropriate for information about progress or the need for the toilet, for example, but using such a person to give complicated information or information relating to a diagnosis, prognosis or the future can be inappropriate.

Essential steps when using an interpreter

1. Establish the purpose of the interaction that requires an interpreter.
2. Schedule and book an appropriate time for everyone required for the interaction. It is important to organise an interpreter in advance. Allow time to brief the interpreter concerning the purpose of the interaction before the commencement of the interaction with the person seeking assistance. Interpreters can be late for good reason so briefing them by telephone may be necessary.
3. Prepare the questions and information for discussion. When using an interpreter it is easy to forget a point or deviate from the original plan. It is therefore important to organise the points carefully to ensure coverage of all necessary information.
4. Clarify any areas of uncertainty in the mind of the interpreter. It is important to establish a signal to indicate when an item of information is too long. All people involved in the interaction should know the meaning of this signal.
5. Introduce everyone. Remember the health professional and the person requiring assistance are the focus of the interaction. Take care to concentrate on developing rapport with the person not the interpreter. Introduce the purpose of the interaction to the person seeking assistance.
6. Speak to the person not the interpreter. It is important that the interpreter connects with the person seeking assistance; however, development of a relationship between them is unnecessary and may detract from the purpose of the interaction. They may have an immediate rapport because they share a common culture and this will assist the person to relax, but it is important to focus on the purpose of the interaction because the interpreter is available for a limited time. Maintain control of the interaction – the interpreter is there to assist not to conduct the interaction.
7. Use small chunks of information not long sentences. Make the point clear and minimise jargon or colloquialisms to avoid misinterpretation or reinterpretation of the content. It is important to keep a mental note of what has been covered and what is yet to be covered as the interaction progresses.
8. Observe the non-verbal reactions of the person carefully.
9. Ask questions in response to these non-verbal reactions, for example, *You appear unhappy about that – am I right? What do you need to know or how can we help you to feel happier?* Because it is often difficult to know exactly what has been communicated, asking questions to clarify and verify understanding throughout the interaction is essential when using an interpreter (Harms 2007).
10. Remember to ask the person seeking assistance to summarise the information to demonstrate their understanding. Include time to answer any unrelated questions or address any concerns. Remember the importance of disengagement in the development of a therapeutic relationship with the person.

DISCUSSION

- Consider the reasons for and against using a family member as an interpreter.
- When might it be appropriate to use a family member? (e.g. when asking about matters such as improvement in symptoms, or the need for toothpaste!)
- When might it be inappropriate to use a family member? (e.g. when giving bad news)

The culture of each health profession

Individual health professions have underlying philosophies, values, assumptions, beliefs, expectations and habits specific to that profession. These generate particular knowledge and behaviours in the everyday activities of each health profession. Thus, each health profession has a 'culture' specific to that profession. These cultures generate differences between health professions. Each profession has a particular concept of the person seeking their assistance and the role of the person and the profession in the healing process (Milliken & Honeycutt 2004). Each profession has a particular understanding of various concepts (e.g. pain, disability, illness, health, wellbeing) and each has a particular role when relating to these concepts relevant to the particular profession. While there are variations in values and beliefs, many professions value family/person-centred practice and all share the common value of mutual respect.

REFLECTIVE ACTIVITY

Consider the particular perspective of your health profession and write a brief outline of that perspective for at least three of the following concepts. State the role of your profession when relating to each of these concepts.
- The concept of the person and their role in their own healing
- The concept of family/person-centred practice
- The concept of health and illness
- The concept of pain
- The concept of disability

The culture of disease or ill-health

The culture that may be the most difficult to understand unless experienced personally is the culture of disease or ill-health, whether chronic or acute, sudden or gradual. During their working week, health professionals consistently relate to people who live in this culture. Achieving appropriate communication that accommodates this culture is challenging but as rewarding as communicating appropriately with individuals from other types of cultures.

ACTIVITY

- What is your experience with disease or disability?
- Which diseases or disabilities cause you the most discomfort when you consider working with people who have that disease or disability? Consider both physical and psychosocial diseases and disabilities, for example, someone who is dying, someone with schizophrenia and someone with an intellectual disability.

Chapter summary

Culture refers to the values and beliefs of a particular group that generate patterns of behaviour. While a health professional can never understand a culture completely unless they are part of it, it is important that they are open to and accepting of the different cultures encountered during practice. Culturally appropriate communication can be achieved through investment of time to negotiate meaning and achieve mutual understanding. Where this requires the use of an interpreter, there are particular steps required to ensure effective communication.

Complete the following:
1. What must a health professional who is committed to culturally appropriate communication understand?

_____

_____

_____

2. Define 'culture'.

_____

_____

_____

3. What are some of the differences that affect culturally appropriate communication?

_____

_____

_____

4. How do members of a culture express the cultural characteristics of the culture?

_____

_____

_____

5. List three factors that affect culturally appropriate communication and give examples of each factor.
   i.   _____
   ii. _____
   iii. _____
6. What promotes openness to cultural diversity in a health professional?

_____

_____

_____

7. List some strategies that assist health professionals to avoid applying their personal cultural biases when communicating with culturally different people.

_____

_____

_____

8. Outline the ten steps for effective communication while using an interpreter.

    i. _____

    ii. _____

    iii. _____

    iv. _____

    v. _____

    vi. _____

    vii. _____

    viii. _____

    ix. _____

    x. _____

9. List some of the values and beliefs of your health profession and give a behavioural example of each listed value.

    _____

    _____

    _____

10. Outline your experience with the culture of disease or disability. Indicate how this experience, if any, assists your understanding of this culture.

    _____

    _____

    _____

References

Bowe H, Martin K 2007 Communication across cultures: mutual understanding in a global world. Cambridge University Press, Melbourne

Brill N I, Levine J 2005 Working with people: the helping process, 8th edn. Pearson, Boston

Dean R 2001 The myth of cross-cultural competence: families in society. The Journal of Contemporary Human Services 86:623–630

Devito J A 2007 The interpersonal communication book, 11th edn. Pearson, Boston

Egan G 2007 The skilled helper, 8th edn. Thomson, Belmont CA

Goddard C 2005 The lexical semantics of culture. Language Sciences 27:51–73

Harms L 2007 Working with people: communication skills for reflective practice. Oxford University Press, Melbourne

Higgs J, Sefton A, Street A et al 2005 Communicating in the health and social sciences. Oxford University Press, Melbourne

Holli B B, Calabrese R J, O'Sullivan Mailett J 2003 Communication and education skills for dietetics professionals, 4th edn. Lippincott, Williams & Wilkins, Philadelphia

Holliday A, Hyde M, Kullman J 2006 Intercultural communication: an advanced resource book. Routledge, London (Original work published 2004)

Miller J, Donner S, Fraser E 2004 Talking when talking is tough: taking on communications about race, sexual orientation, gender, class and other aspects of social identity. Smith College Studies in Social Work 74:377–393

Milliken M E, Honeycutt A 2004 Understanding human behavior: a guide for healthcare providers, 7th edn. Thomson Delmar, New York

Mohan T, McGregor H, Saunders S et al 2004 Communicating as professionals. Thomson, Melbourne

Parbury N 1986 Survival: a history of Aboriginal life in NSW. Ministry of Aboriginal Affairs, Sydney

Purtilo R B, Haddad A 2002 Health professional and patient interaction, 6th edn. Saunders, Philadelphia

Stein-Parbury J 2006 Patient and person: interpersonal skills in nursing, 3rd edn. Elsevier, Sydney (Original work published 2005)

Tyler S, Kossen C, Ryan C 2005 Communication: a foundation course, 2nd edn. Pearson, Prentice Hall, Frenchs Forest, Sydney

Verderber K S, Verderber R F 2004 Interact: interpersonal communication concepts, skills, and contexts, 10th edn. Oxford University Press, New York

Wilcock A A 2006 An occupational perspective of health, 2nd edn. Slack, Thorofare NJ

Wosket V 2006 Egan's skilled helper model: developments and application in counselling. Brunner-Routledge, London

Communicating with indigenous peoples

16

CHAPTER OBJECTIVES

Upon completing this chapter, students should be able to

- Appreciate the importance of using terms appropriately when communicating with indigenous peoples
- Apply the general principles of effective communication when communicating with indigenous peoples
- Analyse and recognise the importance of cultural identity
- Analyse the relevance of the pre- and post-contact states of indigenous peoples
- Appreciate and synthesise the factors affecting the establishment of cultural safety when working with indigenous peoples
- Apply specific communication principles relevant to indigenous peoples
- Recognise potential barriers to effective communication when communicating with indigenous peoples.

Note regarding terminology: It is not possible to be an expert in all the cultural practices of others. The author is not an expert and nor is this chapter able to make experts of the readers. However, it can begin the exploration of what it might be like to work with and assist those who have different practices to oneself, whether because of individual, family or cultural differences.

This chapter will begin the journey for some and continue it for others in understanding and embracing the communication needs of people who were the original inhabitants of a region or country, that is, indigenous peoples.

Correct use of terms

History and attitudes dominate relationships with indigenous groups around the world. This often means that non-indigenous colonists and their descendants demonstrate attitudes and use terms that are discriminatory and offensive to the relevant indigenous peoples. It is important then that health professionals avoid causing offence by ensuring they understand the current terms that are appropriate when relating to indigenous peoples. While this is not always true of every country, in Australia the terms used to describe Aboriginal and Torres Strait Islander Peoples evolve constantly (NSW Department of Health 2004). This provides a challenge for every Australian health professional to know the most current descriptive terms, as the appropriate use of terms is essential for the development of therapeutic relationships and family/community-centred practice. Using the current terms also contributes to positive experiences that will ensure indigenous peoples continue to seek assistance from health services.

GROUP DISCUSSION

How might a health professional ensure appropriate use of terms and avoid offending an indigenous person when communicating with them?

There is no definitive formula for relating to indigenous peoples. Recognition and application of the general purpose of health professionals when communicating will assist in achieving effective communication and positive outcomes. Also, there are specific principles useful in all communicative circumstances that will therefore be beneficial when communicating with indigenous peoples. Before exploring these principles, it is important to consider the reality of cultural identity.

The complexity of cultural identity

Cultural identity is complex because each individual is a member of many different groups that have a unique culture. In each of these groups, every individual has a particular identity that is unique to that group (Holliday et al 2006; see Ch 15). The nationality of the individual provides a particular cultural identity that comes with values, traditions, beliefs and expectations (of self and others) specific to that nation. Membership of other groups – families, clans (in New Zealand *iwi* = tribe and *hapu* = sub-tribe), communities, sporting groups, religious groups, educational groups, employment groups, and political groups – creates additional cultural identities that relate to and affect the national and/or cultural identity of each person. Membership of each group provides a connection through common experiences and expectations that are unique to the group. This phenomenon means that each individual has a unique cultural identity based upon national identity and moulded by membership of multiple groups.

Indigenous persons are no different. They each have a unique identity that reflects their original group or nation. Their connection to the values, beliefs, traditions and expectations of that group influences their cultural identity and their appreciation of that identity. Levels of identity and connection vary for many indigenous persons. If an individual has lived their entire life with their kinship group at a traditional birthplace, their cultural identity will strongly reflect their national group. Traditional knowledge and customs will guide the daily life of that individual. If an individual was separated from their birthplace and kinship group at some point, their cultural identity may reflect other influences as well as the influence of their national origin. An indigenous person who lives in a large metropolis may or may not take pride in their cultural identity. They may have only vague expectations of adhering to cultural traditions and customs, although they may acknowledge particular spiritual and relational values and beliefs. In Australia, although the cultures of Aboriginal and Torres

Strait Islander Peoples are different, there are common core values shared across the country. These values include family and kinship, caring and sharing, and a spiritual connection with and love of the land (*Country*). While Maori have less variation in their distinctive groups, they share a sense of connection to space and belonging. This is reflected in *Tūrangawaewae* – a place to stand, a place to belong to, a seat or location of identity.

In most countries there is a broad range of connection with and adherence to traditions among indigenous peoples. In Australia, for example, many rural Aboriginal and Torres Strait Islander Peoples have replaced walking with horses or motorised forms of transport. However, the same people continue to value the land (*Country*) and their traditional ceremonies and singing. In New Zealand, many Maori have absorbed 'ways' from the dominating culture of the colonists. However, they still believe in and use traditional remedies to augment or replace the health practices of the dominant culture. In the Pacific, various indigenous peoples may use modern equipment to fulfil the traditional occupation of fishing. However, the same people continue to make traditional mats for use in their houses and for particular occasions. In many places in Asia, indigenous peoples use mobile phones to communicate but still plough their fields using buffalo. In many places in northern Canada, the skidoo has replaced the traditional use of the dog sled for transport and sometimes even hunting. However, the same people still create unique clothing that reflects membership of their particular kinship group. It is important to remember that the culture of all indigenous peoples is neither static nor uniform. Each culture and individual within that culture is continually changing and adapting to the influences upon themselves or their community.

The complexity of cultural identity means it is important that health professionals recognise the factors influencing that identity. It is also essential that health professionals acknowledge there are variations within indigenous peoples that prohibit the stereotypical labelling of any individual because of their nationality. Aboriginal and Torres Strait Islander Peoples clearly exemplify this fact, as they are two distinct groupings. The Torres Strait Islander Peoples have an origin, culture and identity distinct from the many Aboriginal groups that originated in the mainland and Tasmania. These many Aboriginal groups also have languages, cultures and identities that are distinct from each other and from those of the Torres Strait Islander Peoples.

There is a long history of stereotyping of many indigenous peoples. Indigenous peoples may also stereotype non-indigenous people and sometimes even other indigenous individuals or groups. It is the responsibility of the health professional to consider their own tendency to stereotype and adjust their knowledge and attitudes to avoid stereotyping any indigenous person. It is also important that the health professional behaves in a manner that will reduce the tendency of some indigenous peoples to stereotype non-indigenous health professionals.

Principles of practice for health professionals when working with indigenous peoples

Creating cultural safety for indigenous peoples

Understanding the concept of cultural safety is essential when relating to indigenous peoples from any country. Practice that respects, supports and empowers the cultural identity and wellbeing of an individual produces cultural safety (Nursing Council of New Zealand 2002). Such practice is more than mere awareness or sensitivity. It requires action that results from critical reflection about personal values (Stein-Parbury 2006) and evaluation of the attitudes and beliefs of the individual health professional. Culturally safe practice also requires awareness of and reflection about the culture and values of the particular health service. It is important that the health professional evaluates how their values, attitudes and beliefs affect the indigenous peoples they assist (Fenwick 2001). It is equally important for health professionals to evaluate the quality and outcomes of the assistance indigenous peoples receive from their health service. Such evaluation requires awareness and appreciation of the lives and perceptions of indigenous peoples, their kinship groups and their communities. These perceptions develop while receiving assistance, whether past or present, and should contribute to any evaluation of a health service. The histories of the relationship of indigenous peoples with the Europeans who have colonised their country also affect these perceptions. The result of such reflection and evaluation should be the achievement of cultural safety for indigenous peoples because of adjustments and improvements in the health service and the practice of the health professional (Fried 2000).

In contrast, lack of cultural safety exists when any individual behaves in a manner that diminishes, demeans or disempowers the cultural identity and wellbeing of any individual within a health service (Nursing Council of New Zealand 2002).

CASE STUDY

Emily is a 5-year-old Australian girl with blonde hair and blue eyes who has come to you for assistance. You have developed a good relationship, based on respect, trust and rapport, with her mother, Jillian. Your assessment of Emily indicates the choice of school will be significant and could affect her learning and thus her future.

Her mother feels safe and comfortable with you and discusses the pros and cons of the local schools with you. She indicates that one school, a distance away, has extra funding for children with an Indigenous background. You are unsure of the meaning of this comment – you have not noticed any indication of Emily's heritage on her record/file and, looking at Jillian and her three children, you assume there is no Indigenous background. You assume Jillian is concerned that if Emily attends that school she will not have the assistance she requires because of the presence of an Indigenous cohort. You say it would not be good for Emily to experience reverse discrimination because of her ethnicity (i.e. to miss out because she does not have an Indigenous background).

Jillian bristles and coldly explains that she was taken from her family post-contact with Europeans and did not know she had an Aboriginal heritage until recently. She states that she was raised by a family that was discriminatory against people with her background and thus she now has to adjust to the fact that she is one of the people about whom she previously thought negatively. While her husband, who married her before she discovered this fact, says it makes no difference to him, she struggles to establish her identity and often avoids disclosing her heritage. This makes her reticent to place Emily at the school that has specific funding for children with an Aboriginal background, despite her eligibility.

You are generally an accepting person and have good friends who have an Indigenous background. You regret your assumptions and offensive comment. You are aware that you could have been assisting Jillian to resolve her struggle, experience acceptance and establish her cultural identity.

REFLECTION

- What could you have done to ensure cultural safety for Jillian and her three children?
- What will you do now to retrieve the relationship and encourage her to continue bringing Emily for assistance?

Note: When treating children it is essential that the health professional assists the *family*, not just the individual child, because it is the context of the family that usually dominates the development of the child. In addition, it is the parents who know the child better than anyone and are invaluable in providing a true picture of the child and their abilities.

There are a number of factors contributing to the creation of cultural safety for indigenous peoples that require examination.

The importance of history

Awareness and understanding of pre- and post-contact history is a factor that contributes to the creation of cultural safety. For many indigenous peoples (particularly those who are older) it is highly significant, because historical factors have created negative perceptions and mistrust of non-indigenous or mainstream health systems (Australian Government Department of Health and Ageing 2004). Thus, pre- and post-contact history requires close consideration.

Pre-contact history

Pre-contact with Europeans, many indigenous groups in various places around the world existed in harmony with their spiritual and physical environments and in varying levels of harmony with each other for generations upon generations. Each group had their own traditional languages; culture; specific identity including dress; spiritual explanation of their existence; rules of behaviour including expectations of the individual and the group; kinship rules; remedies; methods of artistic expression; methods of providing food and water; and laws governing their everyday lives. The groups had designated leaders or groups of leaders who understood their values, traditions and laws. As protectors of these values, traditions and laws, these leaders had particular levels of wisdom and understanding and, thus, were often the decision-makers for the group and the individuals within the group.

In Australia pre-contact there were around two-hundred-and-fifty distinct groups of Aboriginal and Torres Strait Islander Peoples with their own language, culture, identity, kinship rules, boundaries and laws for relating to other groups (Australian Government Department of Health and Ageing 2004). Aboriginal groups had inhabited Australia for approximately 50,000 years pre-contact. These groups did not always relate well to each other and some still experience tension today.

In New Zealand pre-contact there was one Maori language. However, more than one group existed and these groups did not always experience harmonious relations. The Maori inhabited New Zealand for approximately 300 years before the arrival of Europeans. While there was a treaty *(te Tiriti O Waitangi: The Treaty of Waitangi)* in 1840 between the Maori and particular non-indigenous people, that treaty was not ratified by the non-indigenous colonial government of the time. This meant that the rights of the Maori were not recognised, although their organised existence became impossible to ignore. This resulted in post-contact stress that in many ways results in inequality today.

Post-contact history

In many cases, when European contact occurred with the indigenous peoples of a region or country, the indigenous groups were not structured or organised in ways recognisable to the non-indigenous people. In many places 'contact' resulted in violence, devastation through introduced diseases or deliberate attempts to kill and/or control these groups. This control often placed members of 'non-compatible' groups together in reserves or missions. Lack of understanding, multiple incorrect assumptions and misplaced social theories (Harms 2007, Smith 2001) by non-indigenous people post-contact often resulted in histories that established negative expectations in the minds of the affected indigenous peoples. For example, in Australia there was deliberate segregation in society that also occurred in hospitals. Hospital staff often placed Aboriginal and Torres Strait Islander Peoples on the verandah or in unneeded areas of the hospital to keep them separate from non-indigenous people. Many older Aboriginal and Torres Strait Islander Peoples still remember such actions, which contribute to current negative expectations. These expectations continue in many places today because of continued discriminatory attitudes and behaviour by many non-indigenous people. In many sectors of Australian society, however, there has been a slow awakening and recognition of the social, emotional, spiritual and cultural damage caused post-contact to Aboriginal and Torres Strait Islander Peoples. In New Zealand there has been a similar awakening reflected in the *Treaty of Waitangi Act 1975*, which recognises the effects of colonisation on the Maori and has resulted in various changes for the benefit of the Maori.

Knowledge and understanding of pre- and post-contact history is important in the creation of cultural safety. However, genuine synthesis of the history and an appropriate response (including awareness of the personal bias of the health professional) to this history is essential when communicating with indigenous peoples.

Other factors

Many factors affect feelings of cultural safety; some of these factors relate to cultural differences. Some have greater impact on health service delivery than others but all are significant in the creation of cultural safety. The following points in this section have been adapted from the Australian Government Department of Health and Ageing 2004.

- It is important to understand that **communication styles** vary. For example, the use of eye contact for some Aboriginal and Torres Strait Islander Peoples and for Maori (Metge & Kinloch 1978) is a sign of disrespect rather than a sign of attentive listening. However, others may avoid eye contact if they feel ashamed or feel they are being patronised. Some indigenous peoples may feel it is unnecessary to answer a question when the answer is obvious. Some may also consider it impolite to answer a question immediately and thus they will pause before answering a question. The use of direct questions in some cultures (not just indigenous cultures) is rude and thus when requesting personal information it is best to ask open questions (see Ch 4). In many cases telling a story of someone with a particular difficulty may elicit information about the needs of the person seeking assistance. It is important to accept and accommodate differences in communication style wherever possible.
- It is important to understand that many indigenous peoples define the **notion of family** differently to non-indigenous people. For example, Aboriginal and Torres Strait Islander Peoples, Maori and many Pacific Islanders may call and consider someone a brother, sister, uncle or auntie when they are only distantly related in a non-indigenous context. In some indigenous groups a community Elder may have such a place (name) within a family group.

- Equally important is understanding there are differences in **concepts of spirituality** among indigenous peoples. For many, spirituality includes a special relationship with the land or with nature. It is possible for each indigenous person to have unique spiritual requirements that are integral to the provision of healthcare, whether the requirements are related to a special custom or the expectation of particular behaviour when someone is ill. For example, a particular person in the 'family' is expected and expects to care for a relative with a life-limiting illness. This person may consider caring for this relative more important than employment and thus if they are unable to continue working while caring for this ill person they will resign from their employment without a second thought.

- It is important to understand that **kinship obligations** (for Maori reflected in the concept of *whanaungatanga*, an obligation of giving and receiving) may result in large numbers of people either visiting or accompanying the person requiring assistance. Accommodating this factor may mean provision of a particular area or room for the indigenous peoples accompanying the person seeking assistance. Expectations of particular behaviour may also relate to kinship obligations. For example, when a mother is ill among the Aboriginal and Torres Strait Islander Peoples, most often the eldest daughter expects to fulfil the role of carer.

- Also important is the reality that indigenous peoples experience **differences in life circumstances**, family histories and community. Many indigenous peoples live in imposed poverty with living conditions that a non-indigenous person would not tolerate. Therefore, many indigenous peoples experience diseases related to poverty. Life expectancy may be shortened in many indigenous communities, and general levels of health below the average for the non-indigenous population. For example, in Australia the Yawuru people of the West Kimberly country (Western Australia) commonly experience a premature death of one of the members of the community, often on a weekly basis (ANTaR 2007). Aboriginal and Torres Strait Islander Peoples typically have life expectancies that are 20 years less than the total Australian population. The death rates in the 35–54-year age group are five-to-six times higher than in the general population (Australian Bureau of Statistics & Australian Institute of Health and Welfare 2003). Such facts exist for many indigenous peoples (for facts relating to Maori see Durie 1998) and often result in unresolved grief and a sense of loss, for both past and present, in indigenous communities. Recognition of this reality is important for the creation of cultural safety.

- It is important to remember that indigenous peoples will **react differently to people and the healthcare environment**. Some indigenous peoples find it difficult to seek assistance, or to continue to seek assistance, due to factors such as separation from the people in their communal group; arrangement of the environment and rooms in health services and thus restrictions on particular types of behaviour; and unfamiliar people who apparently do not understand or want to understand their customs and their previous experiences with health services. This can affect the creation of cultural safety.

- Any person with a different cultural background will be affected by differences in **education and language**. For many rural and remote indigenous peoples English is a second, third or sometimes fourth language and thus they may require an interpreter (see Ch 15), preferably from an organisation dedicated to that particular indigenous group. If there is no known organisation dedicated to the appropriate indigenous group it is essential to remember that the indigenous person will have their own sociolinguistic and sociocultural expectations that will affect the interaction (Bowe & Martin 2007). It is also important to note that many indigenous peoples have their own dialect of the language of the non-indigenous colonists. In Australia, Aboriginal and Torres Strait Islander Peoples have a particular dialect of English that is in many cases a significant part of their cultural identity (Aboriginal English in the Courts 2000). The use of their own dialect without an interpreter may contribute to pauses of varying lengths as the person silently translates the message into their dialect to facilitate understanding. Acceptance of variations in the dialects of English may be important for creating cultural safety.

- Understanding that indigenous peoples may have **different attitudes, understanding and approaches to illness**, health, death and disability contributes to establishing cultural safety. Some indigenous groups in Asia believe particular disabilities are a punishment for wrong behaviour and thus disability brings shame. Generally, it is unacceptable for individuals with disabilities to relate in public in such cultures. Some indigenous groups in the Pacific and Australia attribute disease and death to sorcery or curses rather than biomedical causes. It is interesting to note that the word 'health' does not have a direct equivalent in the languages of the Aboriginal and Torres Strait Islander Peoples. For Aboriginal and Torres Strait Islander Peoples, 'health' is about **wellbeing**. Wellbeing is not related to illness, but rather to connection with kinship groups and, for many, connection with traditions and the land.

- For many indigenous peoples, having the **same gender health professional** to assist them contributes to their cultural safety. In many cases the indigenous person may not attend repeat appointments if they have a health professional of the opposite gender assisting them.

- Establishing cultural safety for indigenous peoples requires an understanding that **different values and 'ways of doing and caring'** in rural and remote areas may result in behaviours that seem foreign and sometimes unacceptable to the values and ways of the non-indigenous health professional. These ways of caring have been practised for thousands of years and if accepted and creatively accommodated rather than rejected can produce cultural safety and remove a reluctance to access non-indigenous services.

- Another cultural difference that affects cultural safety is **traditional methods of managing illness** and death (Healing Our Way 1999). Such methods are often foreign to non-indigenous health professionals. However, inclusion of such practice in the care of indigenous peoples (e.g. the use of traditional healers and foods) can contribute to their spiritual, emotional, psychological and often physical comfort.

- The impact of the **imbalance of power** in the relationship between the health professional and the indigenous person is a crucial factor affecting the creation of cultural safety. This imbalance occurs even when there is no cultural difference, because of greater familiarity of the health professional with the health system and the particular health profession. When assisting indigenous peoples, however, this imbalance is heightened in many cases because of social, economic and educational advantage on the part of the health professional. Previous government policies relating to indigenous peoples have influenced the expectation of a power imbalance from the perspective of indigenous peoples. This in turn influences the potential development of therapeutic relationships and the creation of cultural safety. It is important that the health professional behaves in a manner that respects and accommodates cultural differences in order to create a collaborative balance of power rather than a dominating one.

- Appropriate **training** in understanding cultural differences for all staff in a health service contributes to achieving cultural safety.

- **Investing time** to learn about cultural differences and discovering ways to accommodate these differences and include them in practice will contribute to cultural safety and positive outcomes.

All the above factors affect the creation of cultural safety for indigenous peoples. They require consideration and accommodation when providing health services for indigenous peoples from both the southern and northern hemispheres. These factors provide a foundation for the principles that guide the practice of a health professional when assisting a person with an indigenous background.

REFLECTION

Which of the factors on pp 205–207 do you feel is most important to you?

GROUP ACTIVITY

- In groups of four, divide the factors on pp 205–207 among the group to ensure consideration of all the listed factors.
- Suggest ways that your health profession or health service might accommodate each factor.
- Suggest ways that an individual health professional might accommodate each factor.

Factors contributing to culturally safe communication with indigenous peoples

Many of the factors that contribute to the creation of cultural safety also influence the effectiveness of communication. However, the following factors relate specifically to communication with indigenous peoples.

- The **direct and confident 'professional' manner** encouraged in non-indigenous health professionals may be offensive to some indigenous peoples, especially when discussing sensitive information. In such situations, a softly spoken, informal manner is more appropriate. An established relationship based on respect and rapport encourages effective communication with indigenous peoples.
- When referred a person with an indigenous background, it is important to consider the **correct people to approach** before initial contact or to include if giving important information about the future of the person receiving assistance. Include all appropriate people in discussions about the intervention plan and where appropriate the discharge plan. As mentioned, when a mother is ill it is often the eldest daughter who needs to know the medication or intervention regime, not the person herself. It may be important to approach a **local Elder** (Kaūmatua [male] or Kuia [female] Maori Elder) before initiating contact or have an Elder present when discussing future intervention or discharge (Clarke et al 1999).
- Establish how to **contact the local community Elder** or **relevant organisation** connected specifically with the cultural background of the person seeking assistance. Establish communication links with the specialist organisation, either at an institutional level or a personal level, depending on the situation. Asking advice from such organisations can assist the health professional in understanding and accommodating the communication and cultural needs of the person.
- Avoid **making assumptions** based on appearance, living conditions, people present and commitment to traditional beliefs and customs.
- Remember the person who is entitled to give consent may not be present despite the presence of a close relative.
- Use an interpreter or an indigenous medical liaison officer from the **particular indigenous group** if communicating complex information or bad news. Clarify with the interpreter

before the discussion the appropriate terms for particular concepts. For example, death and dying are words that may not be used in some indigenous communities.

- **Open communication** that embraces differing communication styles contributes to culturally safe communication. It is important to avoid any temptation to correct the spoken expression of indigenous peoples, including children, because this indicates lack of acceptance of their particular dialect and a desire to impose the dialect of the health professional.

- **Ask** about the **cultural background** of the person/family and community. Ask for information about specific **communication behaviours** and relevant **cultural needs**. Accommodate these differences where possible. Explain the requirements of the health service and remain open to possible ways of complying with these requirements while accommodating the cultural needs of the person/community.

- Sometimes the **questions** asked by health professionals are **offensive** to an indigenous person because of the nature of the questions or the gender of the person asking the questions. Questions may appear **silly** if the answers seem obvious. It is important for health professionals to state the need to ask many questions in an apologetic, concerned manner. **Explain** that everyone seeking assistance from this health service usually answers these questions and the information will not affect their access to services. Reassure them of privacy and confidentiality of the collected information.

- **Listen**. Skills in listening are essential when communicating; however, many indigenous peoples feel that non-indigenous people do not take the time to listen (Clarke et al 1999, Harms 2007). This reality may originate in the different uses of silence and questions/answers in some indigenous cultures.

- Consider the method of providing information that will maximise understanding. Many indigenous cultures use **story-telling** as a means of sharing information. Using a story about a person with a particular condition or difficulty may allow the indigenous person to understand the requirements of the health professional or to recognise their own condition and related needs. For example, telling a story about someone with conjunctivitis and their experience of the relevant intervention may allow the indigenous person to see they too have conjunctivitis and to understand how to control that condition.

- Allow sufficient **time for processing of information**. Verify understanding of the information given and seek clarification where required about that information from an indigenous member of staff or person from the relevant indigenous organisation (Australian Government Department of Health and Ageing 2004). Remember some indigenous peoples may be translating the information into their own dialect or language and thus may require longer to process information.

- **Invest time to establish trust** and a therapeutic relationship with the person and the members of the community who care for them. Many indigenous peoples are accustomed to non-indigenous people talking and filling the silences (Harms 2007, Metge & Kinloch 1978). Therefore, establishing a relationship may require investment of time to sit quietly and listen.

- Provide **time for discussion** and explanation during all stages of the assistance process. Include an indigenous medical liaison officer of the same cultural background where possible.

- **Observe and validate non-verbal cues.** Where direct questions are not the cultural norm, suggest a possible interpretation of the non-verbal cues and wait for a response. For example, if an indigenous person has their eyes averted or head turned away, the health professional might ask a specific question in a non-confronting, non-patronising manner. For example, *I can see you are not happy (frightened etc); are you feeling pain?*

This manner of questioning validates their feelings and allows them to feel and agree or disagree with the assumption. For some indigenous peoples, however, if the health professional has made the correct assumption about the cause of the non-verbal cues they will not answer because the answer seems obvious.

- **Silence** has a particular role in many indigenous communities. It is a positive element of communication that allows learning about a person through thought and observation. Silence is an acceptable part of communicating. It allows time for processing information, 'feeling' those around them and understanding the environment.
- Indigenous peoples may **communicate discomfort through silence** and this has particular implications for a health professional. The silence may indicate physical pain. However, it may also indicate that it is inappropriate to respond to particular questions or comments from a person of the opposite gender. As mentioned, silence may also represent translation time.
- **Lack of response** may indicate an inability to physically hear the message and this requires particular action on the part of the health professional.

REFLECTION

Which of the above factors affecting communication are least familiar to you?

GROUP ACTIVITY

Choose the five factors least familiar to the group and decide how a health professional might accommodate each factor.

Barriers to culturally safe communication

Many indigenous peoples have experiences that suggest most non-indigenous health professionals have limited knowledge of or lack of interest in indigenous cultures and are generally not interested in accommodating indigenous cultures. These experiences often result in indigenous peoples avoiding seeking assistance from non-indigenous health services. They may also result in the indigenous person not returning for repeat assistance.

The following are causes of culturally unsafe communication identified by indigenous peoples and provide barriers to effective communication.

- The presence of **stereotypes** and preconceptions may govern the behaviour of both the health professional and the indigenous person.
- Failure to **explore the actual meaning of words or behaviours** is a barrier to effective communication because words may have a different meaning for the indigenous person. For a non-indigenous person, 'home' may mean a house, but for an indigenous person they are at home when they are with their kinship group, whether or not that group is in a house. Failure to explore the meaning of words can limit communication in the same way that failure to explore the meaning of particular behaviour can limit communication. For example, exploration of the meaning of silence, averted head and/ or eyes, non-attendance, repeated attendance after discharge, or failure to complete the required at-home tasks may assist the health professional to provide appropriate assistance and develop rapport.
- Failure to **understand** that some indigenous peoples provide the answer they think the health professional desires is a barrier to effective communication. Indigenous peoples

may do this because they do not understand the request or because of multiple repeats of the same question.

- Failure to **listen** patiently and quietly prevents effective communication.
- Failure to **observe and explore non-verbal behaviours** in a culturally appropriate manner is a barrier to effective communication.
- Failure to **clarify understanding** limits communication.
- Responses that are **clichés** or automatic and therefore do not acknowledge the cultural needs and differences between the indigenous person and the non-indigenous health professional may result in miscommunication.
- Use of **inappropriate pamphlets or written information** creates barriers to communication. Using written information with visual images and no jargon or technical terms is important when communicating with most people seeking assistance, and especially with indigenous peoples. It is important to seek the advice of indigenous medical liaison officers when preparing any written information for indigenous peoples.

Chapter summary

Many factors affect communication with indigenous peoples. These factors arise from separate and shared experiences of indigenous peoples and non-indigenous people. It is important that health professionals consider the relevant factors when communicating with indigenous peoples to ensure effective communication and family/community-centred practice.

Complete the following:

1. What is the purpose of using appropriate terms to describe their groups when relating to indigenous peoples?

   _____

   _____

   _____

2. Explain why each individual has a unique cultural identity.

   _____

   _____

   _____

3. Define cultural safety.

   _____

   _____

   _____

4. List the five main steps that create culturally safe practice when working with indigenous peoples.

   i. _____

   ii. _____

   iii. _____

   iv. _____

   v. _____

5. Identify eight factors that contribute to the creation of cultural safety for indigenous peoples. Give original examples of how a health professional might accommodate each of these factors in practice.

    i. _____

    ii. _____

    iii. _____

    iv. _____

    v. _____

    vi. _____

    vii. _____

    viii. _____

6. Choose and explain ten factors that contribute to the creation of culturally safe communication for indigenous peoples. Give examples of ways of communicating that will create effective communication with indigenous peoples.

    i. _____

    ii. _____

    iii. _____

    iv. _____

    v. _____

    vi. _____

    vii. _____

    viii. _____

    ix. _____

    x. _____

7. List seven barriers to the creation of culturally safe communication.

    i. _____

    ii. _____

    iii. _____

    iv. _____

    v. _____

    vi. _____

    vii. _____

8. Describe how a health professional might overcome at least four of the barriers to culturally safe communication.

    i. _____

    ii. _____

    iii. _____

    iv. _____

References

Aboriginal English in the Courts 2000 Department of Justice and Attorney-General, Queensland Government. Available: www.justice.qld.gov.au 24 March 2008

ANTaR: Australians for Native Title and Reconciliation 2007 Liyarn Ngarn (Feature film with Patrick Dodson, Peter Postlethwaite, Archie Roach and Shane Howard) ANTaR, Australia

Australian Bureau of Statistics & Australian Institute of Health and Welfare 2003 The health and welfare of Australia's Aboriginal and Torres Strait Islander Peoples. Commonwealth of Australia, Canberra

Australian Government Department of Health and Ageing 2004 Providing culturally appropriate palliative care to Aboriginal and Torres Strait Islanders: resource kit. Commonwealth of Australia, Canberra (The Mungabareena Aboriginal Corporation assisted in the preparation of this resource kit)

Bowe H, Martin K 2007 Communication across cultures: mutual understanding in a global world. Cambridge University Press, Melbourne

Clarke A, Andrews S, Austin N 1999 Lookin' after our own: supporting Aboriginal families through the hospital experience. Aboriginal Family Support Unit, Royal Children's Hospital, Melbourne

Durie M 1998 Whaiora: Maori health development, 2nd edn. Oxford University Press, Auckland

Fenwick C 2001 Pain management strategies for health professionals caring for central Australian Aboriginal People. Australian Government Department of Health and Aged Care, Canberra

Fried O 2000 Providing palliative care for Aboriginal patients. Australian Family Physician 29:1035–1038

Harms L 2007 Working with people: communication skills for reflective practice. Oxford University Press, Melbourne

Healing Our Way: Aboriginal Health and Community Protocols 2005. Discipline of Aboriginal Health Studies, Faculty of Health and Medical Sciences, The University of Newcastle, Australia (Learning Production Group Education Services, USD CD-ROM 1999 release)

Holliday A, Hyde M, Kullman J 2006 Intercultural communication: an advanced resource book. Routledge, London (Original work published 2004)

Metge J, Kinloch P 1978 Talking past each other: problems of cross-cultural communication. Victoria University Press, Wellington

NSW Department of Health 2004 Communicating positively: a guide to appropriate Aboriginal terminology. NSW Department of Health, Sydney

Nursing Council of New Zealand 2002 Guidelines to cultural safety, the treaty of Waitangi, and Maori health in nursing and midwifery education and practice. Nursing Council of New Zealand, New Zealand

Smith L T 2001 Decolonizing methodologies: research and indigenous peoples. University of Otago, Dunedin

Stein-Parbury J 2006 Patient and person: interpersonal skills in nursing, 3rd edn. Elsevier, Sydney (Original work published 2005)

Further reading

Child and Youth Health Inter-government Partnership (CHIP) 2005 Healthy children – strengthening promotions and prevention across Australia: national public health strategic framework for children 2005–2008. Australian Government Department of Health and Aged Care, Canberra

Ellis R, Simms S (eds) 2005 Indigenous health promotion resources: a national information guide for Aboriginal and Torres Strait Islander health workers, 5th edn. Aboriginal and Torres Strait Islander Health Worker Journal, Matraville, Australia

Hazlehurst K 1996 A healing place: Indigenous visions for personal empowerment and community recovery. Central Queensland University Press, Rockhampton

Rolfe S A 2002 Promoting resilience in children. Australian Early Childhood Association, Watson, Australia

Social Health Reference Group for National Aboriginal and Torres Strait Islanders 2004 Social and emotional wellbeing framework for Aboriginal and Torres Strait Islander Peoples' mental health and social emotional wellbeing: 2004–2009. Australian Government Department of Health and Ageing, Canberra

Useful and reliable Australian websites

www.yarrahealing.melb.catholic.edu.au
www.aiatsis.gov.au
www.justice.qld.gov.au/AboriginalEnglish.htm
www.natsiew.nexus.edu.au (see *Topics: Health*)

Misunderstandings and communication

17

CHAPTER OBJECTIVES

Upon completing this chapter, students should be able to
- Define and explain a misunderstanding
- Explain the factors contributing to understanding
- Describe some possible causes of misunderstandings
- Develop useful strategies to reduce misunderstandings
- Explain the steps for resolving misunderstandings effectively.

Communication that produces misunderstanding

It is essential to remember the characteristics of effective communication when experiencing misunderstandings. All health professionals must learn to manage communicative interactions where there is a failure to understand or interpret words or events correctly, and to do so in a reasonable and calm manner (Holli et al 2003). Interactions involving misunderstandings are often uncomfortable. They may produce feelings of anxiety and regret, and, if serious enough, feelings of guilt and unfair judgement. Everyone experiences feelings of discomfort, anxiety and regret because of misunderstandings. Guilt, while a self-defeating emotion, is a typical reaction if lack of care on the part of the health professional causes a miscommunication. If inappropriately blamed for a misunderstanding, however, the health professional may feel misjudged. Both the health professional and the person seeking assistance may experience negative emotions because of misunderstandings.

It is interesting to note that communicating with care and the best intentions do not guarantee understanding (Bowe & Martin 2007, Tyler et al 2005). The perspective of the other person may affect the interpretation of a kind intention. For example, assisting someone after observing them struggling to complete a task may produce anger rather than expressions of thanks if the person was intent on proving they could complete the task themself. Conversely, not assisting a struggling person may also elicit anger. A means of avoiding such situations is to use a question or gesture designed to establish the desire or lack of desire of the person for assistance. Similarly, if a person seeking assistance expects a particular intervention that is outside the role of the health professional, this may cause miscommunication and requires immediate clarification. Misunderstandings decrease levels of trust and may severely affect the therapeutic relationship. This has implications for the health professional, the person seeking assistance and the ultimate outcome of the assistance.

REFLECTION

Consider a time when you experienced a misunderstanding.
- What was the cause of the misunderstanding?
- Were you the person who failed to communicate clearly or were you the person who failed to clarify the meaning?
- What were the consequences?
- How did you feel?
- Did you feel tempted to blame the other person?
- What could you have done to avoid the misunderstanding?
- What did you learn from this experience?
- What will you do next time to avoid a misunderstanding?

It is clear that a misunderstanding might generate negative emotions, but the various factors that contribute to misunderstandings are not always clear. However, it is important to comprehend the various factors affecting mutual understanding in an attempt to prevent misunderstandings.

Factors affecting mutual understanding

Many factors affect the ability of communicating individuals to achieve mutual understanding. Some of these factors include language, word usage, assumptions about meaning, context and the time invested in negotiating meaning. The possibility of misunderstanding increases if communicating individuals come from different cultures. However, misunderstandings may also occur between individuals from the same cultural groupings.

Mutual understanding increases, although is not guaranteed, if the interacting individuals can communicate competently in a common language. Understanding is enhanced when individuals share the same meanings for particular words. Difficulties can arise if one person does not know the various meanings of a word used (see Ch 1) and thus does not recognise that word in a particular context. Lack of word recognition prevents understanding. In many languages, sounds and/or words can carry multiple meanings (Harms 2007, Nunan 2007), and this can make it difficult to understand the sound or word in an unfamiliar context. This may occur with the use of professional jargon or technical words but can also occur when communicating with a person who has learnt the language of the interaction as an addition to their first language.

Mutual understanding is also influenced by assumptions individuals make about meaning. Assumptions can develop because of previous experience, knowledge and understanding of the situation and context. The probability of achieving mutual understanding may be decreased if some of the individuals communicating are unfamiliar with the context of the communication, or communicate outside the expectations of the context (Nunan 2007).

Of the factors that limit the achievement of mutual understanding, it is necessary to consider which of these are relevant to the health professions. Health professionals relate regularly to individuals from different cultures (see Ch 15). Misunderstandings between people from different cultures may occur because of expectations as well as the meaning of particular behaviours and words. Openness, understanding and acceptance of the differences will assist those communicating to achieve mutual understanding. It is the responsibility of the health professional to demonstrate openness and acceptance because of the vulnerability of the person seeking assistance.

Among health professionals there is not always a common language. A health professional who specialises in a particular area may use jargon that a health professional from a different specialty might struggle to understand. For example, someone working in medical radiation science may not understand the terminology used by a person working in occupational rehabilitation. Individuals seeking assistance, even when they speak the local language, may not understand any health-specific jargon. If they are unable to recognise a particular word in the health context they may misinterpret the meaning. The individual struggling to understand a word will often assume the meaning if they feel uncomfortable about asking for clarification. Similarly, some Aboriginal and Torres Strait Islander Peoples will not express an inability to understand because experience tells them the health professional will not listen. In all situations the health professional has responsibility to negotiate mutual understanding. If misunderstandings do occur it is important that the health professional takes responsibility to repair the misunderstanding, regardless of the cause. Misunderstandings occur wherever people interact and thus the health professional will benefit from considering such events carefully to understand the causes and how to avoid them in the future (Higgs et al 2005).

Causes of misunderstandings

The factors affecting mutual understanding – culture, language, word meanings, assumed meanings and context – can also contribute to misunderstandings. There are additional factors that can cause misunderstandings, however, and these are examined in this section.

Attitudes

Misunderstandings can occur because of the attitudes of the interacting individuals. Judgemental attitudes communicated non-verbally may assume greater strength for the person seeking assistance than is felt by the health professional holding the attitude. This can create misunderstandings. It is important that the health professional through reflection and self-awareness fosters an attitude of openness and acceptance towards individuals who might not meet their criteria of what is acceptable. For example, vulnerable individuals from a different culture must experience the same attitude from the health professional regardless of the language they speak and the differing values of the health professional. It is important that an attitude of respect, empathy and inclusion, as well as an attitude that focuses on the goals of the vulnerable individual, saturates every encounter between the health professional and the person seeking assistance. Health professionals with such underlying attitudes will naturally communicate to avoid misunderstandings.

It is difficult to control the attitudes of those around the health professional. However, maintaining a positive and accepting attitude can influence the attitudes of others. A health professional with an appropriate attitude will positively affect the person seeking assistance, contributing to avoidance of misunderstandings and fulfilment of positive outcomes.

Emotions

Emotions can both positively and negatively influence the outcome of communication. It is easy to interpret feelings of frustration, intolerance, impatience and anger in another person and such emotions can significantly compromise communication (Mohan et al 2004). Unresolved emotions – whether in the health professional or the person seeking assistance – can negatively affect any communicative interaction. Failure to give adequate attention to emotions both before and during interactions can cause misunderstandings. When attempting to repair or resolve a misunderstanding, it is important for the health professional to give appropriate consideration to the emotions behind the misunderstanding.

REFLECTION

Consider an interaction in which your negative emotions limited your ability to concentrate or understand. Perhaps you reacted emotionally to something that was said and were unable to hear the rest of the conversation, resulting in misunderstanding.

Relevance of context to determine meaning

The use of context to determine meaning varies from culture to culture, and this cultural variation can cause misunderstandings. Some cultures use verbal and non-verbal messages to construct meaning, while other cultures construct meaning using these messages as well as context. In such cultures the context refers to the circumstances (including the circumstances of the interacting people) or events that form the environment within which the communication occurs. In these cultures the context may have greater weight than the verbal or non-verbal messages. In cultures that rely on context to determine meaning, the speaker, their role, their manner of communicating and their relationship to the listener(s) combine to influence the communication outcome; the actual words spoken may be irrelevant to the meaning of the message. Still other cultures use varying combinations of context and constructed messages to determine meaning. Hall (1997) refers to high-context and low-context cultures according to their use of context to establish understanding. It is important to understand that some cultures use context to determine meaning because this affects the communication style of people from such cultures and may explain any misunderstandings.

GROUP DISCUSSION

- What is important when relating to a person who uses context to determine meaning?
- Should the health professional adjust their manner of communicating? Explain why or why not.

Expectations of styles of communication

Styles of communication vary across cultures and families. This reality rarely requires consideration unless communicating with individuals who expect a different style. Some cultures expect information to be organised in particular ways with the major points clearly expressed first (more direct). Others seem to avoid the major point initially, only reaching it after extensive circular discussion (indirect) (Bowe & Martin 2007). Thus confusion may result between individuals from cultures that organise information in different ways.

REFLECTION

- How could direct and indirect communication styles influence understanding in the practice of the health professional?
- How could the health professional compensate for either style?

Another style of communicating relates to the tolerance of ambiguity (Bowe & Martin 2007). This tolerance is higher in people who have a tendency towards an indirect style of communication. Some cultures, societies and families communicate through implied meaning – one person suggests an implied perception of a concept or idea and another then implies similar or alternate perceptions. This style of communicating is difficult to grasp if it is not the style of the culture of the health professional. However, while to a novice this style appears circular and difficult to follow, the communicators are able to achieve mutual understanding. In contrast, a less ambiguous style of communicating involves explicit statement of points and exploration of these points. The words used to communicate directly reflect the meaning. In this style, unless there is an unconscious agenda, the communicators say exactly what they think, feel and desire. Some cultures and families use both implicit and explicit (some call them ambiguous and clear) styles of communicating, depending on the circumstances. The health professional does not necessarily need to adjust their style to that of their communication partner. However, it is beneficial to be aware of the style of the person seeking assistance, acknowledge that style and explicitly explain the style that will govern the communicative interactions with the health professional. This may reduce the possibility of misunderstandings.

GROUP ACTIVITY

- Decide what style of communication your culture uses – an implicit style, explicit style or combination of both.
- Give examples of each style. State the conditions and the type of subject that regulate the use of each style.

Expectations of the event or procedure

The expectations an individual might have of a health service will influence their understanding within that service. For example, if an individual expects to receive something that will immediately remove their symptoms, it may be distressing to learn they must have further investigations. It is important that health professionals clearly explain their service and the expected results of and reasons for particular procedures and events (see Chs 15 & 16). The vulnerable individual may not understand the situation or the procedures well enough to know which questions to ask. Therefore, it is the responsibility of the health professional to explain rather than assume the person knows how and why something might happen. For example, everyone involved in a family conference should understand the purpose of and the usual process employed during a family conference. This allows the person to clarify their expectations and/or to demonstrate their understanding of the procedure. Clear explanations will assist in avoiding misunderstandings due to particular expectations.

GROUP ACTIVITY

- List the characteristics of a clear explanation.
- Choose one of the following health service contexts: acute, rehabilitation, community, health promotion, occupational rehabilitation or private practice.
- Write a clear explanation of the context and the kinds of 'events' that occur in that context.

Expectations governed by cultural norms

Every culture and society, and most families, have norms that affect communicative behaviours. Such norms govern what is said and when it is said according to particular situations. Lack of understanding of cultural norms can cause miscommunication. It is not possible for any health professional to learn every norm for every culture (Dean 2001), society or family. However, it is important that health professionals are aware of the existence of cultural norms related to communication. This understanding can explain variations in communicative events and empower the health professional to make allowances for these variations. Particular cultures, social groups and families have norms that govern the topic of social conversation in particular situations. Some freely discuss politics, salaries and sex, and openly ask the age of a person, while others avoid these topics. Some freely discuss spiritual beliefs and values while others avoid discussing spiritual or religious topics. Some freely express emotions while others avoid expression of emotions.

Some cultures use specific combinations of words to fulfil a social function. For example, in English, *How are you?* fulfils the function of acknowledging and greeting a person. In most cases it is not a request for information about the health of a person but simply says hello. In Chinese, *Where are you going?* or *Have you eaten?* fulfils the same function. Understanding that different combinations of words may fulfil different functions is important and can assist the health professional to avoid misunderstandings.

Strategies to avoid misunderstandings

There are specific communicative behaviours that can assist in avoiding misunderstandings. Most individuals have a desire to share meaning with those communicating (Bowe & Martin 2007) and will usually concentrate and struggle, if necessary, to understand. This is both an encouragement and a warning to the health professional. It is encouraging because it indicates that those seeking their assistance will want to understand and in many cases will try to understand. The warning is that in a service with limited resources the health professional may not invest the time required to achieve adequate understanding. The temptation to provide information quickly and allow the person seeking assistance to assume the meaning, especially when they are striving to achieve this meaning, is dangerous. This action does not guarantee mutual understanding.

Reducing the incidence of misunderstandings

The following are suggestions that will reduce the incidence of misunderstandings (Bowe & Martin 2007, Tyler et al 2005).

- Plan and prepare for the interaction. Read reports, records and relevant research related to the condition and needs of the person. It is important when referring to reports, records or referrals to avoid the creation of assumptions and opinions about the needs of the person. Remember the overall aim of the health professional is fulfilment of family/person-centred goals and practice.
- Understand the communication expectations of the person involved in the interaction.
- If communicating with a person from another culture, become familiar with the needs, cultural expectations and language level of the person. Schedule an interpreter if necessary (see Ch 15).
- Know and understand the information for discussion and organise it clearly and carefully.
- Speak clearly and avoid a rapid rate of speech.
- Minimise misunderstandings of words and sentences.
  - Be specific. Avoid words that do not communicate specific information (e.g. this, that, then, things, some, many, over there).
  - Choose the words carefully, giving consideration to other possible meanings and anticipating potential assumptions and conclusions.
  - Avoid using jargon or technical terms without a clear explanation of such words.
  - Avoid using colloquialisms or everyday sayings specific to a local dialect or language (e.g. *He's on the road, Go with the flow, A lot, Take it easy*).
- Observe the effect of the information on all communicators, including the health professional, throughout the interaction.
- Ask for confirmation of understanding throughout the interaction.
- Ask for a summary of the information to determine the level of understanding. Give explanations if misunderstandings are apparent.
- Reflect upon the interaction after completion. Reflection can assist health professionals to understand themselves, the other person and the components of the communication. It can assist the health professional to prepare for future communicative interactions and avoid future misunderstandings.

Misunderstandings are inevitable wherever individuals interact. It is important that the health professional understands the causes of misunderstandings and develops confidence to manage misunderstandings. Such confidence will develop through experience, reflection, discussion and understanding of possible management strategies.

Resolving misunderstandings

The experience of misunderstanding affects individuals in different ways. As a health professional, the major concern is the effect of misunderstandings on the emotions of those seeking their assistance. It is also important for health professionals to take care of themselves;

however, resolution of the emotions of the health professional must occur separately to the resolution of the emotions of the vulnerable person. The control of any frustration, impatience or intolerance on the part of the health professional is essential when there is a misunderstanding. Vulnerable individuals receive and interpret such emotions quickly, which may contribute to further misunderstanding. In situations of misunderstanding, clarification of the information may resolve the negative emotions associated with the misunderstanding. Resolution of the emotions resulting from the misunderstanding may accelerate the ability of the vulnerable person to understand the information previously misunderstood. It is important that the health professional decides which to consider first – the resolution of the emotions or the understanding of the information. The existence of a therapeutic relationship will facilitate this decision. The major aim of the health professional at this point is to resolve the misunderstanding.

It is important in every communicative interaction to remember the components of effective communication. If the health professional communicates according to these components, their action will achieve appropriate resolution of any miscommunication. Restoring communication is essential for achieving the ultimate purpose of the health professions – fulfilment of family/person-centred goals.

REFLECTION

Refer to the 'Reflection' section at the beginning of this chapter: 'Consider a time when you experienced a misunderstanding'.
- Was that misunderstanding resolved?
- Was it resolved satisfactorily? If so, outline the steps used to resolve it.
- Could you use these steps in every situation? How could they be adapted for use in any situation?

Steps to resolving misunderstandings

The following are steps that will assist the health professional in resolving misunderstandings.

1. Be aware that there is a misunderstanding. This is not always immediately obvious. However, as soon as it becomes obvious the health professional has a responsibility to act to overcome the cause of the misunderstanding and thus achieve effective communication.
2. Control any negative emotions associated with the misunderstanding. If possible, resolving negative emotions before restoring communication is the most appropriate option. Time constraints may make this difficult or impossible, however, and thus learning to control negative emotions is beneficial. The major emotions for the health professional to communicate are regret that the communication failed and a desire to achieve effective communication.
3. Take responsibility for the misunderstanding regardless of the cause or problem. It is more probable that the vulnerable person will accept the actions of the health professional if the health professional willingly assumes responsibility for the misunderstanding.
4. Understand what caused the misunderstanding. Understanding the cause will assist the health professional to compensate and avoid further misunderstandings because of that cause. It may also assist the health professional to consider and predict other possible causes. Preparation and planning should assist the health professional to avoid

further misunderstandings. It is essential to understand that isolating the cause of the misunderstanding is not a substitute for action to resolve the misunderstanding (Brill & Levine 2005).

5. Make a conscious decision to restore mutual understanding. This will assist the health professional to persevere to overcome the barriers to understanding. It will resolve the misunderstanding and restore trust and effective communication.

6. Focus on the restoration of understanding, not on the cause of the misunderstanding. If the health professional focuses on restoring communication it will assist in controlling the negative emotions associated with the misunderstanding.

Chapter summary

Misunderstandings may occur for many reasons, including the expectations of the person seeking assistance and the limitations of the role of the health professional. Commitment to the components of effective communication will empower the health professional to successfully manage misunderstandings and restore effective communication.

Complete the following:

1. Define 'misunderstanding'.

_____

_____

_____

2. List the factors that affect mutual understanding.

_____

_____

_____

3. Give examples of how each of these factors can affect communication.

_____

_____

_____

4. Give original examples of each cause of misunderstandings.

_____

_____

_____

5. In your own words, list four ways to reduce the incidence of misunderstandings.

i.   _____

ii. _____

iii. _____

iv. _____

6. List the six steps that will assist the health professional to resolve misunderstandings. Suggest reasons for the importance of each step.

   i. _____

   ii. _____

   iii. _____

   iv. _____

   v. _____

   vi. _____

References

Bowe H, Martin K 2007 Communication across cultures: mutual understanding in a global world. Cambridge University Press, Melbourne

Brill N I, Levine J 2005 Working with people: the helping process, 8th edn. Pearson, Boston

Dean R 2001 The myth of cross-cultural competence: families in society. The Journal of Contemporary Human Services 86:623–630

Hall E T 1997 Beyond culture. Anchor Books, New York

Harms L 2007 Working with people: communication skills for reflective practice. Oxford University Press, Melbourne

Higgs J, Sefton A, Street A et al 2005 Communicating in the health and social sciences. Oxford University Press, Melbourne

Holli B B, Calabrese R J, O'Sullivan Mailett J 2003 Communication and education skills for diatetics professionals, 4th edn. Lippincott, Williams & Wilkins, Philadelphia

Mohan T, McGregor H, Saunders S et al 2004 Communicating as professionals. Thomson, Melbourne

Nunan D 2007 What is this thing called language? Palgrave Macmillan, Basingstoke

Tyler S, Kossen C, Ryan C 2005 Communication: a foundation course, 2nd edn. Pearson, Prentice Hall, Frenchs Forest, Sydney

Remote communication

18

CHAPTER OBJECTIVES

Upon completing this chapter, students should be able to

- Define and discuss remote communication
- List types of remote communication typically used in the health professions: written reports, databases, telephone, video/teleconferences and the internet
- Describe the characteristics of remote communication
- Explain the advantages of remote communication
- Justify the principles for use of remote communication
- Develop strategies for appropriate use of remote communication including written information, telephones, video/teleconferences, email, search engines and professional chat rooms.

Remote communication involves communication that is *not* face-to-face or that occurs over large distances. Over the past 50 years health professionals have consistently used written reports and telephones as common forms of remote communication. Written reports and telephones traditionally communicated information about appointments, expectations, interventions, results, needs, future plans and various other issues related to people seeking assistance. Today, however, worldwide technological changes allow health professionals to communicate electronically through video/teleconferences and the internet (Higgs et al 2005, Mohan et al 2004, Purtilo & Haddad 2002). Such electronic forms of communication are called computer-mediated communication (CMC).

While there are advantages and disadvantages of new and old forms of remote communication, it appears that remote communication is a permanent feature of the twenty-first century.

- Consider the amount of time you spend using remote communication. How many hours a day do you spend communicating via telephone calls, text messages, the internet (email and chat rooms) and Skype (or other forms of instantaneous remote video interaction and typing)?
- Why do you use these particular forms of remote communication?
- Which of these forms of remote communication experience the most disruption that is out of your control?
- Do you think everyone in your town or city would spend a similar amount of time each day using remote communication?
- Do you think most people have access to the technical forms of remote communication?
- With which form of remote communication do you feel most comfortable? Why do you think this is so? Does everyone you know feel the same?

Societies, professions, families and individuals respond differently to remote forms of communication. Remote forms of communication potentially increase the convenience and speed of communication (De Ville 2001), however these are not the only factors that determine responses to remote forms of communication. Each form of remote communication has specific characteristics that influence responses to it. These characteristics include convenience, control, speed of delivery, preparation time, level of formality and thought required, reusability, the presence of non-verbal cues to complement meaning, irreversibility, legal implications, security and access to appropriate technology. Many of these characteristics are desirable for health professionals, however, some have implications worthy of consideration (Mohan et al 2004).

Characteristics of remote forms of communication for the health professional

There are a number of characteristics of remote forms of communication for the health professional that require consideration (see Table 18.1).

It is interesting to consider the characteristics of each form of remote communication typically used in the health professions. The often-popular electronic forms are not as available nor as reliable as many suggest (Devito 2007). Many countries and rural areas do not have technological resources available, or such resources may be unreliable. Thus it can be difficult to achieve effective communication when relying on electronic forms of remote communication in the health professions.

- List the advantages and disadvantages of each of the remote forms of communication typically used in the health professions.
- Suggest ways to overcome the disadvantages.

Convenience, immediacy and cost are factors increasingly important in health services due to rising demand for, and in many places decreases in, resources and funding. Most

Characteristics of remote forms of communication for the health professional				
Characteristic	Telephone	Video/tele-conference	Email	Report
Convenience	Y	Y	Y	S
Control for caller/sender	Y	Y	Y	Y
Immediate delivery time	Y	Y & N	Y	N
Quick preparation time	Y	N	Y	N
Formality required	S	S	N	Y
Thought required	S	Y	S	Y
Reusability	Y	N	Y	Y
Permanent record	N	S	Y	Y
Non-verbal cues present	S	Y	N	N
Legally binding	S	S	Y	Y
Availability	Y	S	S	Y
Reliability	Y	S	S	Y
Security	S	N	N	Y
Privacy	Y	N	N	Y

TABLE 18.1 Key: Y = definitely a characteristic; S = sometimes a characteristic, depending on the situation; N = not usually a characteristic.

health services adopt practices that increase efficiency and improve outcomes. Thus, many are adopting electronic methods for storing and accessing records, sharing techniques, and communicating within and beyond the health service (i.e. internal and external email) (Brill & Levine 2005). Many health services and professions promote electronic forms of networking for support and professional development of employees (Ellis et al 2004). However, the nature of the health professions suggests that direct personal contact will always be a necessary component of remote communication.

GROUP REFLECTION AND DEBATE

Explain why the following statement is or is not so:
'Direct personal contact is a necessary component of remote communication.'

There is discussion about the 'paperless' modes of communicating because some health professionals still prefer hard copies of information (Purtilo & Haddad 2002). It is interesting but difficult to predict the preferred form of remote communication for the health professionals of the future.

Principles that govern professional remote communication

There are important principles that govern remote communication among health professionals (see Table 18.2). These principles relate directly to the characteristics of an effective health professional (see Ch 6), but are sometimes forgotten in remote (especially email) forms of communication (Devito 2007, Ellis et al 2004, Higgs et al 2005, Mohan et al 2004, Tyler et al 2005).

Principles that govern professional remote communication	
Use:*	Avoid:*
• Polite forms of words and constructions • Formal language and expression • Clear explanations of any jargon or technical terms** • Correct spelling and grammar – always check before sending • Concise, accurate and clear statements – one idea to one sentence	• Abrupt, impolite messages • Colloquial or everyday expressions • Unexplained use of jargon • Spelling and grammatical errors • Long and rambling sentences

TABLE 18.2 *While 'use' and 'avoid' statements are repetitive and directive, they attempt to clarify meaning and avoid misunderstandings. **Technical terms are words that may have one meaning in everyday use but assume a different meaning in the context of professional communication.

The principles governing remote communication are especially important in health services that do not have support personnel to assist with preparation of documents. When individual health professionals compose and prepare written forms of remote communication, it is beneficial to ask a colleague to proofread the document (for spelling and grammatical errors, appropriate levels of civility and formality, and clarity and accuracy) before sending.

These principles or 'points to remember' govern all types of remote communication. In combination with these principles, the following strategies guide the use of the types of remote communication commonly used within the health professions.

Documentation: Written reports, medical records and letters

Consider the audience/reader

When writing in the health professions it is essential to consider who will read the completed document. If a report or letter is for several 'audiences' it is appropriate to use language and constructions suited to the individual least familiar with the health professions. Thus, if a specialist and the person seeking assistance will both receive copies of a document, it is important to explain all jargon and technical terms. If the document will be read only by other health professionals it is beneficial to explain only those terms that are not commonly known or are specific to a particular health profession. It is important to remember that some medical records may be required in court.

Abbreviations

Abbreviations commonly occur in documents in the health professions because they reduce the time required to complete a report or entry. Abbreviations specific to the health professions are common in medical records (e.g. Ax = assessment, Rx = treatment). It is important to use only commonly known abbreviations. Different health services may use variations of such abbreviations. Some have prepared lists to be used by employees of that health service and thus it is important to become familiar with the abbreviations specific to a particular health service. Not all abbreviations used will be specific to the health professions. A common form of abbreviation not restricted to use in the health professions is an acronym (e.g. CMC). When using an acronym it is essential to also write the full meaning of the letters the first time the acronym appears. In some cases health professionals can invent previously unknown acronyms (e.g. therapeutic use of self = TUOS) and thus it is important to document such meanings clearly.

Formatting

It is important to comply with the requirements of the particular health service when formatting any written document. A report or letter should be printed on the letterhead of the health service. The advantage of this convention is that the contact details of the service will automatically be included on the paper. Reports and letters should include

- The date
- A salutation (e.g. *Dear.......*); use the family name of the person to avoid offence
- A clear reason for the letter (e.g. *Re: Name of person or reason*) before the first paragraph – something to draw the attention and focus of the recipient (Mohan et al 2004)
- A clear statement of the reason for the letter or report in the first paragraph
- Well-organised points. Separate each new point into paragraphs or use bullet points or numbers to make the report or letter easy to read. Use examples of behaviours or needs to validate and verify the stated points (Higgs et al 2005).
- A concluding paragraph that indicates required future action or details of future events
- An appropriate signature related to the tone of the letter (e.g. *Yours sincerely, Thanking you*).

Points to remember

- It is important to distinguish between fact and opinion in all written records. The results of a standardised assessment tool do not require qualification, however, it is important to use appropriate words to indicate the recording of opinion based upon observation (e.g. *It appears…, It seems…*).
- Do not forget to read, correct and photocopy all reports and letters before sending them.
- Remember to sign a letter before sending it.

Databases

Many health services use electronic forms of notes, records and files (databases) for recording information about the people seeking assistance. It is important that the health professional learns and conforms to the expectations and requirements of the health service regarding databases. It is also important for the health professional to remember the principles for recording information presented in this chapter.

Telephones

A telephone conversation allows the use of suprasegmentals – the non-verbal features of the voice – for negotiation of meaning. It is best to avoid using the telephone to deliver bad news, explain a complicated procedure or solve a complicated problem (Purtilo & Haddad 2002). There are important strategies that will assist in the achievement of effective telephone communication.

Strategies for using a telephone

- Prepare for the call – gather all appropriate documents, a pen and a piece of paper or diary before making the call.
- It may be beneficial to compile a list of points (checklist) for coverage during the call to avoid wasting time.
- State your name and place of work, the purpose of the call and the name of the required person for the conversation.
- Exercise patience if there is a delay in locating the required person; it may be helpful to do something that is not demanding while waiting. When connected, ensure the delay does not affect your attitude or tone of voice (Mohan et al 2004). (If receiving a call apologise for any delay caused and maintain pleasant responses if the caller is a little impatient.)
- If the person is unknown it is advisable to begin with a formal tone and reduce the formality with the development of rapport.
- Articulate carefully to produce clear speech.
- Avoid talking when the other person is talking.
- Clarify all points and confirm understanding of important points.
- Listen carefully.
- Give feedback to indicate understanding, whether agreement or otherwise.
- Remember there is only the voice to influence meaning and therefore the conversation may require verbalisation of any non-verbal behaviour (Ellis et al 2004, Mohan et al 2004).
- Allow time for discussion of additional points if required by the other person.
- Remember to thank the person when finished and say goodbye.
- It may be important to provide written confirmation of the conversation (Mohan et al 2004).

Strategies for using an answering service or voice mail

When leaving a telephone message it is important to

- State your name and place of work, the purpose of the call and the name of the required person for the message. State the return phone number carefully – perhaps twice – to allow easy transcription of the message (Mohan et al 2004).
- Articulate carefully to produce clear speech.
- Avoid speaking rapidly or running words together.

When receiving a recorded telephone message it is important to

- Write the message in a particular place (e.g. diary or phone message book). Avoid pieces of paper because they are easily lost.
- Phone the person to indicate receipt of the message (Purtilo & Haddad 2002). Indicate action taken by marking the received message in some manner.

Video/teleconferencing

Video/teleconferencing involves the use of technical devices that allow either a simultaneous video or telephone connection for multiple people from multiple sites. These connections allow communication without individuals leaving their workplace (Ellis et al 2004). A teleconference is not particularly anxiety provoking because it simply requires people to sit and talk. However, a videoconference uses a camera and this can produce consternation for some individuals. Such consternation usually reduces with exposure to the videoconferencing process.

Benefits

Video/teleconferencing is beneficial for

- Networking
- Health professionals in remote settings
- Saving time
- Reducing travel costs
- Allowing non-verbal behaviours to establish meaning
- Sharing ideas with previously inaccessible individuals
- Receiving assistance for problem solving
- Sharing new procedures with remote sites.

Strategies for using video/teleconferencing

- When conducting a video/teleconference introduce each site. If the interacting individuals are unknown to each other, allow time for the individuals to introduce themselves and their roles. If the individuals are known, name those present and restrict introductory details to new people.
- When conducting a teleconference remember to have the individuals identify themselves each time they speak.
- When conducting a videoconference it is essential to include all the connected sites in the discussion and the presentation of ideas or procedures.
  - Ask for confirmation of visual, auditory and cognitive understanding.
  - Ask for comments or questions from all sites.
- When conducting a videoconference it is important to repeat anything not in range of the microphone. This is especially important during question time.
- When finishing a video/teleconference say goodbye to each site separately.

The internet

Email

People often forget that email is neither private nor secure (Brill & Levine 2005). It is possible to forward any email anywhere. As an email passes through a server, a copy appears on that server. There are also problems of access relating to email. Not all sites or individuals have the technology for email, and such technology may be unreliable.

Despite these drawbacks, people often prefer email because it allows the sender and receiver control of their time and ideas (Tyler et al 2005). There are important strategies and 'points to remember' that will assist in the achievement of effective email communication.

- Decide on the purpose of the email.
- Use the appropriate tone for the audience; the tone and content of professional emails should be different to that of personal emails (Mohan et al 2004).
- Remember that every email is a legal document.
- Include a title in the subject box. The title indicates the content of the email and can capture the attention of the recipient.
- Use a salutation (e.g. *Dear.....*). The use of a given name will depend upon the purpose of the email and the relationship with the recipient. Use *Hi.....* thoughtfully in professional emails.
- Use well-constructed sentences to assist the person reading the email.
- Explain critical comments carefully and politely.
- Use careful constructions to avoid appearing abrupt and even rude (Devito 2007).
- Use careful constructions to avoid ambiguity (Tyler et al 2005).
- Describe any emotions because these are unseen (Higgs et al 2005).
- Describe any relevant non-verbal cues because these are also unseen.
- Avoid capital letters because they are considered equivalent to SHOUTING!
- Compose requests for clarification politely, giving reasons for the need for clarification (Higgs et al 2005).
- Avoid abbreviations (Higgs et al 2005) or emoticons (Devito 2007) in professional emails.
- Write what you mean and proofread before sending (Ellis et al 2004).
- Use a signature appropriate to the tone and purpose of the email (Tyler et al 2005). A computer-generated signature is beneficial for professional emails because it ensures that role, position and contact details accompany every sent email.
- Ensure the email is going to the right person before sending!
- Use an explanatory sentence when including an attachment to confirm the contents of the attachment.
- Reduce the size of large attachments by saving them in a compressed format. When creating or saving an attachment in a particular format remember that the recipient may not have the software required to access the attachment (Tyler et al 2005).
- Check for correct address if an email is undeliverable. Undeliverable emails may also mean that the inbox of the recipient is full.
- Reply to every email that is not a mass 'company' email; acknowledgement of receipt is polite and reassuring for the sender.

Email is convenient and in many cases immediate. It allows control and is beneficial in augmenting face-to-face contact with those who interact with the health professional (De Ville 2001). However, there are disadvantages that require careful consideration when using the email form of remote communication.

ACTIVITY

- Using the above bullet points, compile a list of advantages and disadvantages of using email.
- Suggest realistic ways of overcoming the disadvantages.

Search engines

The use of search engines to locate information and practice-related research is common in the health professions where there is appropriate technology. The value of a search engine lies in the number of websites to which it can connect the searching individual. Locating the required websites can be frustrating until an appropriate word or combination of words typed into the search engine provides a satisfactory connection. It is important to consider the reliability of a website when sourcing information from that site (Tyler et al 2005). It is relatively simple to construct a website and thus there are multitudinous websites with particular agendas and biases. When seeking evidence for practice or assessment tasks it is possible to access websites that are less than reliable and not always reputable. Thus it is important for health professionals and students to exercise care when using any information obtained from a website.

Professional chat rooms

There are particular protocols that govern all internet-based chat rooms; the basis of these protocols is a desire for and commitment to respectful communication. Professional chat rooms allow worldwide exploration of alternative protocols, procedures and management strategies. When relating to health professionals from other cultures through chat rooms it is important to remember the factors affecting culturally appropriate communication (see Chs 15 & 16).

Chapter summary

Remote communication is a permanent fixture in the health professions. There are both advantages and disadvantages that require consideration when using remote communication. It is important for health professionals to use remote forms of communication appropriately and politely to benefit from the advantages.

Answer the following:
1. Using your own words define remote communication.

_____

_____

_____

2. List the types of remote communication typically used among health professionals.

_____

_____

_____

3. State the advantages of remote communication.

_____

_____

_____

4. Suggest ways of overcoming the disadvantages of remote communication.

_____

_____

_____

5. Focus upon written documents:
   - Explain why it is important to consider the recipient of written information.

     _____

     _____

     _____

   - Provide original examples of the two major types of abbreviations.

     i. _____

     ii. _____

   - Outline an effective written report or letter.

     _____

     _____

     _____

   - List the things to remember before sending a report.

     _____

     _____

     _____

6. Focus upon using a telephone:
   - What is important when preparing to communicate professionally over the telephone?

     _____

     _____

     _____

   - Briefly, describe an effective telephone conversation.

     _____

     _____

     _____

   - List the things to remember when using an answering service.

     _____

     _____

     _____

7. Focus upon video/teleconferencing:
   - Outline the benefits of video/teleconferencing.

     _____

     _____

     _____

   - Briefly, describe an effective videoconference.

     _____

     _____

     _____

8. Focus upon email: Categorise each point listed in the 'Email' section of this chapter into one of three categories:

Civility	Practicality	Reality

References

Brill N I, Levine J 2005 Working with people: the helping process, 8th edn. Pearson, Boston

Devito J A 2007 The interpersonal communication book, 11th edn. Pearson, Boston

De Ville K A 2001 Ethical and legal implications of e-mail correspondence between physicians and patients. Ethics Health Care 4(1):1–3

Ellis R B, Gates B, Kenworthy N 2004 Interpersonal communication in nursing, theory and practice. Elsevier, London

Higgs J, Sefton A, Street A et al 2005 Communicating in the health and social sciences. Oxford University Press, Melbourne

Mohan T, McGregor H, Saunders S et al 2004 Communicating as professionals. Thomson, Melbourne

Purtilo R B, Haddad A 2002 Health professional and patient interaction, 6th edn. Saunders, Philadelphia

Tyler S, Kossen C, Ryan C 2005 Communication: a foundation course, 2nd edn. Pearson, Prentice Hall, Frenchs Forest, Sydney

FOUR

THE FOCUS OF COMMUNICATION IN THE HEALTH PROFESSIONS: PEOPLE

Introduction

Most government health departments list the rights of people seeking assistance from health services, including the right to experience effective communication. The *Communication Bill of Rights* (www.scopevic.org.au) developed in Victoria, Australia, is an example of a document about this right. While this bill is introduced in the context of communication with people who have a hearing or intellectual impairment, it is applicable to all people regardless of their abilities, race, gender, status, religion, sexual orientation, condition, emotions, stage of life and role. There are various versions of a communication bill of rights in different countries and hemispheres.

In the health professions the rights of every communicator are based upon the steps that contribute to family/person-centred practice (see Ch 2). They include the right to understand and be understood, express, learn, choose, interact and contribute, along with the right to say *no*. Health professionals will practise according to these rights if they conform to the code of conduct relevant to their particular health profession or to the relevant government health department (see Ch 11).

The aim of Section Four is application of knowledge and consolidation of the skills required by health professionals for effective communication. This section can facilitate exploration and application of the principles and skills discussed in the first three sections of this book.

Health professionals communicate with people from diverse backgrounds who have multifaceted issues and varying needs. There are basic elements of healthcare that provide the foundation for dealing with any person a health professional might see in a working week (see Figure 2.4). These practices should be familiar at this stage in the book and are hopefully like 'old friends' to anyone intending to be a committed health professional who practises effective communication.

A health professional must consider the whole person including the environmental constraints on the person. People seeking assistance may experience factors that require particular consideration to ensure effective communication; these are i) strong emotions; ii) stages of the lifespan; iii) particular roles; iv) particular conditions; and v) particular contexts.

This section examines the factors of strong emotions, stages of the lifespan, particular roles, particular conditions and particular contexts in terms of

- The meaning of these factors
- The behaviours related to these factors
- The individuals most susceptible to these factors
- The emotions typically associated with these factors, which can precipitate difficulties when relating to a health service
- Possible reasons for these emotions
- Principles to remember when communicating with people who have these particular factors
- Suggestions for ways to communicate with such people
- Scenarios, which allow role-playing, discussion, and development of strategies for communicating with people experiencing these factors.

Small group activity

Exploration of Chapters 19–23 should begin with around 15 minutes of small group discussion that considers the points listed above in relation to the topic of the chapter (e.g. strong emotions). The group can later note any extra information learnt while working through the chapter.

Scenarios

Section Four contains twenty different scenarios that represent typical people and situations a health professional may encounter in their practice. When considered in depth, these scenarios can prepare the health professional for practising effective communication in similar situations. Each scenario presents guidelines for exploration during problem-based tutorials or group discussions.

Each section within Chapters 19–23 concludes with two scenarios, one considering each gender. Most scenarios can be examined through role plays; however, discussion points have been included for scenarios in which it seems inappropriate or difficult to play the roles. The contributions of group members can be invaluable if they are comfortable to share their knowledge and experience. The role plays or discussion points should occur after exploration of the scenarios to ensure participants are well informed and able to relate to the details of the scenarios.

Procedure if using role plays

- In small groups assign the roles to group members and role-play at least one of the scenarios.
- The people playing the roles consider the communication strategies that will best achieve effective communication.
- The observers note the
  - Words used and their effects
  - Non-verbal behaviours of all communicators and their effects
  - Style of communication used and the effects
  - Characteristics of communication that were the most effective.
- Then, as a group
  - Discuss the results, noting both successes and elements that require improvement. Check that the 'actors' were aware of their non-verbal behaviours.
  - Note whether different people interpreted the non-verbal behaviours and the effects of communication differently. Discuss the implications of any variations in interpretation.
  - Consider the feelings of each person in the role play. Explore what caused their feelings. If the feelings were resolved, consider what caused this resolution.
  - If possible, repeat the role play with different people playing the roles until everyone has played the person seeking assistance.
- When everyone who desires to participate has completed the role play, discuss and devise strategies to assist effective communication in a similar situation.

Procedure if using discussion points

- Establish the meaning of jargon-specific words before the discussion.
- Decide the most appropriate course of action for the health professional.
- Together devise strategies that will assist effective communication in a similar situation.
- Small groups might discuss one scenario and then share their ideas with a group that has discussed a different scenario.

To conclude the exploration of each scenario it may be useful to summarise in point form the appropriate strategies for communicating with a person experiencing the particular emotion, stage of the lifespan, role, condition or context.

Note: The scenarios are fictitious and thus if any of the scenarios cause discomfort and emotions of identification it is essential to seek assistance and resolution. Resolution of discomfort will ensure a consistent ability to provide the best care for both 'self' and those who seek assistance.

Reference

Compic & Scope. Communication Bill of Rights. CAN 004 280871. Communication Resource Centre, Compic, Scope, Box Hill, Melbourne. Available: www.scopevic.org.au/bill%20of%20 rights.pdf 26 Mar 2008

People experiencing strong emotions

19

Health professionals assist vulnerable people who experience a range of emotions. This chapter considers three strong emotions that may be a barrier to effective communication: **aggression**, **extreme distress** and **reluctance to engage or be involved in communication or intervention**.

SMALL GROUP ACTIVITY: STRONG EMOTIONS

Aggression
Extreme distress
Reluctance to engage or be involved in communication or intervention

- Decide what it means to be experiencing these strong emotions.
- List the specific behaviours that might indicate the presence of these strong emotions.
- List the individuals most susceptible to feeling these strong emotions.
- Decide the possible events or environments that might produce the strong emotions and explain why.
- List principles for effective communication to remember when communicating with a person experiencing these strong emotions. Give reasons for the need to remember these principles.
- Suggest strategies for communicating with a person who is experiencing these strong emotions. Decide why you might see such a person in your particular health profession.
- Check your answers against the information below, noting any additional thoughts or ideas.

A person who behaves aggressively

(Key words: aggressive, assertive, violent, angry)

Definition of aggression

Consider anger at one end of a continuum and violence at the other end, with aggressive behaviour in between. A person who behaves aggressively may demonstrate anger initially and violence ultimately.

A person who behaves aggressively is someone who

- Exhibits apparently unprovoked behaviours that threaten those around them
- Feels vulnerable and out of control
- Wants their 'own way' and will intimidate or threaten to fulfil their desires
- May confuse aggression with assertion
- May believe aggressive behaviour is the only way they can 'win' or achieve their desired results
- … and so on (this list is not exhaustive).

Behaviours related to aggression

An aggressive person might

- Be verbally abusive and loud when interacting
- Threaten (verbally or in writing) to physically harm someone or something
- Use non-verbal gestures to indicate feelings of aggression.

Individuals most susceptible to behaving aggressively

A common belief suggests that individuals who behave aggressively are found mostly in mental health settings. This is not always true because aggressive behaviour can occur anywhere.

Individuals may be susceptible to behaving aggressively because of

- Eroded self-esteem
- Emotional trauma (e.g. disappointment, loss, frustration, bewilderment)
- Unresolved anger or frustration
- Stress
- Unfulfilled desires.

People who behave aggressively may have an emotional reason (e.g. unfulfilled desires) to which they respond with aggressive behaviour. However, such people do not always behave aggressively in the environment that provides the trigger for their emotions.

Possible stimuli for aggression

Individuals may become aggressive due to

- Loss of something important (e.g. family, job, health)
- Unexpected events
- Excessive use of addictive substances or withdrawal from addictive substances
- Reaction to medication

- Chronic pain
- Forgetting to take or deciding not to take medication.

Principles for effective communication with a person who behaves aggressively

When communicating with a person who behaves aggressively it is important to

- Respond with patience and understanding
- Empathise with the person, not necessarily with their feelings
- Use active listening and careful observation
- If appropriate, focus on the problem and possible solutions
- Avoid responding to the aggressive statements or threats with aggression – do not retaliate
- Demonstrate interest, attention and concern through non-verbal behaviours
- Remember the principles of assertive communication (see Ch 14); however, some people may become more aggressive if you attempt to discuss what they are expressing at that time
- Validate if appropriate
- Avoid confronting if they are violent
- Always remember safety of self and others
- Position self closest to the door
- Use emergency call buttons or duress alarms if necessary and available.

If there is a risk of violent behaviour it is important to

- Inform the immediate supervisor of the possible risk
- Wherever possible have another health professional present
- Ensure the health service knows the exact whereabouts of the health professionals who work with the person, whether on or off site
- Plan the interaction carefully considering the safety of all involved individuals
- Be alert for the safety of everyone involved and if necessary remove self and others from the scene
- Stay close to the door or exit
- Avoid attempting to physically connect with the person
- Call the police if necessary.

Strategies for communicating with a person who behaves aggressively

- Remain calm to maximise observation and problem-solving skills.
- Ask them to 'tell you their story' to explain their strong emotions. This may allow them to calm themselves.
- If the person is still in control, state they are being inappropriately aggressive. This may stop the behaviour, potentially providing an opportunity to become calm.
- Be aware of non-verbal behaviours and remove yourself if the person is becoming overly agitated. Among group members, brainstorm ways to respond verbally so you can remove yourself safely.
- Engage the person in consideration of their plans for the future and how they might fulfil these plans.

ROLE PLAYS

Role-play the following scenarios. Before acting the roles you may wish to decide what type of assistance Person 1 requires. If it is not possible to role-play these scenarios, consider and explore the possible responses and communication strategies that will achieve effective communication and family/person-centred practice.

Scenario one: The male and the health professional

Person 1: Your name is John. You are a 35-year-old man who had an accident at work 5 years ago. You have been experiencing chronic lower back pain since that time. You were on modified duties for 2 years and have not been employed full-time during the past 3 years. You have seen four doctors and several physiotherapists, chiropractors, podiatrists, massage therapists and rehabilitation providers. You are very frustrated and fail to see how this recent referral will achieve anything different. You feel your divorce a year ago was a result of your pain over the past 5 years. You want to see more of your two children but your pain makes this difficult.

Person 2: You are the health professional. The referral indicates this man is prone to aggressive behaviour. You want to avoid aggressive behaviour in order to develop a therapeutic relationship and some appropriate goals.

Scenario two: The female and the health professional

Person 1: Your name is Jessi. You are a 16-year-old girl who always passively allows other people to have what they want, regardless of what you may want. You do this because you desperately want to have a 'place' in a particular group at school. However, now you cannot control the emotions resulting from repeated hurt, frustration and bewilderment because of your non-assertive responses to those around you. You now respond aggressively to everyone, even your closest friends and family.

Person 2: You are a health professional doing a routine assessment/check-up with Jessi. Her responses are aggressive and rude.

- How should you complete the check-up?

GROUP DISCUSSION

As a large group discuss the observations, emotions and outcomes of the role plays. Suggest possible alternative strategies that may increase the effectiveness of the communication in a similar situation.

A person who experiences extreme distress

(Key words: overwhelming emotion, fear, anxiety, grief, frustration)

Definition of extreme distress

An extremely distressed person is someone who is experiencing overwhelming negative emotions including sadness, anxiety, fear and loss.

Behaviours related to extreme distress

An extremely distressed person might

- Express the depth of their emotions silently through non-verbal behaviours
- Express emotion uncontrollably through paralinguistic means (e.g. crying or sobbing)
- Withdraw from contact with others, depending on their personality.

Individuals most susceptible to extreme distress

Individuals may be susceptible to extreme distress because of

- Strong emotions, including fear, anxiety and grief
- Chronic situations such as war
- Conditions such as chronic arthritis or chronic pain that cause strong emotions
- Post-traumatic stress disorder
- Loss, including loss of control over their circumstances.

Possible stimuli for extreme distress

Individuals may become extremely distressed due to

- The impending death of a child, sibling, spouse or parent
- An accident
- An attack
- Physical or psychological abuse.

Remember there are cultural variations in the expression of emotion. A particular culture might consider extreme emotional expression to be an appropriate response to something that another culture might consider a minor event.

Principles for effective communication with a person who is extremely distressed

When communicating with a person who is extremely distressed it is important to

- Empathise and validate
- Listen actively – encourage them to say whatever they need to say
- Be silent if appropriate
- Comfort in an affirming and encouraging way that does not fulfil the needs of the health professional.

Strategies for communicating with a person who is extremely distressed

- Be willing to sit in empathic silence.
- Avoid mind-reading.
- Be aware of the use of touch.
- Consider whether gender-specific care might be important (i.e. male to male and female to female).
- If a young person, remember environmental factors (see Ch 8) when communicating. Young people are often more susceptible to situations that cause distress and can have less ability to control their emotions if distressed.
- If an indigenous person, involve an appropriate indigenous liaison officer.
- Remember to debrief confidentially if required to maintain 'self'.

ROLE PLAYS

Role-play the following scenarios. Before acting the roles you may wish to decide what type of assistance Person 1 requires. If it is not possible to role-play these scenarios, consider and explore the possible responses and communication strategies that will achieve effective communication and family/person-centred practice.

Scenario one: The male and the health professional

Person 1: Your name is David and you are a 40-year-old father of three children. Your eldest son is in the final stages of leukaemia. No-one really knows when he will die. The emotions you feel make it difficult to continue working and supporting your wife, who is also overwhelmed by the situation. You are extremely distressed but desperately trying to appear OK whenever you are with your son or with members of your immediate family. The energy involved in maintaining this appearance is exhausting, but you feel it is necessary. You are now sitting in a waiting area, waiting to see a health professional for an unrelated reason. Although it is only 8.30 a.m. you can only sit with your head in your hands. You would really like to cry, but are not accustomed to crying in public places.

Person 2: You are the health professional. You have a busy day ahead and the first person for the day is someone who is new to your service. When you enter the waiting area and see a man sitting with his head in his hands, you wonder what is wrong and why he looks like that at 8.30 a.m. You wonder whether this person works night shifts or is unwell. You discover this man is the person you are scheduled to see. How will you respond?

Scenario two: The female and the respite volunteer

Person 1: Your name is Cindy. You are a 14-year-old girl who watched your father try to murder your mother a few months ago. Your father is now in prison, your mother is in hospital with fractured C3 & C4 vertebrae and your grandparents live in the UK. The foster family you currently live with are caring, but you miss your mother. You visit her in hospital daily and she always appears pleased to see you, but she is not able to relate to you because of immobility, pain and emotional shock. Whenever you try to sleep at night you see the attempted murder scene all over again and usually cry yourself to sleep. At school you keep to yourself because you do not want anyone except the principal and two teachers to know. You find your situation embarrassing because anything makes you burst into tears. Therefore you isolate yourself, which means you try to keep control of yourself by avoiding relating to anyone.

↳

Person 2: You are a trained volunteer assigned to give foster families respite. You usually enjoy this role and develop very good relationships with the adolescents for whom you provide respite. However, Cindy is very difficult to relate to – she is either emotionally withdrawn or crying whenever you are with her. The foster family indicate they feel this experience is not the first distressing experience for Cindy, but she will not talk to them about her previous life. You have a day scheduled with her and want to find out what she wants to do with the day.

GROUP DISCUSSION

As a large group discuss the observations, emotions and outcomes of the role plays. Suggest possible alternative strategies that may increase the effectiveness of the communication in a similar situation.

Some health services offer services for distressed people and thus the health professionals working in such services will often encounter extremely distressed people. However, it is possible for all health professionals to encounter distressed people in the course of their working life, regardless of the particular context of the health professional. When relating to such people it is challenging but essential to communicate in a manner that fulfils the needs of the individual(s) and considers all the people communicating.

A person who is reluctant to engage or be involved in communication or intervention

(Key words: uncertain, avoidant, reluctant, resistant)

Definition of reluctance to engage

A person who is reluctant to engage or be involved is someone who is
* Unwilling to be or do in a particular situation, environment or context
* Unsure about the situation, environment or context
* Unsure about something particular in the situation, environment or context
* Unsure about someone in the situation, environment or context.

Behaviours related to feeling reluctant to engage

A person who is reluctant to engage or be involved might

* Verbally refuse to engage, be involved or collaborate
* Deny there is a problem
* Take action that appears cooperative, but resist non-verbally
* Express themselves through aggression and sometimes violence
* Avoid looking at the health professional by turning their head away
* Withdraw as far from the health professional as possible.

Individuals most susceptible to feeling reluctant to engage

Individuals who may be susceptible to feeling reluctant to engage or be involved include

* Children
* The elderly
* Individuals scheduled for complicated procedures
* Individuals attending a health service for the first time
* Individuals who are unfamiliar with something or someone in the health service
* Individuals with inability in some area(s).

Possible stimuli for reluctance to engage

Individuals may be reluctant to engage or be involved due to

* Unfamiliarity with the situation, environment or context, which creates apprehension
* Feeling afraid about possible events in the situation, environment or context
* Previous experience of negative emotions in that particular situation, environment or context, or in a similar one
* Experiencing pain or discomfort and that causes reluctance to move
* Not being in the situation, environment or context by choice, but because i) of an emergency or forced admission (Community Treatment Order) into a mental health institution or ii) their family might be 'pushy'
* Not accepting their need
* Feeling unsure about the expectations of the situation, environment or context
* Not understanding what they are being asked to do or say

- Not understanding the particular role or expectations of the health professional
- Feeling they are unable to perform the required tasks or requested actions
- Being physically unable to perform the required tasks or requested actions.

In common with all people requiring assistance from a health professional, people who feel reluctant are feeling vulnerable for many different reasons.

Principles for effective communication with a person who is reluctant to engage

When communicating with a person who is reluctant to engage or be involved it is important to

- Make introductions
- Listen actively
- Validate
- Question sensitively
- Provide information
- Confront false beliefs and attitudes (if appropriate) to emphasise reality.

Strategies for communicating with a person who is reluctant to engage

- Remain calm.
- Check they understand the language you are speaking.
- Consider your non-verbal behaviours – avoid overbearing or intimidating body language.
- Clearly explain the reasons why something is happening.
- Clearly explain the expectations or expected events.
- Ask if they do or do not want something and if possible do that to reassure them.
- If violent, indicate their behaviour is inappropriate and call for assistance.

ROLE PLAYS

Role-play the following scenarios. Before acting the roles you may wish to decide what type of assistance Person 1 requires. If it is not possible to role-play these scenarios, consider and explore the possible responses and communication strategies that will achieve effective communication and family/person-centred practice.

Scenario one: The male and the health professional

Note: When working with children it is important to remember that the parents and siblings are part of their environment and thus must be considered when gathering information. The parent is usually the expert in terms of knowledge about the skills and behaviour of their child.

Person 1: You are a 10-year-old boy called Carl and you need assistance from a health professional. As you arrive with your mother for the first appointment you are reminded of the last time you went to see a health professional. That person was not friendly – they kept talking to your mother not to you and they hurt you. You do not want to relate to the health professional because they look just the same as the last one. You stand behind your mother and cling to her, hiding your face in her back. You refuse to look at the health professional or respond to any of their attempts to talk with you.

Person 2: You are Carl's mother. You are very surprised at Carl's behaviour because he does not usually behave like this and you have no idea why he is clinging to you. You have no idea how to respond to promote a relationship between Carl and the health professional.

Person 3: You are the health professional. You know 10-year-old boys do not usually relate in this manner and you would like to tell him to 'get over it' and act his age! However, you remember the three steps in effective communication and wish to apply these to this boy and his mother who are seeking your assistance.

Scenario two: The female and the health professional

Person 1: You are a 79-year-old lady who prefers to be called Mrs Jones. You love attending for treatment and try to be very cooperative despite the discomfort you sometimes feel because of the treatment. You often require assistance to find the toilet and are easily disoriented when trying to find the exit after treatment. One day you could not actually find your car in the parking lot. You are anxious to hide the fact that you have been experiencing more confusion lately because you do not want to be made to leave your home, where you have lived for 30 years. You always say you are fine when you are at home – that there really is not a problem – whenever the health professionals suggest they contact the home care organisation. You do not want anyone in your house – you just want to be able to stay there and be independent.

Person 2: You are the health professional. You have noted the regular disorientation Mrs Jones exhibits when attending for treatment. You note that Mrs Jones appears to take pride in her appearance because she is always clean and well dressed. But you are wondering whether her appearance is an attempt to pretend that things are OK. You are concerned about her safety and think Mrs Jones might require some assistance at home. You ask her if she would like you to contact the appropriate organisation to arrange some assistance with cleaning and meals at home.

GROUP DISCUSSION

As a large group discuss the observations, emotions and outcomes of the role plays. Suggest possible alternative strategies that may increase the effectiveness of the communication in a similar situation.

There are many reasons for reluctance to engage on the part of the person seeking assistance. A health professional may require more than a warm, friendly persona to achieve positive outcomes. The health professional may require specific communication skills and strategies to encourage the person who is reluctant to engage in order to achieve family/person-centred practice.

People in particular stages of the lifespan

20

CHAPTER OBJECTIVE

Upon completing this chapter, students should be able to apply knowledge and consolidate the required skills to communicate effectively with people in three particular stages of the lifespan.

People who represent three of the different stages of the lifespan – **children**, **adolescents** and **people who are older** – present with particular attitudes and associated needs. When assisting people in these stages of life it is important to remember the abilities and events that are typical of these stages.

SMALL GROUP ACTIVITY: STAGES OF THE LIFESPAN

Children
Adolescents
People who are older

- Define these stages of the lifespan.
- List some of the specific behaviours that might occur during these stages of life.
- List the individuals most susceptible to experiencing difficulty when seeking assistance from a health service during these stages of life.
- List possible negative emotions someone in these stages of life might experience when seeing a health professional and explain why.
- List principles for effective communication to remember when communicating with a person in these stages of life. Give reasons for the need to remember these principles.
- Suggest strategies for communicating with a person who is in these stages of life and experiencing issues related to that stage. Decide why you might see such a person in your particular health profession.
- Check your answers against the information below, noting any additional thoughts or ideas.

A child

(Key words: child, children, childhood, dependent, under-age)

When assisting children it is essential to remember the parent is the expert about the child. They are familiar with the skills and abilities of the child and if they indicate the child can do something you do not witness, they will probably be correct. It is important to avoid talking about children when they are present. Whether the child can understand the words or not, they are able to understand non-verbal cues and thus will respond with an appropriate emotion or behaviour.

Definition of a child

For the purpose of this chapter, a child is a person aged 0–16 years.

Behaviours related to being a child

The behaviour of a child will depend on their age, their personality, their culture, the experiences of their upbringing, the stability at home, their sense of security, the reason for the referral and the presence of a significant adult.

A child might be

- Quiet and non-engaging
- Shy and hiding
- Crying and clinging
- Happy but initially untrusting
- Looking to their parent for assurance
- Angry and aggressive
- Curious and wanting to explore.

Children most susceptible to experiencing difficulties when attending a health service

Children susceptible to experiencing difficulties when attending a health service include those who

- Have a history of experiencing trauma
- Are very young and are not accustomed to separating from a parent
- Are from a different cultural background
- Are unfamiliar with healthcare settings
- Are experiencing physical or emotional pain
- Are very ill
- Have a previous negative experience with a health professional
- Are a victim of an accident, attack or natural disaster
- Have communication difficulties
- Have a visual or auditory impairment.

Possible emotions a child might experience

A child might experience emotions related to

- Fear and anxiety
- Physical or emotional 'pain' from any source, causing frustration and despondency
- Boredom
- Isolation and displacement
- Awareness that they are different to other children
- Lack of familiarity with the environment, people and procedures, causing uncertainty and discomfort
- Difficulties at home, school or in the neighbourhood.

Principles for effective communication with a child

When communicating with a child it is important to

- Make introductions
- Demonstrate empathy
- Carefully observe the responses of the child
- Validate their perceptions (it may be necessary to validate the perceptions of the parent if the child is unable to validate)
- Make appropriate use of non-verbal behaviour – if there is no common language, non-verbal or visual communication is essential to develop rapport and a therapeutic relationship
- Monitor the language level – use simple explanations and indicate upcoming events
- Touch only if appropriate
- Establish boundaries and expectations for behaviour
- Relate consistently with consistent expectations
- Practise holistic communication
- Disengage
- Ensure family-centred practice.

Strategies for communicating with a child

- Talk directly to the child.
- Avoid talking about the child with the child present.
- Explore toys and activities that are meaningful to the child and use them to engage, comfort and relax the child.
- Provide a safe environment.
- Understand the culture of the child.
- Understand the familial, developmental, social, physical, cognitive, cultural and spiritual background of the child.
- Tell the child what will happen and when it will happen. Give adequate warning about when the session will finish to facilitate smooth transition from the completion of the session to leaving the room.
- Respond to the non-verbal behaviours of the child with verbal questions or reflective comments about the observations.
- Avoid touching the child wherever possible or ask permission to touch the child from the child and the parent.
- Avoid distractions and use silence if appropriate to encourage concentration and focus.

ROLE PLAYS

Role-play the following scenarios. Before acting the roles you may wish to decide what type of assistance Person 1 requires. If it is not possible to role-play these scenarios, consider and explore the possible responses and communication strategies that will achieve effective communication and family/person-centred practice.

Scenario one: The male and the trained volunteer

Person 1: You are Mohammad, a 12-year-old Sudanese boy whose family has taken refuge from the Sudan. You have learnt some English, but still do not understand many of the behaviours of those around you and you cannot read or write English yet. Your older brother was killed just before your family left the Sudan. Your father does not have a job yet and your mother works until late at night for little pay washing dishes in a Chinese takeaway shop. You do not feel accepted at school, even by the other Sudanese who have been there longer than you and often tease you in Arabic. Your little sister seems happy and has friends with whom she plays. You have been feeling angry and you have begun to verbally abuse teachers and the other boys from the Sudan at school. You do not enjoy relating to anyone other than your family.

Person 2: You are a trained volunteer for the local multicultural centre and you run a group for 'at-risk' boys with refugee status. This afternoon is the first time you will meet Mohammad. You know he is sometimes violent, but that is all you know. Many of the at-risk Sudanese boys are violent.

Scenario two: The female and the health professional

Person 1: Your name is Elise and your 2-year-old daughter, Jenny, has just been diagnosed with an intellectual disability. She is your only child and has been a joy to your immediate family. You are confused and unsure. You are afraid of the future and while you wait to see the health professional you become sad and teary. You watch Jenny play on the floor at your feet. What does this mean for her future? She is so beautiful and you had such wonderful plans for her future.

Person 2: You are the health professional who must assess Jenny's abilities. When you enter the waiting area you call Jenny's name and notice a woman flinch and look up. She smiles at you and lifts Jenny from the floor. How will you relate to Jenny and Elise in this initial session? What are your communication priorities?

- Elise does not want Jenny to leave her lap and nor does Jenny want to leave it. How will you encourage them both?

GROUP DISCUSSION

As a large group discuss the observations, emotions and outcomes of the role plays. Suggest possible alternative strategies that may increase the effectiveness of the communication in a similar situation.

Children are often the focus of a specialty health service. However, health professionals from many contexts may need to relate to children. It is both challenging and rewarding to work with children, for whom particular skills are required to ensure effective communication and family-centred practice.

Note: There are many groups and associations that provide information and support for parents of children with particular conditions (e.g. Autism Association, Royal Institute for Deaf and Blind Children).

An adolescent

(Key words: adolescence, adolescent, teenager)

Definition of an adolescent

An adolescent is someone who is

- A youth
- Between childhood and maturity
- Growing up or maturing
- Experiencing physical changes in their body that indicate development to maturity
- Experiencing emotional insecurity, social and cognitive challenges, and often spiritual independence.

The age of maturing varies depending on gender and ethnicity. In some cultures there are expectations of particular genders at a certain age. Once these expectations are met, the individual takes the role and responsibilities of an adult and is considered an adult in all aspects of their existence.

In most western cultures age determines the arrival of adulthood. Individuals regardless of gender assume some of the responsibilities of adulthood from 14 years onwards (e.g. paid employment at 14.9+ years, driving a car at 16–17 years) but are not considered adults until they reach 18–21 years (when they can purchase cigarettes and alcohol). It is not the emotional, intellectual and social maturity of the individual that officially indicates the arrival of adulthood, but rather age.

Behaviours related to being an adolescent

An adolescent may

- Engage in high-risk behaviours
- Exaggerate their actions (act out) to gain attention
- Withdraw and keep to themselves
- Behave in ways that create direct conflict with their values in order to maintain a position in a social group
- Be verbally abusive and argumentative
- Experiment with various substances
- Behave in a happy and carefree manner.

Adolescents most susceptible to experiencing difficulties when attending a health service

Adolescents susceptible to experiencing difficulties when attending a health service include those who

- Are different to their peer group
- Do not want to receive assistance from a health professional
- Are from a different cultural background
- Are unfamiliar with healthcare settings
- Have difficulties adjusting to the changes occurring in their body
- Experience physical or emotional pain

- Have a previous negative experience with a health professional
- Are a victim of an accident, attack or natural disaster
- Have a visual or auditory impairment
- Have an intellectual disability.

Possible emotions an adolescent might experience

Emotional responses in adolescents are complex and often unpredictable for both the individual and those around them. An adolescent may experience extremes of emotion including

- Anger
- Loneliness
- Confusion
- Isolation
- Restlessness
- Conflict and stress
- Dissatisfaction

- Feelings of inadequacy
- Hatred of their appearance
- Insecurity
- Anxiety
- Feelings of unimportance
- Boredom
- High energy.

Possible reasons for these emotions

An adolescent undergoes complex changes in their physical, emotional, cognitive, social and spiritual self during adolescence. An adolescent may experience extremes of emotion because of

- Hormones
- Social pressures
- School pressures
- Home pressures
- Cultural differences
- Focusing on their own needs
- A dominance of social needs
- Their friends.

Principles for effective communication with an adolescent

The principles of effective communication apply to all individuals seeking assistance. However, it may be more difficult to communicate using these principles when relating to an adolescent unless the health professional is aware of the needs of the adolescent and self-aware about the effects of their own experience of adolescence.

When communicating with an adolescent it is important to

- Be self-aware – of own experiences, values and beliefs
- Practise holistic communication
- Understand and be sensitive
- Demonstrate unconditional positive regard
- Demonstrate respect
- Adhere to ethical boundaries
- Accommodate cultural differences
- Confront inappropriate self-talk, values and beliefs
- Observe their non-verbal behaviours.

Strategies for communicating with an adolescent

- Aim at family/person-centred practice.
- Establish a safe environment, both emotionally and physically.
- Use of a holistic approach is vital because the physical symptoms may be covering underlying needs.
- Be aware of personal limitations – the health professional does not need to meet all the needs of every adolescent seeking their assistance.
- Relate consistently with consistent reactions and explanations.
- Be committed to and compassionate for the person, not necessarily their behaviour.
- Demonstrate understanding and interest through the use of activities the person finds meaningful.
- Be aware of the non-verbal behaviours of all individuals communicating.
- Explicitly state the expectations of behaviour.
- Establish clear boundaries.

ROLE PLAYS

Role-play the following scenarios. Before acting the roles you may wish to decide what type of assistance Person 1 requires. If it is not possible to role-play these scenarios, consider and explore the possible responses and communication strategies that will achieve effective communication and family/person-centred practice.

Scenario one: The male and the health professional

Person 1: Your name is Jake. You are 17 years old and in your final year at school. You have found adolescence difficult. It has been difficult to concentrate and therefore learn at school. You are not sure why your parents insisted you stay at school because you rarely pass your exams. The teachers do not really understand you and only one or two seem to care. You have some great friends and do outlandish things together – not life-threatening things, just 'out-there' fun things. Recent assessments indicate you have attention deficit-hyperactivity disorder (ADHD) and you have begun to take medication for this. You do not like the medication because although it makes you calm and gives you greater control, you no longer feel you are yourself. You love working outside in gardens and have begun working in the grounds of a local health service, mostly during your school holidays.

Person 2: You are a health professional who often has lunch in the grounds of the health service. You have begun chatting with one of the new grounds-people, Jake, and find he lacks confidence and a sense of self-worth. While this is typical of many adolescents, you feel there is more about Jake than typical adolescence. You have decided to befriend, encourage and affirm him so you often have lunch with Jake.

- Do you need to be able to encourage and affirm Jake? Why?
- How can you encourage and affirm him?

↳

Scenario two: The female and the health professional

Person 1: Your name is Ruth and you are a well-known local 15-year-old with a promising career in surfing. You are the leading junior female surfer in the country. You were excited when you signed a contract with an international surfing label for sponsorship and promotions. You are popular with teachers and students and your parents tell you often how proud they are of you. You have applied yourself at school and at the local surf club. You love surfing and at every opportunity you are at the beach on patrol or on your board.

In a recent and unusual shark attack you lost your right arm below the elbow. The experience was very traumatic, but you have other things to concern you. What about the contract you have with the surf label? And your surfing career – what happens now? You are devastated because surfing is your life and you cannot image surfing without your lower arm and hand. You were hoping to be school captain in a few years but think no-one would nominate someone without an arm. You are right-handed and you cannot image how you will ever write without your right hand. You are sure that boy you like in the surf club will not even look at you now. You were looking forward to driving; you often imagined driving up the coast with your board on top of the car and not a care in the world. How will you ever drive a car without your right hand? You have so many questions and fears. All your parents can say is *You're alive – that's all that matters!*

You wish you could find someone who understands your fears and could answer your questions. However, you do not enjoy talking about or feeling negative emotions, so you need convincing to openly discuss your feelings.

Person 2: You are a health professional and also a senior member of the surf-lifesaving club of which Ruth is an active member. You have been mentoring Ruth for some years and while you are devastated by the attack, you know Ruth has greater needs than you. You have been spending time with Ruth but feel helpless. You know of another young woman who surfs without an arm because of a car accident and you have contacted her to organise a time to meet with Ruth. You go to see Ruth to tell her about the other woman and arrange a time to meet, but first you want to be sure that Ruth is willing to talk about her experience and associated feelings.

GROUP DISCUSSION

As a large group discuss the observations, emotions and outcomes of the role plays. Suggest possible alternative strategies that may increase the effectiveness of the communication in a similar situation.

Adolescence can be an uncomfortable time for most people, both the adolescent and those around them. Adolescents feel vulnerable because of their stage of development. If an adolescent requires the assistance of a health professional, their feelings of vulnerability may multiply exponentially and thus the health professional must communicate using all of the principles of effective communication.

An adolescent values their peer group and thus, wherever possible, it can be beneficial to include individuals of the same or similar age in the assistive process. Adolescents with similar experiences can be very therapeutic for an adolescent who requires assistance from a health professional.

A person who is older

(Key words: ageing, elderly, senior, over 65, frail-aged)

Definition of an older person

An older person may be someone who

- Experiences the constraints of 'age' when moving, thinking, relating or feeling, regardless of their chronological age, joint stiffness or hair colour
- Has reached the age of retirement
- Is eligible to join a senior's organisation.

Behaviours related to being an older person

An older person – like any person – might exhibit idiosyncratic behaviours typical of their personality, interests, culture, upbringing, generation and life experiences. Older people may not exhibit age-related behaviours of any kind – they may live full, independent and meaningful lives.

However, older people who require the assistance of a health professional might

- Insist on doing a task without assistance and without fear for their safety, regardless of their ability
- Request assistance even when they are able to complete something independently
- Request information repeatedly due to difficulty hearing or remembering
- Request glasses and/or written information in large print
- Repeat the same information on different occasions
- Attempt to monopolise the time of the health professional with complex new needs at every session
- Be uncooperative and sullen
- Be well-adjusted and enjoy attending the health service.

Older people most susceptible to experiencing difficulties when attending a health service

Older people susceptible to experiencing difficulties when attending a health service include those who

- Have negative experiences of health services
- Have never experienced a health service before
- Are experiencing some cognitive or hearing loss
- Deny they require assistance
- Have limited function and participation
- Are in pain
- Have recently experienced loss of someone or something close to them.

Possible emotions an older person might experience

An older person might experience emotions related to

- Fear and anxiety about the future
- Fear and anxiety about death and dying

- Grief and sadness
- Confusion and deteriorating abilities
- Depression
- Chronic diseases and/or multiple conditions
- Pain
- Previous negative experiences
- Feeling that they want to die
- Feeling that they do not belong anywhere and cannot offer anything anymore.

Principles for effective communication with an older person

When communicating with an older person it is important to

- Make introductions
- Demonstrate respect
- Demonstrate empathy
- Provide clear written information with pictures if necessary to clarify meaning
- Listen actively
- Provide encouraging comfort
- Confront inappropriate beliefs and thoughts where appropriate.

Strategies for communicating with an older person

- Use a holistic approach.
- Ask them what they would like to be called – they might prefer to be addressed as Mr, Mrs or Miss rather than their given name until they feel the health professional is not a stranger.
- Treat an older person as an equal, regardless of their age, gender, cultural background or abilities.
- Listen to and remember their story.

ROLE PLAYS

Role-play the following scenarios. Before acting the roles you may wish to decide what type of assistance Person 1 requires. If it is not possible to role-play these scenarios, consider and explore the possible responses and communication strategies that will achieve effective communication and family/person-centred practice.

Scenario one: The male and the health professional

Person 1: Your name is Ron and you are an active 78-year-old man who swims every morning. Since your wife died you have independently cared for yourself and even assisted in caring for your two granddaughters. You have recently had a fall while doing the shopping and currently you require regular treatment for a knee injury. You are not enjoying the change in your functioning and are anxious to return to swimming every day. During your treatment you are polite but do not really enjoy requiring the assistance of anyone. You are accustomed to assisting others, not having them do things for you. This young health professional is very nice but too young to know very much about anything.

Person 2: You are the health professional. You have developed a working relationship with Ron and have been attempting to establish how he feels about his recent fall, because you would like to refer him to another health professional who can give him some information about avoiding falls in the future.

↳

Scenario two: The female and the health professional

Person 1: Your name is Elsie. You are an 84-year-old woman who lives alone. Despite a coccygeal fusion, osteoporosis of the upper vertebrae of your spinal column and bilateral arthritis of the hands you have continued to spin, knit and sew. Until recently you were very active – you attended line dancing and played bowls several times a week. However, you pulled a muscle in your leg while line dancing 6 months ago and have not been the same since. You had to stop line dancing and playing bowls. Then, a month ago, just as you were recovering from your leg injury and thinking about returning to line dancing, you pulled a muscle in your shoulder while cleaning your light fittings. You are fiercely independent and despite having a gold card with the Department of Veterans' Affairs (DVA) you have never thought of using it for assistance. You see a physiotherapist at present who has asked you to consider a home-care assessment to determine whether you might benefit from assistance with your housework and washing.

Person 2: You are a health professional who knows Elsie very well and have been asked to convince her to accept home-care for her safety.

GROUP DISCUSSION

As a large group discuss the observations, emotions and outcomes of the role plays. Suggest possible alternative strategies that may increase the effectiveness of the communication in a similar situation.

People who are older bring a wealth of experience and wisdom to every interaction. Unless experiencing cognitive decline, they do not usually require variation in the style of communication. As for all individuals, effective communication with an older person requires respect, empathy, rapport, empowerment, collaborative involvement in their treatment and, of course, person-centred practice. These characteristics should be evident in the relationship of the health professional with every older person, regardless of any decline in the physical, social, cognitive or emotional competence of that person.

People in particular roles

21

CHAPTER OBJECTIVE

Upon completing this chapter, students should be able to apply knowledge and consolidate the required skills to communicate effectively with people in particular roles.

Individuals may fulfil many roles during their lives, for example, **carer**, **colleague**, **parent**, **single parent** and **student**. These roles make particular demands upon the individual, which may have a variety of effects depending on their stage of life. One role most individuals fulfil at some stage in their life is the role of **group member**. Health professionals experience various groups in their role and thus the last scenario in this chapter is about the groups found in the health professions. This scenario is unique and thus there are unique steps to follow for the small group activity that occurs at the end of the chapter.

SMALL GROUP ACTIVITY: PARTICULAR ROLES

Carer
Colleague
Parent
Single parent
Student

- Define these particular roles.
- List some of the specific behaviours that might be typical of a person fulfilling these particular roles.
- List the negative emotions individuals fulfilling these roles might experience when relating to a health service.
- List possible explanations for the emotions someone fulfilling these roles might experience when relating to a health professional.
- List principles for effective communication to remember when communicating with a person fulfilling these particular roles. Give reasons for the need to remember these principles.
- Suggest strategies for communicating with a person who fulfils these particular roles. Decide why you might see such a person in your particular health profession.
- Check your answers against the information below, noting any additional thoughts or ideas.

A person who fulfils the role of carer for a person seeking assistance

(Key words: carer, legal and informal, long-term, caregiver, guardian)

Definition of a carer

A carer is someone who cares for a person with atypical health full-time or for more than a designated number of hours each day. (The designated number of hours varies according to legislation.)

Carers might be

- Spouses, daughters, sons, siblings, close friends of the same or opposite gender and sometimes neighbours
- A person who is paid to provide care, by either the government or the family of the person who requires care.

Behaviours related to being a carer

The behaviours of a carer will vary according to the age of the carer and the condition of the person requiring assistance. A carer might

- Act as an advocate for the person, always indicating their needs and desires
- Be constantly doing things for the person, regardless of the abilities of the person
- Exhibit non-verbal behaviours that appear opposite to their verbal messages.

Possible emotions a carer might experience

A carer might experience emotions related to

- Fear
- Anxiety
- Confusion
- Depression
- Grief
- Anger

- Inadequacy
- Desperation
- Loneliness
- Denial of the problem
- Hopelessness.

Possible reasons for these emotions

A carer might experience these emotions because of

- Spending all their time caring for the person
- Social isolation
- Responsibility and stress
- Limited knowledge about and skill in caring
- Loss of hope
- Confusion about the implication of recent needs that have resulted in seeking assistance from a health professional
- Fear of and anxiety about the future.

Principles for effective communication with a carer

When communicating with a carer it is important to

- Demonstrate empathy and sensitivity
- Make introductions
- Listen actively
- Give encouraging comfort
- Validate
- Answer any questions clearly and honestly
- Provide clear and well-organised information about the health service and any services or organisations that will provide assistance and support.

Strategies for communicating with a carer

- Do not avoid the issues – be prepared to respond to the obvious and stated needs of the carer.
- Be prepared to respond to the non-verbal behaviours of the carer – they may send a different message to their words.
- If necessary, refer the carer to other appropriate health professionals or organisations.
- If appropriate, confront the fears and feelings of the carer.

ROLE PLAYS

Role-play the following scenarios. Before acting the roles you may wish to decide what type of assistance Person 1 requires. If it is not possible to role-play these scenarios, consider and explore the possible responses and communication strategies that will achieve effective communication and family/person-centred practice.

Scenario one: The male and the health professional

Person 1: Your name is Steve. You are 39 years old and married to Marie, who was diagnosed with multiple sclerosis (MS) 7 years ago. You have recently reduced your hours of work to assist Marie with the maintenance of the house, her personal care and mobility, as well as your two children. Marie was falling at home while you were at work, so you reduced your hours to be with her when she most requires assistance. You accompany Marie to every appointment with the health professionals and you know them all quite well. You sit in the waiting area, feeling tired and distressed by Marie's recent deterioration. You are not sure but you think you need to resign from work and live on your savings and a carer's pension. You find it increasingly difficult to fulfil all the roles you have and you are not sure how you will manage when Marie finally dies. You stop, shocked at the thought – you would rather call it 'passing on'. Your religious beliefs have been very important to how you manage your emotions and friends from church have been supportive, often cooking meals, doing housework and mowing the lawns for you. However, you are very tired and feel like you need a rest.

Person 2: You are the health professional responsible for the needs of Marie, a person with MS. Marie is being seen by a health professional with different expertise today and you have decided to use the time to talk with her husband, Steve.

↳

Scenario two: The female and the health professional

Person 1: Your name is Genevieve and you are the main carer for your 6-year-old son, Damien, who has cerebral palsy (CP). Damien is a boy with a wonderful sense of humour who is confined to a wheelchair. Although you usually anticipate what he wants, he communicates using sounds, gestures and an augmentative communication system. You are also providing meals and some house maintenance for your ageing father who lives in the next street. You are tired and wondering how you can continue to care for both your son and your father. So much with Damien takes so long; you want to encourage him to feed himself and do some of his dressing himself, but it takes much longer when you give him time to do things for himself and you do not feel you have the time.

Person 2: You are a health professional who has not met Genevieve before, but have been working with Damien on school days. Genevieve has arrived early today and you go to meet her. You are committed to family/person-centred practice and want to find ways to encourage Damien to feed himself at least a few teaspoons of food every day instead of being fed everything.

GROUP DISCUSSION

As a large group discuss the observations, emotions and outcomes of the role plays. Suggest possible alternative strategies that may increase the effectiveness of the communication in a similar situation.

A person who fulfils the role of a colleague

(Key words: team, multidisciplinary team, interdisciplinary)

Definition of a colleague in the health professions

A colleague in the health professions is

- Any other professional whether inside or outside the health service who works with the health professional to assist vulnerable people
- Any other worker who supports the health professional to assist vulnerable people.

Attitudes and/or behaviours expected of a health professional

A health professional should be

- Professional
- Ethical
- Reliable
- Respectful
- Punctual
- Caring
- Interested in people
- Committed to caring
- Sacrificial

- Willing to assist
- Self-aware
- Thoughtful
- Diligent
- Supportive of colleagues
- Reflective
- Reflexive
- Accepting of differences
- Observant.

Attitudes and/or behaviours not expected of a health professional

A health professional should *not* be

- Self-serving
- Self-focused
- Non-reflective
- Personally ambitious
- Lazy
- Judgemental
- Sexist

- Sexually predatory
- Resistant
- Uncooperative
- Slovenly
- Non-reflexive
- Racist.

Possible emotions a colleague might experience

A colleague might experience emotions related to

- Frustration
- Grief and loss
- Disappointment
- Feeling misunderstood

- Betrayal
- Isolation
- Feeling unvalued
- Feeling inadequate.

Possible reasons for these emotions

A colleague might experience these emotions because of

- Personal experiences that occur outside the work context in family or social relationships

- Decisions made by the employing institution
- Their own attitudes and behaviour at particular times
- The attitudes and behaviour of other colleagues
- Unmet expectations
- Accidents either at work or in their personal life
- A person dying either at work or in their personal life
- Attempts to fulfil the unclear expectations of others
- Limited resources and pressure of work.

Principles for effective communication with a colleague

When communicating with a colleague it is important to

- Use holistic communication
- Listen actively
- Validate
- Clarify
- Understand
- Confront
- Show sensitive honesty
- Give encouraging comfort
- Be assertive.

Strategies for communicating with a colleague

- Demonstrate colleague-centred communication.
- Balance acceptance of the colleague with confrontation that empowers them to change inappropriate attitudes and behaviours.
- Do not assume understanding of the behaviour of a colleague.
- Demonstrate unconditional positive regard despite the differences.
- Use 'I' messages to communicate both your negative and positive emotions to a colleague.

ROLE PLAYS

Role-play the following scenarios. Before acting the roles you may wish to decide what type of assistance Person 1 requires. If it is not possible to role-play these scenarios, consider and explore the possible responses and communication strategies that will achieve effective communication and family/person-centred practice.

Scenario one: The male and the health professional colleague
Person 1: Your name is Ian and you are a single parent with three school-aged children. You are often called to emergencies with the children and find it difficult to balance life with work. You love your work as a health professional and have excellent relationships with your colleagues and the people you assist. You work efficiently and always have positive results.
Person 2: You are new to this health service and you are Ian's immediate supervisor. You have noticed that he often arrives late and leaves early without explanation. He works efficiently when he is at work and everyone thinks very highly of him. He appears to have excellent relationships with everyone, as well as positive outcomes. You have a supervision meeting with Ian scheduled for today.
- What are your aims for this session and why?
- Role-play the session when you have established those aims.

↳

Scenario two: The female and the health professional colleague

Person 1: Your name is Paula and you have a very busy day of work scheduled in your health service. A colleague notices your schedule and offers to assist you. You are quite surprised because this colleague often appears to avoid work. Together you agree that they will do some easy administration tasks due today that your supervisor has allocated to you. You clarify when they must be done, how to do them and where to place them upon completion. Throughout the day you notice your colleague chatting and reading a novel and you hope they have done those tasks. You have no time to do them yourself. At the end of an exhausting day, you are with this colleague and your supervisor asks for the tasks the colleague had agreed to complete. You look at the colleague, who looks away, and say you have not had time to complete them. The supervisor is not happy that you have not completed these specific tasks and says they hold you responsible. The colleague listens and says nothing. You are angry because you had no time to complete them today. You are now in the room with the colleague, you feel angry and you....... (decide what to do).

Person 2: You are the colleague who offers to assist then chooses to chat and read instead, thinking that you will get to those tasks later. As the day disappears you think *I can do them tomorrow*. You watch the supervisor talk to Paula but you cannot see the problem – you said you would do them and you will try to remember to do them tomorrow. You find it difficult to understand why Paula is angry.

GROUP DISCUSSION

As a large group discuss the observations, emotions and outcomes of the role plays. Suggest possible alternative strategies that may increase the effectiveness of the communication in a similar situation.

Health professionals have a responsibility to care for themselves, their colleagues and those seeking assistance. Reflection is beneficial in achieving this care in a manner that considers the needs of all communicators within the health professions.

A person who fulfils the role of parent to a child requiring assistance

(Key words: parents, foster-parents, role models, family, legal guardian, uncertain)

Definition of a parent

A parent is someone who

- Has been part of creating the 'child'
- Is legally responsible for the 'child'
- The 'child' views as their parent or parent figure – their protector, provider and model.

A 'child' is someone who has a parent and may be of varying ages.

Behaviours related to being a parent

The behaviours related to being a parent will depend on the age of the child. Such behaviours are often related to the feelings the parent is experiencing.

For a *young* child a parent might be

- Protective and even angry on behalf of the child
- Anxious to understand everything related to the child
- Controlling of the child
- Able to coax the child into engaging and being involved in the process
- Able to reassure the child and provide safety for the child.

For an *adolescent* 'child' a parent might be some of the above and/or

- Protective and overbearing
- Accusatory, depending on the cause of the need for a health professional.

For an *adult* 'child' the behaviour of the parent might depend on the quality of the relationship with the 'child' and the nature of the reason the 'child' is seeking assistance from a health professional.

Parents most susceptible to experiencing difficulties when attending a health service

The parents susceptible to experiencing difficulties when attending a health service may be those who

- Are young
- Have an intellectual disability
- Have addictions
- Are unfamiliar with the health system
- Have unrealistic expectations
- Have children with long-term difficulties
- Have negative experiences of health services.

Possible emotions a parent might experience

A parent might experience emotions related to

- Fear
- Anxiety
- Uncertainty
- Desperation
- Denial
- Shock

- Guilt
- Resignation
- Being lonely
- Feeling inadequate
- Grief.

Possible reasons for these emotions

The possible reasons for emotions in a parent will depend upon the age of the child and the severity of the condition for which the child requires assistance. However, the emotions regardless of their cause are as significant as those of the child and require management by the health professional.

Family-centred practice is particularly relevant to practice associated with children aged 0–16 years. Children exist in the context of the family and should not be assisted without reference to and consideration of that context.

Parents may experience negative emotions because of

- Concern for the continued health, wellbeing, participation, functioning and safety of the child
- Feeling guilt and responsibility for the condition
- Loneliness and isolation
- Fear of and anxiety about the future
- Confusion about the meaning of their life if something happens to the child
- Inadequacy and desperation
- Grief for lost opportunities related to career, friendships, family and siblings, in the case of a long-term condition.

Principles for effective communication with a parent

When communicating with a parent it is important to

- Demonstrate empathy and sensitivity
- Make introductions
- Provide and explain information
- Provide clear and well-organised information about any services or organisations that will provide assistance and support
- Listen actively
- Schedule time for discussion and answers to pertinent questions
- Give encouraging comfort
- Validate
- Disengage.

Strategies for communicating with a parent

- Invest time with the parent as well as the child to develop a therapeutic relationship.
- Clearly explain and clarify their understanding of the procedures and events regularly – avoid assuming they understand everything.

- Respond to their non-verbal messages.
- Acknowledge and use the expertise and knowledge the parent has about the child.

ROLE PLAYS

Role-play the following scenarios. Before acting the roles you may wish to decide what type of assistance Person 1 requires. If it is not possible to role-play these scenarios, consider and explore the possible responses and communication strategies that will achieve effective communication and family/person-centred practice.

Scenario one: The male and the health professional
Person 1: Your name is Theo. You are the 72-year-old father of 48-year-old Christopher who has recently been diagnosed with motor neurone disease (MND). You are anxious about the wellbeing of your eldest son who has managed your concreting business for many years. Christopher has been a great son, especially since your wife, Anna, died 4 years ago. He has provided for his wife and your five grandchildren, managed the business expertly and, like you, loves concreting. You have no idea what MND means and you just want your son to go back to his life of participation and providing.
Person 2: You are the health professional who Theo sees monthly and you have noticed recently that he is not himself. Whatever is troubling him seems to be affecting the way Theo cares for himself so you would like to explore this and see if he requires some form of intervention.

Scenario two: The female and the health professional
Person 1: Your name is Sally. You are a mother of two girls with a husband who is often away for extended periods with his job. Your eldest daughter, Susie, is 8 years old. She seems to have difficulty learning and appears to be aggressive at school. Your younger daughter, Katie, is 6 years old. They both attend the same school and the behaviour of Susie at school embarrasses Katie, who is becoming aggressive towards her older sister at home. You have no idea how to help either of your children and feel desperate. Susie is gentle and loving at home so you cannot understand her behaviour at school. You attend a health service regularly so decide to ask the health professional there for help.
Person 2: You are the health professional who has been seeing Sally for some time and feel you have a positive therapeutic relationship with her. She has always been cooperative and friendly. You have no idea about the difficulties her children are experiencing, but when she explains you decide you would like to help, even though it may not be your area of expertise.

GROUP DISCUSSION

As a large group discuss the observations, emotions and outcomes of the role plays. Suggest possible alternative strategies that may increase the effectiveness of the communication in a similar situation.

Parents of children who require the assistance of a health professional, regardless of the age of the children, require a supportive and therapeutic relationship along with their children. The needs of the parents may or may not be different but the parents are a vital component of the context of the person seeking the assistance of the health professional.

Similarly, when parents are receiving assistance from a health professional the children will have similar needs and emotions to those listed in this section. In such situations the child of the person, whether adult or not, is an integral part of the context of the person and will therefore require consideration and effective communication.

A person who fulfils the role of single parent to a child requiring assistance

Single parent
(Key words: parenting alone, one-person parenting, sole responsibility, unsupported)

Definition of a single parent

A single parent

- Is someone who is attempting to raise the child(ren) alone
- Often has no-one with whom they can share the care of the child(ren)
- Is often working full-time as well as managing the needs of the child(ren), sometimes without the support of extended family.

Characteristics single parents may expect of themselves

Single parents may expect themselves to be

- Competent
- Able to manage regardless
- Good at problem solving
- Determined
- Able to persevere.

Possible emotions a single parent might experience

A single parent might experience emotions related to

- Struggle
- Fear
- Inadequacy
- Anger
- Envy
- Resentment
- Feeling overwhelmed
- Depression
- Loneliness
- Isolation
- Insecurity
- Feeling discouraged
- Frustration
- Anxiety
- Scepticism
- Constant tiredness
- Desperation
- Stress
- Grief
- Exhaustion.

Possible reasons for these emotions

A single parent might experience these emotions because of

- Feeling rejected through divorce or separation
- Any unexpected event
- Responsibilities and stress related to their role
- Demands of the child(ren)
- No respite or rest
- Financial burdens
- Friends appearing to 'have it easy'

- Having no sense of being valued
- Considering the needs of the child(ren) above their own needs.

Principles for effective communication with a single parent

When communicating with a single parent it is important to

- Listen actively
- Encourage
- Give information
- Establish boundaries
- Confront
- Disengage.

Strategies for communicating with a single parent

- Avoid critical comments about their parenting.
- Imagine how you would manage if you were in their situation.
- Set achievable goals.

DISCUSSION POINT

See the Introduction to Section Four for instructions about how to use these scenarios for group discussion.

Scenario one: The male and the health professional

Paul is a single parent to his three children. His wife died 3 years ago and he has managed to care for the children since then. The schools the children attend have after-care facilities but Paul finds this too expensive for three children. Each of the children is allowed one extracurricular activity. Jordan (15 years old) plays soccer, Lara (14) plays the piano and Lacey (10) settled for tap dancing because her father said horse riding was too expensive and too hard to organise.

Paul manages a department store and relies on his eldest child, Jordan, to care for the younger girls until he arrives home from work each day. The younger children, Lara and Lacey, do not enjoy the time before their father returns home from work because Jordan orders them to do chores around the house while he plays computer games or watches television. Their father is always tired when he arrives home and thanks Jordan for the completed chores. Jordan does not say he did not do them and enjoys his father's appreciation. Sometimes one of the girls makes a meal, but often Paul prepares the evening meal and then supervises their homework. They have a routine that allows everyone to fulfil their responsibilities at home, work and school. Organising extracurricular activities and sport is challenging and exhausting, but parents of friends of the children often drive them home.

Today Paul receives a call from Jordan's principal requesting an interview with Paul to discuss Jordan's progress. Two hours after receiving that call, a teacher from Lacey's school rings to say Lacey has fallen at school and needs medical attention. As Paul drives to the school he wishes his wife was alive just so he could have someone with whom to talk. The teacher has assured him Lacey is all right so he is not prepared for the swelling on her forehead or the blood on her arm. He wonders why he thought it was just a scratch and a bruise. Lacey is barely conscious but seems to know he is there.

↳

↳   At the hospital Paul waits quietly by his youngest daughter, holding her hand. He misses his wife especially at times like these because she was so good with sick people. He has no idea how he will manage if Lacey needs extra time and attention, because he only just manages now. He thinks about Jordan. *That 15-year-old needs more attention than I give him*, he thinks. He remembers how hard it was to be 15 and how many temptations there were when he was growing up. He realises he has not had the time to talk with Jordan about this the way his father did when he was about 12. So much of his energy goes in just getting the basic things done each day.

Someone comes to take Lacey for an X-ray; Lacey does not notice that Paul does not go with her. Another health professional arrives to ask a few questions and to see what Paul needs.

- If you were that health professional, what questions would you be required to ask?
- Answers to some of those questions would lead you to ask further questions – what might they be?
- How important might the story of Paul and the children be for achieving the goals associated with Lacey's care?

Scenario two: The female and the health professional
Jenna is a 33-year-old woman who is a single parent to 6-year-old Jonah. Jonah is currently receiving speech pathology, occupational therapy and physiotherapy for delayed speech, attention deficits and gross motor coordination. A podiatrist has made arch supports for Jonah and this has helped his gross motor performance in some areas, but he needs assistance to develop his muscle tone and strength.

Jenna and her husband separated 5 years ago. Jonah always spent the weekends with his father, until recently, when his father moved interstate. Jenna found that the break from caring for Jonah on the weekends helped her manage during the week. It also meant she did not have extra expenses on the weekends because Jonah's father paid for the movies and other expensive activities Jonah liked doing on the weekends.

Since that time, Jenna and Jonah seem tense when they are together and they often yell at each other out of frustration. Jenna says she hates yelling, but she gets so frustrated when Jonah will not listen to her. Jenna says she is really struggling with being alone. She finds it difficult to be responsible for Jonah without a break because he has particular needs all of the time. She is unsure how to manage the frustration and anger she feels most of the time. She is not always frustrated with Jonah, just with their situation.

- If you were a health professional involved with the care of Jonah, how would you approach this situation?
- What are the aims of communication with Jenna?

GROUP DISCUSSION

As a large group share the main points discussed by each small group about these scenarios. Consider various strategies that may increase the effectiveness of the communication in a similar situation.

A person who fulfils the role of a student

Student
(Key words: studying, learning, professional practice, clinical experience, applying theory)

Definition of a student in the health professions

A health professional student is someone who is not fully qualified in their health profession. Students usually visit clinical settings to consolidate theory and learn skills, and may become excellent health professionals in their particular profession. They might be observing, practising or consolidating, but ultimately they are connecting theory with practice.

Being a student means individuals might

- Feel underpaid and overworked!
- Feel isolated if away from family
- Find balancing work and study hard
- Feel pressure to party and abuse alcohol
- Feel inadequate
- Feel pressure to achieve high grades.

Behaviours related to being a student

A student might

- Observe enthusiastically
- Attempt to compensate for inadequacy
- Engage in risk-taking behaviours
- Not ask questions
- Chatter about irrelevant things.

Possible emotions a student might experience

A student might experience emotions related to

- Insecurity
- Loneliness
- Fear
- Lack of confidence
- Disappointment
- Frustration
- Anxiety
- Pressure
- Feeling overwhelmed.

Possible reasons for these emotions

A student might experience these emotions because of

- Lack of knowledge or skills
- Pressure to perform and achieve
- Feelings of inequality
- Social isolation – away from family
- Financial pressure and struggles
- Different learning styles
- Relationship issues

- Peer pressure
- Poor self-management skills
- Imbalance in the activities of life
- Different personality types.

Principles for effective communication with a student

When communicating with a student it is important to

- Make introductions – to *everything*!
- Consider their non-verbal behaviours
- Demonstrate respect and empathy
- Understand
- Be consistent in communication
- Confront when necessary
- Provide information
- Listen actively
- Give encouraging comfort
- Disengage.

Strategies for communicating with a student

- Provide clear and detailed information about the expectations of the student while they are on placement.
- Avoid making assumptions about what they know and their life experience.
- Become familiar with their learning style and manner of managing information.
- Provide immediate and specific feedback in a format that reflects their learning style.
- Communicate positive and negative feedback clearly with suggestions of definite behaviours to improve. Be specific.
- Address the causes of their issues not the symptoms.
- Adjust communication style to be approachable – being friends with students is acceptable.
- Avoid intimidating facial expressions and behaviour.
- Allow them time for processing information.

ROLE PLAYS

Role-play the following scenarios. Before acting the roles you may wish to decide what type of assistance Person 1 requires. If it is not possible to role-play these scenarios, consider and explore the possible responses and communication strategies that will achieve effective communication and family/person-centred practice.

Scenario one: The male and the health professional
Person 1: Your name is Ryan and you are a third-year student completing a 5-week clinical placement. You were punctual and relaxed on the first day but each day since then you have been late and you appear anxious. On the Friday of the first week you lose a medical record required by another health professional. This becomes a major issue because the record for this person is required in court on Monday.

↳

↳

Person 2: You are the supervisor responsible for Ryan and, as such, you are responsible for the lost record. Respond to Ryan to achieve the best outcome for all involved individuals.

Scenario two: The female and the health professional

Person 1: Your name is Sharon and you are a 19-year-old student health professional. You are currently on placement at a health service with five other students from different health professions. This health service provides activities and education for people who are high-functioning but have a history of mental illness. You have been enjoying the placement. You relate well to the various people who attend the service for assistance. You are young, attractive and naturally friendly to everyone. The other students are from other cities and you invite them to the pub after work. A particular male who attends the centre for assistance, Tom, is present when you make the arrangements and assumes he is included in the arrangements. When you arrive at the pub Tom is there waiting for you. You think he is there with his mates. You say *Hi* and then ignore him, not realising he is there to join you. Some of the other students notice he leaves in a distressed state. You do not worry, saying *It's a free world – he can do what he likes and so can I. I meant no harm; he should have known the arrangements were only for the students.*

Person 2: It is Monday morning and you are the student supervisor for this health service. Several qualified staff have heard that Tom was admitted to hospital on Friday night. One of the students feels guilty because she knew Tom was in the room when Sharon arranged to go to the pub and she knew it was not appropriate to make the arrangements in the presence of a person seeking the assistance of the centre. This student has told you everything that happened at the centre and the pub. You ask to speak with Sharon privately to hear her side of the story and to ensure she does not behave in this way again.

GROUP DISCUSSION

As a large group discuss the observations, emotions and outcomes of the role plays. Suggest possible alternative strategies that may increase the effectiveness of the communication in a similar situation.

Student health professionals are the future of their profession. They deserve and require effective communication and specialised assistance to achieve their goal of successful completion of their program.

Groups in the health professions

(Key words: groupwork, group dynamics, group growth)

The health professional might encounter two major kinds of groups during their practising life. The first type of group is one in which they are a member of the team or group of people. Such multidisciplinary or interdisciplinary teams may be found in public or private health services. Such teams aim to help those seeking their assistance. These teams may consist of people with different roles and different skills. The people may work for the same health service or for different services. As a member of a multidisciplinary team, it is important to understand the workings of a group and the possible experiences groups may provide. The second type of group often has therapeutic or educational goals and is one in which the health professional may be the leader or facilitator of the group.

Each of these groups require trust, commitment to group goals and participation in group activities from all participants, whether group members or group leader. Groups have a life of their own and, while beneficial, require particular knowledge and skills to maximise the benefits.

SMALL GROUP ACTIVITY: GROUPS IN THE HEALTH PROFESSIONS

- Decide what types of groups occur in the health professions.
- List the stages of growth in a group.
- List the emotions typically experienced in a group.
- List the expectations of group behaviour (group norms) for a multidisciplinary health professional team, considering the possible needs of group members and the health service.
- List the expectations of group behaviour (group norms) for a therapeutic group, considering the possible needs of group members.
- List principles for effective communication to remember when communicating within a group. Give reasons for the need to remember these principles.
- Suggest strategies for communicating effectively within a group. Relate the strategies to the goals of your particular health profession.
- Check your answers against the information below, noting any additional thoughts or ideas (of the group or from the information below).

Types of groups offered in health services

Health services may offer

- Educational groups
- Therapeutic activity groups
- Life skills groups
- Healthy lifestyle groups
- Condition-specific groups (e.g. stroke groups, autism groups)
- Therapeutic play groups
- Craft groups
- Staff development groups
- Professional development groups

* Support groups
* Seniors' groups
* Leisure groups (e.g. non-professional sporting, music, dancing and drama groups).

Stages of group growth

Groups experience growth and change as group members become familiar with each other. Initially group members experience uncertainty and possibly limited trust, they then experience differing levels of conflict as the members adjust to ways of relating within the group, and finally most groups achieve working relationships that facilitate group cohesion and productivity. Group members establish their roles and patterns of interrelating as they develop an understanding of self and of other group members. The development of trust and 'working' group relationships facilitates fulfilment of group goals. Various theorists describe the stages of group growth (see Table 21.1). Some describe groups with psychosocial goals and others describe groups with task-oriented goals.

Each of the theorists referenced in Table 21.1 describe group stages using words that indicate groups will experience tension followed by ease of relating that facilitates positive outcomes. It is important to remember these stages whether a member of a group or the leader of a group.

Stages of group growth		
Tuckman (1977)	**Schutz (1973)**	**Mosey (1996)**
• Forming • Storming • Norming • Performing • Mourning	• Inclusion • Control • Affection	• Orientation • Dissatisfaction • Resolution • Production
TABLE 21.1		

Johnson & Johnson (2006) describe a group as having a leader who guides the group into productivity. The stages they describe often occur when the group is task-oriented. However, being a task-oriented group does not mean the group will be free of tension because time is required to establish mutual understanding and commitment to the goals of the group. The stages take place as follows (Johnson & Johnson 2006):

* Defining and structuring procedures
* Conforming to procedures and getting acquainted
* Recognising mutuality and building trust
* Committing to and taking ownership of the goals, procedures and other members
* Functioning maturely and productively
* Terminating.

Emotions typically experienced in a group

Yalom & Leszcz (2005) describe the therapeutic factors of groups that create particular emotions for all group members. While the dynamic of interdependent relationships within groups is challenging, Yalom & Leszcz (2005) indicate that therapeutic factors occur because of the existence of the group and because of the complex interplay of the experiences typical of group membership. They highlight eleven primary factors that create particular emotions and demonstrate the therapeutic nature of groups. These therapeutic factors include the instillation of hope and the feeling of universality, both of which develop from the fact that other group members have similar experiences. Another therapeutic factor occurs because of feelings that arise from regular expression of experiences and feelings (catharsis) and the sharing of various types of information. Groups allow members to relate with selflessness (altruism) as they develop understanding of the feelings and needs of others through interpersonal learning. This provides opportunity to develop socialising techniques through observing and imitating the positive behaviour of other group members. Groups provide opportunity for positive group experiences that contribute to group cohesiveness and override possible negative experiences of family groups. They provide opportunity to understand existential factors relating to responsibility, because group membership requires particular behaviour to avoid unpleasant consequences.

Overall group aims

There are always overall goals for the existence of a group, whether the group is a health professional team or a therapeutic group. It is important that each group member understands and is committed to these goals. Health professional teams may have mission statements and therapeutic groups will always have an overall aim. Clear explanation of the overall aim(s) is important to ensure appropriate expectations and behaviour from all group members. Both types of groups assemble for meetings which have particular goals that contribute to the overall aim of the group. A therapeutic group may have a specific number of meetings and thus a limited group life.

Events of specific group sessions and associated emotions

Each group session contributes to the growth of the group and thus the movement through the stages of group development. The events within each session will elicit particular emotions for group members. The structure and preparation of each session will assist in management of any negative emotions associated with the session.

The events typical of a group session are as follows:

- **Welcome and aims:** Discussing the aims of the particular session allows group members to leave the events of everyday life and focus on group members and the forthcoming group events. This stage is important because it relaxes group members and allows them to remember their 'place' in the group and the 'place' of the other group members.
- **Warm-up:** A warm-up allows group members to re-connect with the group norms and goals, and with other group members.
- **Main activities:** The main activities usually fulfil the aims of the overall purpose of the group and the aims of the particular session.
- **Warm-down/wrap-up:** A wrap-up allows group members to reflect upon the events of the group and their relative success in achieving the aims of the session. It allows group members to reflect on the effect of the group session upon themselves and other group members. It also allows disengagement from the group members until the next group session.

Group norms: Expectations of group behaviour

Group norms are the values that govern behaviour within a group. They are essential in any group because they promote cooperation and cohesion between individuals with different personalities, skills, knowledge and opinions. A group norm is the shared agreement and acceptance of rules that govern behaviour within a group. Norms include expectations regarding acceptable appearance when attending the group, punctuality, expression of emotions, acceptance of group members and confidentiality. A norm can also govern the rate, quality and method of producing outcomes if the group has a task focus. Explicit discussion of group norms in the initial stages of the group process facilitates openness concerning the expectations of particular behaviour within the group.

Principles for effective communication within groups

When communicating within groups it is important to

- Remember that non-verbal behaviour is very powerful in a group and can be easily misinterpreted
- Give non-judgemental encouragement to all members
- Respect, accept, encourage, and use all other elements of effective communication.

Strategies for communicating as a group leader

- Be well prepared, with the required equipment and material to facilitate the group effectively and efficiently.
- Clarify and clearly state the group goals. The goals must be relevant and easily implemented, create positive interdependence, and encourage commitment from group members.
- Establish and state group norms and revisit them whenever necessary.
- Encourage open and accurate expression of ideas and feelings without judgement.
- Encourage participation, inclusion, acceptance, support and trust of each group member.
- If appropriate, share the leadership among all group members.

DISCUSSION POINT

See the Introduction to Section Four for instructions about how to use these scenarios for group discussion.

Scenario one: A 2-day team development group
A health service has about twenty-four staff members who work full-time and part-time within the service. The person in charge has noticed there are difficulties in the relationships among many of the staff. They have organised a 2-day team-building experience to attempt to develop trust and cohesion among the staff. They expect everyone to attend, including the administration staff, the cleaners, the people who work in the grounds and all health professionals.

There is a mixed reaction on the first day because some people feel the cleaners should not be there and others feel the administration staff should not be there.
- Decide who should be there and explain why.
- How do you think the person in charge should manage these responses, which are contrary to the purpose of the 2 days?

Scenario two: An education group
A group educates its members about their condition and how to manage the condition. It runs for 6 weeks for 1½ hours each week. You facilitate the group and have other health

↳

↳
professionals attend at different times to provide a holistic consideration of the particular condition.

- Choose a condition relevant to your health profession that could require an educational group.
- Using the specifications listed above (i.e. 6 weeks for 1½ hours/week) decide upon the overall goals of such a group, the possible aims of each session and the content.
- Indicate whether you will include any other health professionals in the overall program. If so, devise the information and instructions you might give them as a guide for their involvement in the group.

GROUP DISCUSSION

As a large group share the main points discussed by each small group about these scenarios. Consider various strategies that may increase the effectiveness of the communication in a similar situation.

References

Johnson D W, Johnson F P 2006 Joining together: group theory and group skills, 9th edn. Allyn and Bacon, Boston

Mosey A C 1996 Psychosocial components of occupational therapy. Lippincott-Raven, Philadelphia

Schutz W C 1973 Elements of encounter. Joy Press, Big Sur, California

Tuckman B W, Jensen M A C 1977 Stages of small group development revisited. Group and Organisation Management 2(4): 419–427

Yalom I D, Leszcz M 2005 The theory and practice of group psychotherapy, 5th edn. Basic Books, New York

Further reading

Cohen M B, Mullender A (eds) 2003 Gender and groupwork. Routledge, New York

Finlay L 2002 Groupwork. In: Creek J (ed) Occupational therapy and mental health, 3rd edn. Churchill Livingstone, London, p 245–264

Greif G L, Ephross P H (eds) 2005 Group work with populations at risk, 2nd edn. Oxford University Press, New York

Haight B, Gibson F 2005 Burnside's working with older adults: group process and techniques. Jones & Bartlett, Sudbury MA

Malekoff A 2004 Group work with adolescents: principles and practice, 2nd edn. Guilford Press, New York

Preston-Shoot M 2007 Effective groupwork, 2nd edn. Palgrave Macmillan, Basingstoke

People with particular conditions

22

CHAPTER OBJECTIVE

Upon completing this chapter, students should be able to apply knowledge and consolidate the required skills to communicate effectively with people with particular conditions.

This chapter considers the communication needs of people presenting with particular conditions: **decreased cognitive function**, **life-limiting illness**, **mental illness**, **hearing impairment** and **visual impairment**.

SMALL GROUP ACTIVITY: PARTICULAR CONDITIONS

Decreased cognitive function
Life-limiting illness
Mental illness
Hearing impairment
Visual impairment

- Define these particular conditions.
- List some of the specific behaviours (and emotions if relevant) that might be typical of a person with these conditions.
- Choose one of three options:
  - List the emotions a person experiencing a life-limiting illness might experience when relating to a health service, *or*
  - Consider which level of cognitive loss (mild, moderate or severe) may cause the most difficulty for an individual relating to a health professional, *or*
  - Consider which individuals may be most susceptible to experiencing a mental illness, hearing impairment or visual impairment.
- List possible reasons that might explain the emotions a person with these conditions might experience when seeing a health professional.
- List principles for effective communication to remember when communicating with a person with these conditions. Give reasons for the need to remember these principles.

↳

- Suggest strategies for communicating with a person who has these conditions. Decide why you might see such a person in your particular health profession.
- Check your answers against the information below, noting any additional thoughts or ideas.

A person who has decreased cognitive function

(Key words: dementia, Alzheimer's disease, intellectual disability (mental retardation), addictive behaviours)

It is important to note that children with decreased cognitive function due to Down Syndrome or an intellectual disability do not fall into the same category as someone who has lost cognitive function because of ageing, head injury or addictive behaviours. Such children have specific needs but are able to learn and are very able in many areas. Alternatively, in most cases people experiencing a loss of cognitive function find it difficult to compensate for that loss after a particular level of deterioration.

Definition of decreased cognitive function

A person with decreased cognitive function may be experiencing a mild, moderate or severe decrease in cognitive function.

A person with a *mild* decrease in cognitive function is someone who may

- Function independently
- Choose to participate in the activities they perform well and enjoy
- Perform their self-care activities
- Assist others in basic tasks they enjoy performing
- Understand and express themself to facilitate understanding
- Develop and use compensatory strategies to participate and function
- Learn and thus remember with repetition and perseverance
- 'Work' in a structured environment with some support
- Enjoy social interaction.

A person with a *moderate* decrease in cognitive function is someone who may

- Function with some assistance
- Know what they enjoy performing but may have difficulty making choices
- Perform some self-care activities independently (e.g. dressing and toileting; may require a reminder to bathe)
- Not always use words to communicate, but may understand others
- Learn simple tasks with repetition and visual cues
- Be able to 'work' in a supported workplace with repetitive activities
- Enjoy social interaction with particular familiar people.

A person with a *severe* decrease in cognitive function is someone who may

- Require assistance with all personal care needs and with all other activities, except activities relating to mobility
- Require constant supervision if they tend to wander and become lost
- Be incoherent and unable to consistently communicate; however, may respond randomly to particular people, pictures or objects
- Recognise familiar people they see constantly, but not consistently recognise others
- Be repetitive in the sounds they make and in their behaviours
- Be violent
- Be sweet and passive.

Behaviours related to being a person with decreased cognitive function

The behaviours of a person with decreased cognitive function will vary according to the severity of the decrease in function. A person with decreased cognitive function might

* Be illogical, irrational and unpredictable
* Be perfectly happy sometimes
* Repeat particular behaviours
* Ask the same irrelevant questions repeatedly
* Become easily distressed without provocation
* Wander for no reason
* Be violent – although not all individuals with a decrease in cognitive function will be violent
* Behave in socially unacceptable ways.

Individuals with decreased cognitive function most susceptible to experiencing difficulty when relating to a health professional

A person with a moderate decrease in cognitive function is most likely to experience difficulty when relating to a health professional. In groups discuss and explain why.

Possible emotions a person with decreased cognitive function might experience

A person with decreased cognitive function might experience emotions related to

* A change in routine, which can cause confusion and fear
* Unfamiliar environments and/or people, which may cause disturbed behaviour
* A lack of connection with reality.

Principles for effective communication with a person with decreased cognitive function

When communicating with a person with decreased cognitive function it is important to

* Demonstrate respect
* Demonstrate empathy and understanding
* Be consistent
* Have a sense of humour
* Give clear instructions with visual cues if necessary
* Practise holistic communication.

Strategies for communicating with a person with decreased cognitive function

* Invest time to develop a therapeutic relationship.
* Do not take anything personally that the person might say to you or about you.
* Consider the whole person.
* Communicate gently and consistently.
* Avoid expressions of anger and frustration.

- Communicate with patience and a 'go-with-the-flow' attitude.
- Aim to maintain a feeling of safety, happiness and comfort for the person wherever possible.
- Remember they are generally unable to change the way they relate, how they behave and what they say.

ROLE PLAYS

Role-play the following scenarios. Before acting the roles you may wish to decide what type of assistance Person 1 requires. If it is not possible to role-play these scenarios, consider and explore the possible responses and communication strategies that will achieve effective communication and family/person-centred practice.

Scenario one: The male and the health professional

Person 1: Your name is Fred. You are 75 years old and you live alone in a large house. A bus collects you weekly to attend a group. You do not know where your wife has gone and what happened to the custard tarts you were going to eat with your cup of tea.

Person 2: You are the health professional who has Fred in a weekly group. Fred is a friendly man, however, he repeatedly asks you what happened to his wife who died 10 years ago and if you have eaten his custard tarts. Because Fred lives alone, you are very concerned about his safety and his ability to care for himself. You know his daughter visits daily, cleans his house and provides him with a hot meal. However, you are still concerned about his safety. Have a conversation with Fred and decide if he may be safer in the familiarity of his own home than elsewhere.

Scenario two: The female and the health professional

Person 1: Your name is Sarah. Your mother, Irene, is 82 years old and is currently in a rehabilitation unit because she recently had a right cerebrovascular accident (CVA). Prior to the stroke your mother and father, Harry, lived together in their house for 35 years. While your father is frail, he is mentally able and has been successfully caring for your mother with your support. You realise your mother has decreased cognitive function that was present before the stroke and has been worsened by the stroke, and that it might be suitable for her to be placed somewhere for people with her stage of dementia. However, you are worried about how your father will cope emotionally if they are separated.

Person 2: You are Irene and you have little control over your behaviour. You often wander and disappear to be found undressing and trying to get into bed with any man you can find on a bed. Some of the male people seeking assistance think it is amusing, while others find it disturbing.

Person 3: You are Harry. As Irene's husband of 53 years you really want to continue caring for her. You do find her exhausting and are aware that you are not as strong as you have been. You feel you can continue caring for her with the support and assistance of your daughter.

Person 4: You are the health professional who needs to speak with the family including Irene to determine whether she will return home or go to a high-dependency ward of a nursing home.

GROUP DISCUSSION

As a large group discuss the observations, emotions and outcomes of the role plays. Suggest possible alternative strategies that may increase the effectiveness of the communication in a similar situation.

Working with individuals with decreased cognitive function can be challenging but rewarding. However, such work – even on an occasional basis – does not suit all health professionals.

A person who experiences a life-limiting illness and their family

(Key words: life-limiting illness, critical care, terminal illness, death, grief, loss, palliative care)

Facts about people who know they are dying and their families

A person who knows they are dying and the members of their family or circle of friends will experience emotions according to the 'cycle of grief'. Kubler-Ross (1969, 2005) suggested stages of grief; however, it is now recognised that people who know they are dying can experience the emotions typical of a 'stage' at various times throughout the process of the disease. They do not experience them in order, nor do they move through the emotions as though they are stages. They may experience them repeatedly before they reach acceptance. The emotions include denial, rage, resentment, envy, bargaining, depression and acceptance.

It is important to note that an individual experiencing loss of any kind may experience these emotions while attempting to grieve and adjust to the loss. Family members or friends of a person who is dying usually experience the cycle of grief and the related emotions.

People who have a life-limiting illness often receive services from palliative care units. These units generally follow national policies, standards and guidelines specifically developed for palliative care situations (see Palliative Care Australia [www.pallcare.org.au] or New Zealand Palliative Care Strategy [www.moh.govt.nz/moh.nsf/pagesmh/2951]).

The World Health Organization (WHO 2008) states that palliative care is an approach that improves the quality of life of people and their families facing the problems associated with life-threatening illness. This is achieved through the prevention and relief of suffering by means of early identification and impeccable assessment as well as treatment of pain and other problems (physical, psychosocial and spiritual).

WHO (2008) states that palliative care aims to assist people with life-limiting illnesses to experience quality of life until the moment they die. Palliative care should provide relief from pain and other distressing symptoms. It should affirm life but regard death as a normal part of life. Palliative care should neither hasten nor postpone death. Palliative care considers the whole person and integrates psychological and spiritual care for the benefit of the person and their family members. Palliative care is committed to supporting the family during the course of the illness and after death.

Core values of Palliative Care Australia (www.pallcare.org.au)

- Dignity of the person, caregivers and each member of the family
- Respect and empowerment of all of these individuals
- Compassion for all involved
- Equity in access to services
- Excellence of provision of care
- Family-centred practice.

Definition of a life-limiting illness

A person who has a life-limiting illness is someone who has 0–6 months to live. This may be due to

- Cancer
- A progressive neurological disorder

- End-stage cardiac, renal or respiratory disease
- AIDS
- Other degenerative diseases
- Experiencing a serious accident, attack or natural disaster
- Experiencing an unexpected and serious life-threatening medical occurrence (e.g. cerebrovascular accident [CVA] or cardiac arrest [CA]).

Behaviours a person experiencing a life-limiting illness might exhibit

A person experiencing a life-limiting illness will exhibit a range of behaviours that might include

- Acting as though nothing is wrong one day and being totally withdrawn the next
- Being quiet and thoughtful one day and chatty the next
- Forcing themself to do something regardless of their pain or fatigue
- Sleeping excessively because of pain medication, fatigue and depression
- Being unable to sleep and thus being awake all night
- Being short-tempered and dismissive towards carers and health professionals
- Being teary sometimes
- Wanting to discuss spiritual issues or beliefs about life after death.

Possible emotions a person experiencing a life-limiting illness and their family members and friends might experience

A person experiencing a life-limiting illness and their family members and friends might experience emotions related to

- Bargaining (*If I do this it will cure me*)
- Denial
- Rage
- Resentment
- Envy
- Depression
- Anxiety
- Confusion
- Fear
- Despair
- Hopelessness
- Desperation
- Acceptance.

A person experiencing a life-limiting illness may experience physical, emotional, social, cognitive and spiritual distress.

Physical distress may include

- Pain
- Fatigue
- Anorexia
- Restlessness
- Breathlessness
- Oedema
- Disfigurement
- Bladder and bowel disturbances
- Neurological dysfunction.

Psychological or emotional distress may include

- Sadness
- Shock
- Uncertainty
- Fear
- Anxiety
- Depression
- Loss of control
- Role changes
- Loss and grief
- Change in self-esteem
- Change in body image.

Social distress may include

- Isolation
- Lack of support
- Financial issues
- Carer stress

- Family conflict
- Inability to manage social situations
- Inability to manage at home.

Cognitive distress may include

- Negative self-talk

- Decreased cognitive function.

Spiritual distress may include

- Search for meaning
- Crisis in faith
- What is death?
- What will death be like?
- What about my life?

- Religion
- Paranormal experiences
- Review of priorities
- Review of values.

Family members and friends may experience a range of emotions for many reasons possibly related to the components of the whole person.

Principles for effective communication with a person experiencing a life-limiting illness or with their family and friends

When communicating with a person experiencing a life-limiting illness, or with their family and friends, it is important to

- Be self-aware – of own values, beliefs and needs
- Demonstrate respect
- Show empathy and compassion
- Be silent when necessary
- Listen actively
- Be sensitive to non-verbal behaviours and voice
- Touch if appropriate – hugs can be good
- Demonstrate ethical behaviour
- Provide company for the person dying or for a family member or friend
- Use an interdisciplinary approach – you cannot do it alone
- Always behave with integrity and honesty.

Strategies for communicating with a person experiencing a life-limiting illness or with their family and friends

- A family-centred approach is essential when someone is dying.
- A holistic approach is vital when a person is dying.
- Be committed to the quality of life of the person.
- Be willing to discuss the practical aspects of dying.
- Be aware of personal limitations – the health professional does not need to meet the needs of every person seeking their assistance.
- Consider the need for debriefing at various times with other team members.

ROLE PLAYS

Role-play the following scenarios. Before acting the roles you may wish to decide what type of assistance Person 1 requires. If it is not possible to role-play these scenarios, consider and explore the possible responses and communication strategies that will achieve effective communication and family/person-centred practice.

Scenario one: The male and the health professional

Person 1: Your name is James and you are a 47-year-old pastry chef. You love working in your local bakery and have lots of friends who come into the shop. You contracted a virus 8 months ago, which you thought was from walking half an hour to work at 2 o'clock every morning. However, the cough did not improve and you began to lose weight rapidly. After 4 months of having the terrible cough the local doctor sent you for tests. You knew deep down there was something seriously wrong, but you did not want to think about it because it was less than a year since your mother died unexpectedly.

Then, 2 months ago the doctors told you that you have final-stage cancer, an aggressive form of cancer that is in the major organs of your body and in your lymphatic system. You know you have a limited time to live, but you do not know how long. You are home from hospital and you are struggling to get through each day. You try to do something every day – you go for a walk or talk to the neighbours, but you need to sleep a lot. Although you want to remain positive for the sake of your brothers and sister it is very difficult to remain positive and you just want it all to end. You are confused and while you want to think about dying, you are not sure what it means, what it will feel like and what will happen to you when you die. You have questions but no-one who you feel you can ask about them.

Person 2: You are a health professional who lives next door to James. You see him over the back fence most days and try to encourage him to talk about what he is feeling and the things he wants to discuss. You are willing to talk about whatever he wants to, even the spiritual issues he is facing.

Scenario two: The female and the health professional

Person 1: Your name is Janice. Your mother died of breast cancer when she was 42 years old, a few years ago now. She was diagnosed, had treatment, lived for 5 years, then had a relapse and died 4 months after the recurrence of the cancer. The doctor has just told you that you have breast cancer. You are sure there was a mix-up with the pathology sampling and ask for more tests. It just is not true.

Person 2: You are the health professional who has to tell Janice the result of the extra tests is positive – she does have breast cancer.

GROUP DISCUSSION

As a large group discuss the observations, emotions and outcomes of the role plays. Suggest possible alternative strategies that may increase the effectiveness of the communication in a similar situation.

Many individuals who seek the assistance of a health professional experience a sense of grief and loss – not always about their life, but about their ability to function and participate. Health professionals who understand this reality can communicate more effectively with people experiencing a life-limiting illness as well as people experiencing a loss of any kind.

See the end of this chapter for relevant references and further reading in palliative care.

A person experiencing a mental illness

(Key words: mental illness, psychiatric, DSM-IV, mental health)

Definition of a mental illness

A person experiencing a mental illness is someone who for various reasons is unable to manage the demands of life. People with particular conditions require assistance from a mental health service from time to time. Some of these conditions include anxiety, personality disorders, psychosis, paranoid schizophrenia, bipolar disorder, post-traumatic stress disorder, depression, alcoholism, drug addiction, obsessive compulsive disorder, phobias and combinations of the above.

Behaviours related to a person experiencing a mental illness

A person attending a mental health service may behave in a variety of ways depending on their condition, compliance with medication, current stability, the predictability of events in their life and their consistency of participation in health-sustaining behaviours.

A person experiencing a mental illness might be

- Withdrawn with no desire or ability to relate
- Aggressive and sometimes violent
- Repetitive in actions or words
- Behaving in a manner that does not indicate connection with reality
- Perfectly coherent and conversant.

Individuals most susceptible to experiencing a mental illness

The individuals susceptible to experiencing a mental illness include people who

- Have addictions
- Have experienced previous episodes of any mental illness
- Have reduced sense of worth or self-esteem
- Self-harm
- Are suicidal
- Believe someone is attempting to hurt them
- Say they hear voices that tell them what to do.

Possible emotions a person with a mental illness might experience

A person with a mental illness might experience emotions related to

- Rejection
- Hopelessness
- Changing cultures
- Having no place to belong
- Feeling under-valued
- Loss of any kind
- Never being 'able'
- Paranoia
- Cognitive dysfunction
- Having always been told they were not good enough
- Negative self-talk
- Addiction
- Loss and grief
- Hallucinations
- Failure to take medication
- Reactions to medication.

Principles for effective communication with a person experiencing a mental illness

When communicating with a person experiencing a mental illness it is important to

- Make introductions
- Demonstrate respect
- Show appropriate honesty
- Confront if appropriate
- Give clear explanations
- Listen actively
- Accept
- Disengage.

Strategies for communicating with a person experiencing a mental illness

- Understand that the person is vulnerable.
- Remember the person is not always aware of the consequences of their behaviour.
- Do not take comments the person makes personally.
- Do not believe the accusations of the person about anyone else.
- Therapeutic groups can be effective.
- Outline clear and consistent expectations.
- Set clear and consistent boundaries.

DISCUSSION POINT

See the Introduction to Section Four for instructions about how to use these scenarios for group discussion.

Scenario one

Matthew is a 28-year-old man who is addicted to alcohol and currently in hospital for detoxification. He has developed a good relationship with a male student health professional. They have very different backgrounds but are the same age and share common interests. The student visits Matthew one morning to find him writhing in pain, sweat pouring off his brow and looking terrible. Matthew seems desperate and surprises the student by grabbing his wrist. Matthew is trembling and he says that the doctor caring for him has not been assisting him. He pleads for a 'drink', saying all he needs is one – just one would get him through this and he would never touch another drop.

The student feels sorry for Matthew; he knows Matthew has had a very tough life and feels he has suffered enough. He wants to help Matthew to stop him from suffering.

A nurse sees the student leaving Matthew's room and says *You have to be careful of alcoholics when they are at this stage – they will do anything for a drink*. This comment seems unfeeling and callous to the student, who simply thinks that Matthew has suffered enough.
- What would you do?
- What would you think if you learnt the student gave Matthew a drink?
- What would you think if you learnt the student was so disturbed by this situation he over-used alcohol himself that night?
- How would you feel if you were the health professional student?

↳

↳
Scenario two

Rod is a 56-year-old secondary school teacher who loves teaching mathematics. However, he has recently found the behaviour of some of the 15-year-olds upsets him and makes him angry. He is usually patient and understanding and is able to relate well to the needs of young people. He is finding his impatience disturbing and has begun to think it means he is not a good teacher. He begins to feel discouraged about his ability to teach and to relate appropriately to the students. He believes he no longer has the ability to teach successfully and begins to feel he must find another profession. He feels he is too old to retrain so he applies for a curriculum development position, but is unsuccessful. Several weeks after this, his mother and twin brother suddenly die in a car accident. He now often feels hopeless and alone. These emotions continue for over a year. He is constantly tired and finds it difficult to sleep. When asked if he is feeling unwell, he simply states he is tired. His wife, colleagues and friends notice he is withdrawn with limited affect. His wife suggests he seek assistance because he seems depressed. He says he is fine. Several weeks later, he unsuccessfully attempts suicide.

- What do you think? What would you do if you were Rod?
- How would you communicate with Rod?
- What do you feel is important when communicating with people similar to Rod?

Scenario three

Sally is a 20-year-old woman with a history of treatment for anorexia. She is no longer haunted by the thoughts that caused the anorexia and is enjoying studying to be a health professional. She has recently begun to experience what she describes as panic attacks. She says she knows she can successfully complete the courses in the program but finds herself having these attacks whenever she thinks about the amount of work she has to complete. She says she has trouble breathing and her heart races, her palms become sweaty and she wants to vomit. The symptoms usually pass after a few hours, but they are occurring more frequently and lasting longer. She decides to ask a close friend for advice about this.

- What would you say to Sally?
- How would you relate to Sally?
- What elements of communication do you feel are important when relating to Sally?

GROUP DISCUSSION

As a large group share the main points discussed by each small group about these scenarios. Consider various strategies that may increase the effectiveness of the communication in a similar situation. Decide how a health professional should act in similar situations.

There is a particular stigma associated with people who experience mental illness. Both the media and social misconceptions support and sustain this stigma. However, it is not the symptoms and behaviours associated with mental illness that are the focus of the health professions. It is people who are human beings with particular needs and desires that are the focus of all health professions.

A person experiencing a hearing impairment

(Key words: hearing loss, deafness, hard of hearing, deaf, industrial deafness, Auslan, New Zealand Sign Language, American Sign)

Definition of a hearing impairment

A person with a hearing impairment is someone who

- Finds verbal or aural communication difficult because of an inability to hear.
- Finds comprehension of cultural cues difficult to understand because of a hearing impairment.

Behaviours related to a person with a hearing impairment

A person with a hearing impairment will exhibit different behaviour according to the age at which they developed a hearing impairment, whether they grew up in the Deaf community or a hearing population, whether they have learnt to lip-read and whether they can read and write.

A person with a hearing impairment might

- Often communicate with strong non-verbal gestures and facial expressions
- Make intense efforts to be understood that may appear aggressive
- Appear rude or inappropriate if they do not hear many auditory cues (the social or cultural cues of hearing people may have different meaning or no meaning to a person with a hearing impairment)
- Demonstrate behaviour typical of mistrust
- Behave in a stubborn manner.

Individuals most susceptible to a hearing impairment

The individuals susceptible to experiencing a hearing impairment are

- Unborn babies with family members who are deaf – hereditary
- Babies who do not develop appropriately in utero – congenital
- Babies who have undetected meningitis
- Premature infants who receive antibiotics with ototoxic side effects
- Individuals who experience trauma to the head or neck
- Individuals who experience an industrial accident
- Children with recurring undetected or untreated ear infections
- Individuals who do not wear earmuffs in areas of high noise
- Older people who experience age-related hearing loss
- Individuals from countries that do not have occupational health and safety standards to protect their hearing
- Individuals from countries or regions within countries that have limited health services.

Possible emotions a person with a hearing impairment might experience

A person with a hearing impairment might experience emotions related to

- Anger
- Frustration
- Rejection
- Fear
- Confusion
- Vehemence
- Isolation.

Possible reasons for these emotions

A person with a hearing impairment might experience these emotions because of

- Seeing what is happening but not being able to hear or understand everything
- Having people shout at them because they think speaking loudly will assist their ability to hear
- People talking too quickly and/or with unclear articulation when they are trying to lip-read
- People talking to the hearing people in a situation but not including the person with a hearing impairment
- People speaking or signing to an interpreter rather than to the individual with the hearing impairment.

Principles for effective communication with a person experiencing a hearing impairment

When communicating with a person experiencing a hearing impairment it is important to

- Show patience and perseverance – keep trying to achieve understanding
- Avoid responding with frustration
- Clarify understanding
- Validate
- Disengage – this is very important
- Avoid using humour, as subtle nuances of language associated with humour are difficult to perceive, understand or explain
- Use predictable and well-articulated speech if the person is lip-reading.

Strategies for communicating with a person experiencing a hearing impairment

- Use alternative methods of communicating if you do not share a common language.
- If working with individuals who have a hearing impairment on a regular basis, consider learning the appropriate sign language for your country (e.g. Auslan [Australian Sign Language] for Australia and some of the Pacific).
- Try to communicate even if you do not understand.
- Use written words or pictures wherever possible.
- If communicating with someone who lip reads, stand directly in front of them, articulate clearly and speak at a steady pace.
- Do not assume they want to hear, because lack of hearing may be part of their identity.

DISCUSSION POINT

See the Introduction to Section Four for instructions about how to use these scenarios for group discussion.

Scenario one

Simon is a 10-year-old boy who was diagnosed with a severe hearing impairment at the age of 6. The hearing impairment was discovered during a routine medical checkup at school. By that time Simon had been labelled as having a behaviour problem, because he would never sit still to listen in class and was always the last to finish any work. His written work was good when he could copy but he was never able to write a story or read words.

Simon has always been a child who loves to move and thus he rarely played games that required hearing. He rarely spoke before attending school but seemed to understand spoken words and instructions. He is a loving boy and has a supportive mother who trained as a teacher's aid to assist him with his school work. He has recently had cochlear implants, which have restored 70% of his hearing in both ears. However, Simon is still behind other children his age with his school work and requires constant assistance with his work.

• How will you relate to Simon?
• What will be your goals in communicating with him?

Scenario two

Rhonda is a 24-year-old beautician. She was born without hearing to parents who could hear. They did not consider that Rhonda should learn sign language and insisted she learn to lip-read and verbalise. They sent her to a non-specialist local school with her siblings. Rhonda learned to read and write as well as lip-read. She is intelligent and thus is able to compensate for her hearing impairment by guessing the meaning of situations if she cannot actually understand. She is determined and studied hard to become a beautician. She is very difficult to understand when she speaks and often repeats words in an attempt to be understood. She is confident but very moody when others are talking without including her. According to the culture of the hearing population, her non-verbal behaviours are exaggerated and often appear rude.

• How will you relate to Rhonda?
• What will be your goals when communicating with her?

GROUP DISCUSSION

As a large group share the main points discussed by each small group about these scenarios. Consider various strategies that may increase the effectiveness of the communication in a similar situation.

There are many different sign languages worldwide. Within Australia there are two main dialects of Auslan. The northern dialect is based on French Sign Language and the southern dialect on British Sign Language. New Zealand Sign Language was adopted as the official sign language of New Zealand in 2006. Sign languages are languages in their own right, unrelated to the spoken language of the people who live in the same country. (Auslan, for example, is not the same as Signed English, which uses a sign to represent each English word.) Users of sign languages use signs to indicate particular meanings and may express a whole concept with one sign, where it might take many words to express the same concept in a spoken language. Each sign language also has alphabet signs for finger spelling. Many use a two-handed method of spelling letter by letter. However, American Sign uses a one-handed finger-spelling system. Alphabet signing/finger spelling is a small component of signing for sign language users, only used if needing to communicate an English name or word, or with people who are not fully competent in the sign language.

Individuals who are born with a hearing impairment into a hearing population have a very different identity to individuals born Deaf into a community of Deaf individuals ('the Deaf community'). The Deaf community believe that being Deaf is part of their identity and are sometimes vehement about maintaining that identity. Thus, they may choose not to have cochlear implants despite the possibility of being able to hear.

A person experiencing a visual impairment

(Key words: visual loss, blindness, blind, visual impairment)

Definition of a visual impairment

A person with a visual impairment is someone who

- Is unable to experience the world visually because of a loss of visual acuity – the ability to see clearly
- Has less than 6/60 corrected visual acuity in both eyes
- Has a field of vision constricted to less than ten degrees of arc around the central fixation in either eye.

Behaviours related to a person with a visual impairment

A person with a visual impairment will exhibit different behaviour according to the age at which they developed the visual impairment – whether they were born with no sight or lost their sight at a later age, whether they experienced special education specifically designed for people with visual loss, and whether they can read and write.

A person with a visual impairment might

- Move confidently with particular self-controlled assistance
- Move timidly when in an unfamiliar environment
- Have limited facial and non-verbal behaviours, depending on the situation
- Show well-adjusted behaviour and ease of mobility.

A person who is losing their vision slowly might

- Walk close to a wall
- Have poor posture
- Move hesitantly or with short steps
- Squint or tilt their head
- Spill or knock over food and other items
- Bump into objects
- Look closely at items such as print
- Request changes in lighting
- Be sensitive to light
- Easily become lost
- Be unable to find items
- No longer recognise people by sight
- Demonstrate altered emotional states, such as anxiety, tearfulness, frustration and embarrassment
- Stop taking care of their appearance
- Stop socialising in a group
- Stop reading or sewing
- Stop participating in activities.

Individuals most susceptible to a visual impairment

The individuals most susceptible to a visual impairment are those who

- Have a family disposition to blindness
- Have degenerative eye conditions
- Have congenital causes
- Experience trauma to the head or face
- Experience an industrial accident
- Have repeated and untreated eye infections
- Are children with poor nutrition
- Are children who live in environmentally deprived situations
- Do not wear goggles in designated work areas
- Are from countries that do not have occupational health and safety standards to protect their sight
- Have diabetes
- Are children with juvenile diabetes
- Are from countries or regions within countries that have limited health services.

Possible emotions a person with a visual impairment might experience

A person with a visual impairment might experience emotions related to

- Interest
- Insecurity
- Confusion
- Frustration
- Fear
- Sadness
- Envy
- Resentment
- Helplessness
- Determination.

Possible reasons for these emotions

A person with a visual impairment might experience these emotions because of

- Other people assuming they know their needs
- Other people assuming they must require assistance because they are blind
- Strangers feeling sorry for them
- Hearing things but being unable to see them
- Hearing threatening sounds to which they cannot respond because they cannot see the cause
- Having limited control when in unfamiliar situations.

Principles for effective communication with a person experiencing a visual impairment

When communicating with a person experiencing a visual impairment it is important to

- Touch – remember to ask permission first
- Validate
- Clarify
- Ensure use of physical contact to demonstrate your presence if using silence
- Provide information – use Braille or computer technology if appropriate
- Disengage.

Strategies for communicating with a person experiencing a visual impairment

- Identify yourself – do not assume the person will recognise you by your voice.
- Speak naturally and clearly. Loss of eyesight does not mean loss of hearing.
- Continue to use body language. This will affect the tone of your voice and give a lot of extra information to the person.
- Use everyday language. Do not avoid words like 'see' or 'look' or talking about everyday activities such as watching television or DVDs.
- Name the person when introducing yourself or when directing conversation to them in a group situation.
- In a group situation, introduce the other people present.
- Never channel conversation through a third person.
- Never leave a conversation with a person without saying you are doing so.
- Use accurate and specific language when giving directions, for example, *The door is on your left* rather than *The door is over there*.
- Avoid situations where there is competing noise.
- Always ask if they require assistance – do not assume they do.
- In dangerous situations say *Stop* rather than *Look out*.
- Relax and be yourself.
- Do not assume you know what they want or what will help them. Ask them.

ROLE PLAYS

Role-play the following scenarios. Before acting the roles you may wish to decide what type of assistance Person 1 requires. If it is not possible to role-play these scenarios, consider and explore the possible responses and communication strategies that will achieve effective communication and family/person-centred practice.

Scenario one: The male and the health professional
Person 1: Ronny lives in a rural area. He is 64 years old and last week received the diagnosis of trachoma after experiencing conjunctivitis for some time. He lives with his extended family. There is only one income to support seven people. He is happy but finds his fading vision disturbing, because he is not as mobile these days and loves watching the local children play in the school-yard next to his house. He finds it difficult to watch television but has it on for company when the others are away.
Person 2: You are the health professional who needs to have a conversation with Ronny and collaborate to set achievable goals. You know that his visual loss may be permanent.
- What is important for Ronny?
- What might you need to know in order to assist him to maintain meaning in his life?

Scenario two: The female and the health professional
Person 1: Your name is Tania and you are a 24-year-old woman with an indigenous background. You are a well-respected early intervention teacher who manages a local preschool. You love everything about your job – the paperwork, the children, the parents, seeing the children develop skills and grow taller, as well as having them proudly display their work before they leave each day. The parents, staff and children say you have excellent skills in observing and interpreting the non-verbal cues of children, parents and staff. However, you have recently lost your vision after an accident and have not been able to

↳

↳ work. Your boyfriend of 4 years – now your fiancé – is supportive but you sense he is afraid and unsure of your future together.

Person 2: You are meeting Tania for the first time and you want to assist her to establish some appropriate short-term and long-term goals.

GROUP DISCUSSION

As a large group discuss the observations, emotions and outcomes of the role plays. Suggest possible alternative strategies that may increase the effectiveness of the communication in a similar situation.

References

Kubler-Ross E 1969 On death and dying. Routledge, London

Kubler-Ross E, Kessler D 2005 On grief and grieving: finding the meaning of grief through the five stages of loss. Simon and Schuster, London

New Zealand Palliative Care Strategy. Available: www.moh.govt.nz/moh.nsf/pagesmh/2951 24 Mar 2008

Palliative Care Australia. Available: www.pallcare.org.au 23 Mar 2008

World Health Organization 2008 Available: www.who.int/cancer/palliative/definition/en/ 23 Mar 2008

Further reading

Life-limiting illnesses

Australia & New Zealand Society of Palliative Medicine www.anzspm.org.au

White G 2006 Talking about spirituality in health care practice: a resource for the multi-professional health care team. Jessica Kingsley, London

Helpful journals

Bereavement Care
Cancer Journal
Critical Care Medicine
Critical Care Nursing Clinics in North America
European Journal of Palliative Care
International Journal of Palliative Nursing
Journal for Community Nurses
Journal of Pain & Symptom Management
Journal of Palliative Care
Nursing and Residential Care
Palliative Medicine
Psycho-oncology
Qualitative Health Research
Topics in Geriatric Rehabilitation

Hearing impairment

Australia

Australian Hearing	www.hearing.com.au
Auslan Sign Bank	www.auslan.org.au
(Royal Institute for Deaf and Blind Children)	

New Zealand

Deaf Association of New Zealand Inc	www.deaf.co.nz
National Foundation for the Deaf Inc	www.nfd.org.nz

United States of America

National Association of the Deaf	www.nad.org
American Sign Language	www.aslinfo.com

United Kingdom

Royal Society for Deaf People	www.royaldeaf.org.uk

Visual impairment

Australia

Vision Australia	www.visionaustralia.org

New Zealand

Royal New Zealand Foundation of the Blind	www.rnzfb.org.nz

People in particular contexts

23

CHAPTER OBJECTIVE

Upon completing this chapter, students should be able to apply knowledge and consolidate the required skills to communicate effectively with people in particular contexts.

Health professionals assist vulnerable people in a range of contexts. This chapter considers people in three contexts that may be a barrier to effective communication: **an emergency, domestic abuse** and **a different language to the health professional**.

SMALL GROUP ACTIVITY: PARTICULAR CONTEXTS

An emergency
Domestic abuse
A different language to the health professional
- Decide what it means to be a person in these contexts.
- Choose one of three options:
  - List the specific behaviours that might relate to being a person who experiences an emergency, *or*
  - List the emotions a person experiencing domestic abuse might experience when relating to a health service, *or*
  - Discuss which individuals may be most susceptible to the emotions associated with not being able to speak the language of the health professional.
- List possible reasons that might explain the emotions a person in these contexts might experience when seeing a health professional.
- List principles for effective communication to remember when communicating with a person in these contexts. Give reasons for the need to remember these principles.
- Suggest strategies for communicating with a person in these contexts. Decide why you might see such a person in your particular health profession.
- Check your answers against the information below, noting any additional thoughts or ideas.

A person who experiences an emergency

(Key words: emergency, near-death experience, accident, disaster, attack, trauma)

Definition of a person who experiences an emergency

A person who experiences an emergency is someone who experiences adverse bodily harm because of an accident, attack or natural disaster.

Behaviours related to being a person who experiences an emergency

A person who experiences an emergency might be

- Impatient and angry, even aggressive
- Irrational and incoherent due to shock
- Chatty and apparently unconcerned
- Quiet and unresponsive
- Frustrated – expressed verbally or non-verbally
- Completely passive.

Individuals most susceptible to emergencies

The individuals most susceptible to emergencies are anyone who lives, breathes and moves, regardless of age, racial group and gender! However, people may be especially susceptible to emergencies if they

- Play sport or do extreme sports (e.g. mountain climbing, abseiling)
- Drive
- Work with machinery, whether in cities or rural areas
- Are involved in violent encounters.

Possible emotions a person who experiences an emergency might experience

A person who experiences physical or emotional harm because of an emergency may feel

- Fear
- Anger
- Shock
- Guilt
- Despondency
- Impatience
- Disbelief
- Frustration from being asked to answer the same questions by different health professionals
- A lack of control over the things being done to them.

Principles for effective communication with a person who experiences an emergency

When communicating with a person who experiences an emergency it is important to

- Demonstrate empathy to build a therapeutic relationship
- Validate
- Make introductions
- Provide and explain information
- Remember that such people are often in pain and may be impatient and angry if asked the same questions repeatedly; instead, make statements to verify the gathered information
- Recognise that shock can affect the cognitive functioning of an individual
- Recognise that the person may respond differently to their actual feelings if medicated for pain
- Verify or clarify the interpretations of perceptions
- Comfort and reassure through encouragement –they may be afraid of the implications of the emergency for their future
- Remember that the person may experience social isolation in hospital if they were airlifted from a rural area
- Remember the person did not intend to have or cause the accident.

Strategies for communicating with a person who experiences an emergency

- Consider the whole person – they will have more than physical needs.
- Observe the non-verbal behaviours of the person closely and ask for verification or clarification of the interpretations of those perceptions.
- Gather information from notes and other health professionals rather than asking the same questions repeatedly. If unsure about the accuracy of the information, make statements and ask for verification; this allows the person to simply nod or affirm in some manner.
- Give non-verbal cues or visual indication of what is happening or what the person needs to do.
- Express sensitivity and compassion regardless of the cause of the emergency.
- Remember the family members of people seriously hurt because of an emergency – they are often terrified and have feelings of helplessness.

ROLE PLAYS

Role-play the following scenarios. Before acting the roles you may wish to decide what type of assistance Person 1 requires. If it is not possible to role-play these scenarios, consider and explore the possible responses and communication strategies that will achieve effective communication and family/person-centred practice.

Scenario one: The male and the health professional
Person 1: Your name is Malcolm. You are a 28-year-old man who shattered your right tibia and fibula playing football. You are no longer in the acute ward but you remember your experience in emergency vividly.

You arrived in an ambulance, were hurriedly transferred to a cubicle in emergency with the curtains drawn and left alone in pain for what seemed like hours. Thirsty and exhausted, you realised you wanted to go to the toilet. You were not comfortable calling for help. Finally, a nurse came in with a tray. Without introducing himself, he asked particular questions and filled in a form. Then, without explaining what he was doing, he rolled up your sleeve. You pulled your arm away, not sure what was coming next. He grabbed the tray and left. As he disappeared through the curtains you quickly said you needed to go to the toilet. You heard the nurse say *The one with the broken leg is uncooperative and wants a bottle*. Some time later a different nurse arrived with a bottle. Every person who came in after that asked you the same questions. There were several hours of waiting and your lower back was hurting. A doctor finally arrived. She examined you and asked the same old questions. She explained you would need surgery, which would take place in about an hour. There were no explanations of anything and no time to ask questions or find out what happened to your expensive football boots. Your parents were an hour away and you had just terminated your relationship with your girlfriend of 5 years. You thought about how you were studying full-time and working part-time doing deliveries. You lay in emergency worrying about how you would pay your rent, drive your car and continue your studies. You felt lonely and unloved.

You are now attending a rehabilitation service and find it difficult to trust most health professionals because of the treatment you received on that first day, the day you broke your leg during that tackle. You are meeting a new health professional today. You are not interested in another change – it will mean more of the same questions.
Person 2: You are the health professional assigned to assess Malcolm. You have heard he is not trusting and although motivated to improve he is often sullen and reluctant to develop a relationship.

Scenario two: The female and the health professional
Person 1: Your name is Rachel and you are a solicitor in a big law firm. You are 40 years old and divorced, with two children aged 12 and 14 who live with you every alternate week. Your parents are ageing and quite frail. While you were driving to work a young driver drove through a red light, hitting the driver's door next to you. You fractured four ribs and your right femur and lost some teeth in the accident. You are now in an emergency department. You are very worried about your children and the future, including paying the mortgage for your recently-purchased beautiful new apartment. You cannot think clearly or remember what has happened since the accident. Fear, anxiety and pain limit your ability to concentrate and understand what is happening around you.
Person 2: You are the health professional who must explain a procedure or future event to Rachel.

GROUP DISCUSSION

As a large group discuss the observations, emotions and outcomes of the role plays. Suggest possible alternative strategies that may increase the effectiveness of the communication in a similar situation.

Not all health professionals relate to people who experience emergencies immediately after the emergency. However, many will communicate with people who remember the experience of an emergency, either as a victim or an observer. Such individuals require communication that considers the various aspects of their lives that influence their everyday roles, participation and functioning.

A person who experiences domestic abuse

(Key words: domestic violence, domestic abuse)

Definition of domestic abuse

Domestic abuse occurs when individuals in a family experience physical or emotional abuse in direct or indirect forms from a member of the same family.

Domestic abuse can take the form of

- Physical aggression, that is, an attack causing physical harm
- Emotional manipulation or accusatory blaming
- Deprivation of needs by controlling money
- Isolation from friends and family
- Constant expectation of explanations of behaviours and whereabouts.

Both men and women experience domestic abuse, however, the majority of people experiencing domestic abuse are women. Domestic abuse can occur in heterosexual and homosexual relationships. Another form of abuse is elder abuse. This abuse may occur in families or aged-care facilities. Elder abuse can be as undetected and destructive as domestic abuse.

Individuals who experience domestic abuse have many needs. They need first to understand that women or men generally and them specifically do not have to submit to abusive relationships. They will not benefit from discussion about suspected domestic abuse until they establish this understanding. Once individuals accept that they do not have to remain in an abusive relationship, they will require particular assistance from an appropriate service. They will require a safe place to live, appropriate care for any children, financial assistance and child support, a means of becoming financially self-supporting and, possibly, legal protection.

Many people who experience domestic abuse find it difficult to leave because they believe the person will change. The abusive relationship usually includes patterns of alternating i) abuse and ii) expressions of love and promises to change and never abuse again. Fear of the abuser committing suicide, of trying to kill them or hurting the children, or fear of being alone, may stop a person from leaving an abusive relationship. If they do actually leave the relationship, they require ongoing counselling to overcome the erosion to their self-image that results from an abusive relationship.

Behaviours related to being a person who experiences domestic abuse

A person who experiences domestic abuse might

- Always act to satisfy the people around them, especially their partners
- Accept any abusive or violent behaviour they experience
- Avoid mentioning their experiences regardless of the associated depth of emotion
- Find it difficult to make decisions
- Be passive in relationships and not mention their own needs
- Show behaviour that is not assertive or acknowledging of their needs
- Always take the blame when things do not go according to plan
- Stay in an abusive relationship because of fear for the children or fear of being alone
- Always be looking at the time – not wanting to be late or away too long
- Blame themselves for having provoked the abuse.

Possible emotions a person who experiences domestic abuse might experience

A person who experiences domestic abuse might experience emotions related to

- Fear
- Uncertainty
- Poor self-esteem
- Feeling deserving of the abuse
- Anger
- Guilt
- Mistrust of men and/or women
- Anxiety
- Feeling unlovable
- Insecurity
- Depression
- Isolation
- Denial of the problem
- Ambivalence.

Possible reasons for these emotions

People experiencing domestic abuse may experience these emotions because of

- Negative self-talk
- Feeling that women deserve abuse
- Their partner using non-verbal behaviour to control
- Their partner often threatening to harm
- Their partner constantly 'putting them down'
- Their partner not allowing access to their money
- Their partner not allowing them to do paid work
- Their partner stating they are not a good parent
- Their partner controlling who they see and what they do
- Their partner destroying their property
- Their partner saying they deserve the abuse
- Their partner threatening suicide
- Their partner threatening to hurt the children.

Principles for effective communication with a person who experiences domestic abuse

When communicating with a person experiencing domestic abuse it is important to

- Be reliable and worthy of trust
- Create a safe place
- Confront inappropriate beliefs
- Listen actively
- Observe their non-verbal communication
- Validate their emotions, not their situation
- Provide clear information.

Strategies for communicating with a person who experiences domestic abuse

- Build rapport – this is essential.
- Be careful with touch.
- Deal with the specific issues.
- Affirm their strengths.
- Communicate to externalise the problems.
- Set achievable goals.
- Use same-gender health professionals.
- Refer to appropriate services.
- Avoid criticism of their skills.

DISCUSSION POINT

See the Introduction to Section Four for instructions about how to use these scenarios for group discussion.

Scenario one

Jan loves wine and often drinks a bottle of wine over lunch and with the evening meal. She is a friendly person whose partner, Greg, gives her everything she wants to keep her happy and away from alcohol. She often screams and swears at Greg and even chases and hits him with whatever she can find at the time. Greg comes in for regular checkups and has just come in for treatment. He has a broken right arm and states he broke his arm falling off a ladder more than a month ago. The next time Greg comes in he has a black eye and a hand shaped bruise on his now-healed broken arm. He states he ran into a door but has no answer when asked about the shape of the bruise on his arm. He quickly covers it with his sleeve.

- How should you relate?
- What should you say?
- Do your goals change?

Scenario two

Alicia lives in a caravan (trailer) park with her three children and husband, who is a labourer at the local ship-building yard. He is often tired and angry when he returns from work. He expects everything exactly as he wants it when he arrives home and regularly hits Alicia if things are not as he wants. She has presented to your health service with a back injury and has bruises on her back that suggest she was hit. She maintains she hurt her back from a fall, but does not remember the details. You suspect domestic abuse.

- How should you relate?
- What are the major aims of relating?
- What do you wish to communicate?

GROUP DISCUSSION

As a large group share the main points discussed by each small group about these scenarios. Consider various strategies that may increase the effectiveness of the communication in a similar situation. Decide how a health professional should act in similar situations.

Health professionals who suspect domestic abuse of adults or children have a duty of care to report this suspicion. It can be beneficial to discuss any suspicion with a more senior or experienced health professional in order to plan strategies for relating and the requirement to report. The realities of domestic abuse are complex and the person experiencing the abuse may believe they deserve the abuse. They may believe that removing themself would have far worse consequences than remaining in the relationship. Counselling to achieve skills in assertiveness may assist, although assertiveness may simply escalate the levels of violence. Communicating with people who experience domestic abuse is challenging. It requires understanding and affirmation of the person to achieve effective communication.

A person who speaks a different language to the health professional

(Key words: speaker of languages other than English [LOTE], non-native speaker [NNS], non-English-speaking background [NESB])

Definition of a person who speaks a different language to the health professional

A person who speaks a different language to the health professional is someone who is unable to communicate verbally or in written form in the language of the health professional.

Behaviours related to being a person who speaks a different language to the health professional

A person who speaks a different language to the health professional might

- Show apparently aggressive non-verbal behaviours
- Demonstrate apparent comprehension even when they do not understand
- Attempt to work problems out alone
- Avoid asking for assistance because of embarrassment
- Sit quietly and avoid indicating they do not understand
- Expect the services to be the same as they are in their own culture.

Possible emotions a person who speaks a different language to the health professional might experience

A person who speaks a different language to the health professional might experience emotions related to

- Fear about communicating in another language
- Confusion and vulnerability, even though they normally understand conversational English
- Inadequacy because they understand general English but not the English of the health professional
- Frustration because of trying to understand but not being sure that they do.

Possible reasons for these emotions

A person who speaks a different language to the health professional may experience these emotions because of

- Regular breakdowns in communication
- Apparently aggressive non-verbal behaviours from those around them
- Regular misunderstandings
- Differences in cultural and social expectations
- Age and gender differences
- Cultural differences.

Principles for effective communication with a person who speaks a different language to the health professional

When communicating with a person who speaks a different language to the health professional it is important to

- Demonstrate empathy
- Respect cultural differences
- Establish rapport to build a therapeutic relationship
- Negotiate meaning to achieve mutual understanding
- Constantly clarify the understanding of the person
- Avoid making assumptions
- Consider the potential meaning of the non-verbal behaviours of the person – do not assume the non-verbal behaviours have the same meaning in both cultures.

Strategies for communicating with a person who speaks a different language to the health professional

- Use an interpreter – remember to speak to the person *not* the interpreter.
- Ask questions about what is appropriate in their culture. You could ask the interpreter or family members who are fluent in your language.
- Avoid using non-verbal or visual cues unless you are certain of their meaning.
- Explain how and why things are done in this health service.
- Wherever possible avoid using family members or friends to interpret.
- Wherever possible use a same-gender health professional.
- Wherever possible provide all information in *translated* written form, ensuring the translation is the correct form of the language of the person.
- Have a known person introduce any new health professionals that will assist the person.
- Learn a few simple words and phrases of the language of the person (e.g. hello, thank you, please, goodbye, how are you?)
- Avoid presuming they understand.
- Avoid presuming the health professional understands.
- Have a sense of humour.

ROLE PLAYS

Role-play the following scenarios. Before acting the roles you may wish to decide what type of assistance Person 1 requires. If it is not possible to role-play these scenarios, consider and explore the possible responses and communication strategies that will achieve effective communication and family/person-centred practice.

Scenario one: The male and the health professional
Person 1: Your name is Ahmed and you are a 45-year-old Middle-Eastern man who requires assistance from a health service. You speak very limited English and feel insecure about this unfamiliar place. Although you do not usually speak to unknown women, especially in public places, you spoke to a woman who was wearing a uniform. You hoped she might speak Arabic and you tried to speak to her. She seemed confused when she looked at you but obviously did not understand Arabic.

↳

↳

Person 2: You must assess and devise some goals for a new person seeking assistance. He is a Muslim man who you think appears arrogant and rude. You observed him speak to the female cleaner who, although she does not speak fluent English, does not speak Arabic either. She appeared shocked and confused and you assume the man was rude to her. However, you are unsure because you may be misinterpreting his non-verbal behaviours or his tone of voice.

Scenario two: The female and the health professional

Person 1: Your name is Kyoko and you are a 20-year-old woman from Japan. You have been studying English and have basic conversational skills. You are planning to become a health professional when you complete your English studies. You would prefer to see the health professionals in Japan but you will not be in Japan for another 10 months so you are sitting timidly in a health service waiting room. You remember the first time you came to this service – you were very embarrassed and distressed that a young male health professional assessed you. Although he explained everything, your English skills were not proficient enough to understand. You remember crying very quietly. The young man, Matt, did not notice until you were leaving, when a lady waiting asked Matt what he had done because you were crying. When he noticed he seemed to be concerned; he thought he had physically hurt you.

The next time you came he introduced a female health professional and an interpreter. You were able to apologise for crying and explain that you would feel more comfortable with a female health professional assisting you if possible. You were able to have all your questions answered. Matt was able to explain everything he did the last time and explain what would happen next time. Since then, you have been seeing Rochelle and she has been helping you.

Person 2: You are Matt. Kyoko is a lovely young lady who has been receiving assistance for several weeks. The beginning was difficult but using an interpreter really helped for her second visit. Having Rochelle work with her also made a difference. However, today Rochelle is away and you have to see Kyoko. You are concerned and enter the waiting area with a little trepidation.

GROUP DISCUSSION

As a large group discuss the observations, emotions and outcomes of the role plays. Suggest possible alternative strategies that may increase the effectiveness of the communication in a similar situation.

Glossary

Aboriginal or Torres Strait Islander Peoples The original inhabitants of the continent of Australia. An Aboriginal or Torres Strait Islander is a person of Aboriginal or Torres Strait Islander descent who identifies as an Aboriginal or Torres Strait Islander and is accepted as such by the community in which they live.

Active listening Listening that responds to the verbal and non-verbal messages sent in a manner that indicates interest and acceptance. It enables the health professional to Assist, Enjoy, Influence, Observe and Understand.

Aggressive communication Communication in which perceptions, opinions and feelings are expressed in a manner that intimidates or attacks the other communicating individual(s).

Alternative communication Non-verbal forms of communication to replace the spoken word, for example, an electronic device using visual communication software.

Ambiguity A situation in which something can be understood in more than one way and it is initially not clear which meaning is intended.

Assertive communication Communication in which perceptions, ideas or opinions are expressed in a manner that respects the worth and rights of others to have and express perceptions, ideas or opinions.

Attitudes Unconscious values and beliefs.

Augmentative and alternative communication (AAC) Systems that allow non-verbal methods of communication, including visual and computer-assisted devices.

Augmentative communication Non-verbal forms of communication that highlight the spoken word through simultaneous gestures, signs, pictures and key-word signing.

Background The environment in which a person grows and matures, and develops their values and beliefs.

Barrier Anything that stops or restricts something from happening; can restrict function and/or participation in a particular area.

Beliefs Principles or doctrines that a person or group considers true.

Bias An unfair preference or dislike of someone or something.

Body language Non-verbal communication that includes gesture, facial expression, posture, eye contact, gait and clothing.

Clan A group of families related through a common ancestor or through marriage.

Clarifying To make something clear, either by asking questions to ensure understanding or by explaining any unclear information.

Cliché A phrase or statement that is overused and does not communicate care or understanding.

Cognition The process of perceiving, processing, storing and retrieving information, as well as thinking and planning with intuitive thought and perception.

Collaborative partnership A partnership that requires the contribution of each person to achieve a satisfactory and appropriate outcome.

Comforting The process used by the health professional to ensure the person seeking assistance feels encouraged, affirmed and empowered to continue meeting the challenges they face.

Community: health profession All people who are qualified in a particular health profession.

Community: health service All people who work in or attend a particular health service.

Community: indigenous Local Aboriginal or Torres Strait Islander Peoples or Maori, or people from their place of birth.

Complementary and alternative medicine (CAM) Treatment that does not usually conform to 'traditional' medicine or the medical model.

Computer-mediated communication (CMC) Electronic forms of communication.

Confidentiality Keeping information within a particular context; involves keeping information private.

Conflict A struggle or clash between two different or opposite ideas, thoughts, people or principles; can be physical, psychological, social or spiritual.

Confronting The act of challenging and sometimes disagreeing with inappropriate attitudes and beliefs in order to clarify and examine these attitudes and beliefs and ultimately change them. It is neither intimidating nor judgemental.

Consent To give permission or approval for something to happen, usually in writing.

Context Surrounding factors that affect meaning; can be situational and environmental.

Control The ability to manage or direct the events in life.

Cross-cultural communication Occurs when people from different cultures interact with the intention of reaching mutual understanding.

Cultural assumptions Opinions about patterns of behaving, beliefs and values that are culturally determined.

Cultural competence To understand the customs, beliefs, values and behaviours of a particular culture.

Cultural identity Characteristics that a person recognises as belonging uniquely to their own culture.

Cultural norms Standard patterns of behaviour that are considered normal in a particular culture.

Cultural safety (security) Achieved through practice that respects, supports and empowers the cultural identity and wellbeing of an individual.

Cultural sensitivity Achieved through practice that accommodates the cultural identity, needs and practices of different cultures.

Culture Traditions and patterns of behaviour that develop in a particular group because of the values and beliefs of that group. It influences every aspect of life.

Culture: disease/illness Individuals with illness experience adjustment to their beliefs, values and daily habits or 'ways of doing'.

Culture: health professions Each health profession has particular values, beliefs, traditions and underlying principles that are unique to that profession.

Cultures: large Cultures with a large membership, or a nation.

Cultures: small Cultures with a small membership.

Customs Actions that people from a particular group always perform in particular ways in particular circumstances.

Defenses (defense mechanisms) Adaptive mental mechanisms that assist the individual to continue functioning, despite the presence of uncomfortable emotions, thoughts, information or wishes, by removing them from the conscious mind. They are a method of managing thoughts and emotions that would otherwise be unmanageable. There are four kinds that occur on a continuum: psychotic, immature, neurotic and mature defenses.

Disengagement Process that leads to the disconnection of the individuals in a communicative act. It involves satisfactory completion of an interaction.

Diversity Variety of something – cultures, opinions, beliefs etc.

Dominant/primary needs Needs that dominate relationships and may negatively impact on the relationship between a health professional and a person seeking assistance.

Efficacy The ability to produce the necessary and desired results with efficiency and accuracy.

Effective communication All people communicating have clearly understood the exact meaning of every message, regardless of the forms of the message.

Effective listening Listening that adapts to the particular individual, their non-verbal cues and the context. Requires active engagement with the person and their message and is a characteristic of a therapeutic relationship.

Effective speaking Requires interest in, enthusiasm for and knowledge about the topic and the 'audience', as well as understanding of the effect of non-verbal behaviours upon the words spoken.

Elders Custodians of cultural laws, ceremonies, practices, traditions and remedies. Often the key decision-makers who provide advice and leadership.

Emotions Feelings that individuals experience because of internal factors that cause negative or positive agitation or disturbance.

Empathy The direct, clear and accurate understanding and expression of the emotions of an individual.

Empower To give the person seeking assistance a sense of confidence to overcome the challenges they face.

Emphasis Stress on a particular word or phrase that may change the meaning.

Environment Factors external to the person which may be physical, emotional, social, financial or spiritual.

Equality Balance of power in a relationship through shared opportunities and mutual demonstrations of an attitude of acceptance.

Ethical communication Requires knowledge of and commitment to the requirements that result in appropriate communicative behaviour while practising as a health professional.

Ethical responsibility Protecting information about the people seeking assistance, whether read or heard.

or

Acting in the interests of the person seeking assistance and in accordance with the appropriate code of ethics or conduct.

Ethnocentric When an individual believes their particular method or way of approaching a situation is superior and indeed the best way.

Explaining To make the meaning of something clear by using words that make it easy to understand.

Eye contact Occurs when communicating individuals look directly into each others' eyes. Not appropriate in all cultures.

Facial expressions A type of body language in which the face is used to communicate meaning.

Family/person-centred practice The needs and wishes of the family or person are the centre of the goals and elements of practice.

Function To perform any activity of choice.

Gestures A type of body language in which meaning is expressed through the use of the arms, hands or fingers.

Health Sound condition of the mind, body, emotions and spirit that allows a person to function and participate.

Health professional An individual who works in a profession that directly affects the health of the people they assist.

Holistic care Considers all aspects of the person and their context, and allows them to have an active part in their healing.

Holistic communication Requires a willingness to communicate about contexts, experiences, thoughts, emotions, needs and desires. Requires understanding of the value and uniqueness of each individual.

Honesty A characteristic that results in an upright disposition and conduct.

Humour The ability to see that something is funny; the ability to laugh at oneself when an error has been made.

Ideal health professional An excellent example of a health professional because of exemplary thoughts, patterns, attitudes, values and behaviour.

Indigenous peoples 'First Nation' people – those who inhabited a country or region before another group came and settled the country or region as though it belonged to them.

Informed consent To give written permission or consent on the basis of real knowledge and understanding of an event or procedure.

Informing Communicating information or knowledge to the person seeking assistance.

Instructing Teaching someone how to do something.

Interpretation: sequential The interpreter translates a small portion of the information and then waits for the next piece of information before they interpret further.

Interpretation: simultaneous The interpreter interprets at the same time as the information is presented.

Interpreter Someone who translates orally or visually what is said in one language into another language to facilitate communication.

Interpreting Translating the meaning of an utterance regardless of the word/sound spoken.

Intervention Action taken by the health professional after collaboration with the person that will change something that is happening for the person in a positive manner.

Introducing Presenting oneself, the role, the environment, the people in the environment and their role.

Jargon Words used in a particular context or profession that gives those words specific meaning known only to those familiar with the context or profession.

Journal A helpful learning tool in which to record answers to questions and thoughts about self and reactions; can promote learning about self.

Judgement An opinion of someone based on personal values and beliefs. May not always be accurate or informed and may negatively affect communication.

Kinship group People related by blood or marriage.

Learning preferences Style of learning that best suits an individual.

Listening barriers Habits that limit the ability to listen, process, remember and respond appropriately to a spoken message.

Mainstream Health services that are provided by and for the dominant cultural group, whether owned by the government or a non-government body.

Maori The people who were the original inhabitants of New Zealand.

Misunderstanding A failure to negotiate meaning; also known as miscommunication.

Model Assists in directing practice.

Mutual understanding All the people communicating understand all the factors that contribute to the meaning of the message.

Nation A community of people who live in a defined area and share a common origin, culture, traditions and language.

National identity The characteristics that a person recognises as unique to their nation.

Non-judging Avoiding forming an opinion in order to ensure positive relations with acceptance regardless of differences between the people communicating.

Non-verbal communication Communication without spoken words.

Non-verbal messages Message sent using body language or suprasegmentals of the voice.

Open communication Accepting and accommodating differences and needs while communicating.

'Other' Any person to whom the health professional relates while fulfilling their role as a health service provider. May include colleagues, other workers in the health service, the person seeking assistance and their family and friends.

Over-identification Occurs when the health professional discusses a similar situation or experience to the person seeking assistance.

Paralinguistic features of the voice (paralanguage) Particular vocal effects that change meaning, including emphasis, timely pauses, tone, laughing, whining, moaning and other non-verbal sounds.

Participation Active involvement in activities of choice.

Passive communication Lack of expression of perceptions, ideas or opinions because the person feels they do not have the right or value to express themself in that situation.

Pauses Paralinguistic features of the voice where the speaker does not produce words; provides opportunity for thought and processing.

Perfection Always being as good and accurate as possible; reaching the highest standard in action and words.

Personal space A comfortable distance between people when communicating or moving past each other; usually culturally determined.

Physical The part of the person that relates to the external and internal parts of the body.

Pitch Frequency of sound, which makes the voice sound low or high.

Prejudice A preformed opinion often of a negative kind, based on ignorance, irrational feelings and uninformed or inaccurate stereotypes.

Processing preferences Style of organising information that best suits the individual.

Prosodic features of the voice Vocal effects including volume, pitch, speed and rate of speech that create the unique rhythm of a language.

Psychology Mental and emotional processes.

Rapport A connection between two people based on trust and awareness that they have a common goal.

Reflection Examination of how the reactions of the self affect interactions; uses the experience and knowledge of the self as well as theory to increase self-awareness and understand the causes of those reactions.

Reflective Describes the revisiting of uncomfortable events in order to understand them and change behaviour in similar situations in future.

Reflexive Considering how the self affects and is affected by particular events in order to evaluate and critique the self; facilitates internal change that benefits relationships with people seeking assistance.

Remote communication Communication that is not face-to-face.

Respect Unconditional positive regard for self and others regardless of weaknesses or failures, position or status, beliefs and values, and material possessions or socioeconomic level. It assumes all human beings have innate worth and value.

Role The expected function of a person given their position or membership in society and the expected behaviour that accompanies that position.

Self-awareness Awareness of the beliefs, values, thoughts, inadequacies and fears that affect and drive thoughts and responses of the self during interactions.

Self-disclosure Sharing own experiences and feelings.

Self-introduction To make the person seeking assistance aware of the health professional and the role of the health professional in that health service.

Sexual Reproductive organs and the responsibilities associated with the use of those organs; also refers to sexual preference.

Silence Absence of speaking.

Social The aspect of a person that relates to others as an individual or a group.

Spiritual The aspect of a person that gives meaning to self, life and the universe. It determines the beliefs and values that motivate and sustain the person.

Status The relative 'importance' of someone in a particular group or in society.

Stereotype An oversimplified idea or image of one person or a group that is usually incorrect.

Suprasegmentals Elements of the voice (not words or body language) that affect the meaning of messages. There are two types: prosodic and paralinguistic features.

Therapeutic relationship A collaborative relationship between the health professional and the person seeking assistance that fulfils the needs of the person and empowers them to overcome any challenges.

Tone of the voice Indicates the feeling, attitude or thoughts of the person about the particular topic.

Touch A non-verbal way of physically connecting with a person by using a part of the body, usually a hand, to connect with a part of their body.

Transliteration The exact translation of each word/sound spoken regardless of meaning; these interpretations often have limited meaning.

Trust Confidence in and reliance upon the health professional to provide quality service that is always in the best interests of the person seeking assistance.

Unsafe cultural practice Practice that diminishes, demeans or disempowers the cultural identity and wellbeing of an individual.

Validation The health professional confirms the existence of particular situations or emotions, whether or not they agree, and indicates that the emotional response is understandable.

Value The measure of worth, importance or usefulness of something or someone.

Verification A health professional explores their perceptions of the person seeking assistance to establish the truthfulness of the perceptions and the appropriateness of the emotions.

Visual Anything that can be seen with the eye.

Volume of a voice Whether the voice is loud or soft; can communicate particular meaning.

Vulnerable Feeling emotionally insecure and unsure about the possibility of experiencing harm.

Wellbeing A sense of feeling comfortable and safe.

Whole person A dynamic system in which every aspect of the individual affects and interacts with the other aspects simultaneously. It consists of five fundamental aspects: the physical; the emotional, including the sexual aspect; the cognitive; the social and the spiritual aspects.

Worth The value of someone – innate and inbuilt in all human beings.

Index

abbreviations, in documents 229
accidents *see* emergency, people experiencing an
active listening 131, 133, 134
addictive behaviours *see* decreased cognitive function,
   people with
adolescents 256–9
AEIOU (listening skills) 131
age of individuals, and effective communication 7
aged people *see* older people
aggressive behaviour 242–4
   response during conflict 180
   see also assertive behaviour
agreements, signed 142
alternative communication 95–6
Alzheimer's disease *see* decreased cognitive function,
   people with
angry behaviour *see* aggressive behaviour
anxiety *see* extremely distressed people
assertive communication 181–2
   response during conflict 180
   see also aggressive behaviour
assumptions, cultural *see* cultural expectations/
   assumptions
attacks *see* emergency, people experiencing an
attitudes
   causes of misunderstandings 217–18
   expected/not expected of health professionals 267
   negative, towards another 178–9
   self-awareness of 192
   unhelpful, confronting 32–3
audiences
   of documents 228
   and effective communication 6–7
augmentative and alternative communication (AAC)
   95–6
awareness
   of different environments *see* environments,
      awareness of different
   of the 'other' *see* the 'other'
   of self *see* self-awareness

background of individuals 79
   and effective communication 7
   information gathering 26
   and meanings of words 5
barriers
   caused by stereotypical judgements 167–8
   to culturally safe communication with indigenous
      peoples 210–11
   to experiencing, accepting and resolving emotions
      48–51
   to listening 67–9, 131–2

beds, rooms with 106
behaviours
   expected/not expected of health professionals 267
   expected of groups in the health professions 281–2
   health 187
   meanings of 210
   related to adolescents 256
   related to aggression 242
   related to carers 264
   related to children 253
   related to extreme distress 245
   related to older people 260
   related to parents to children requiring assistance
      270
   related to people experiencing a hearing
      impairment 297
   related to people experiencing a life-limiting illness
      291
   related to people experiencing a visual impairment
      301
   related to people experiencing an emergency 307
   related to people experiencing domestic abuse 311
   related to people experiencing mental illnesses
      294
   related to people speaking a different language to
      the health professional 315
   related to people with decreased cognitive function
      287
   related to reluctance to engage in communication
      248
   related to students in the health professions 276
beliefs
   health 187
   self-awareness of 192
   unhelpful, confronting 32–3
bias *see* prejudice
blindness *see* visual impairment, people experiencing
body language 156–8
boundaries 145–7

carers for people seeking assistance 264–6
caring, values concerning, and indigenous peoples
   207
children 253–5
   parents to 270–2
   single parents to 273–5
clichés 211
codes of ethics 147, 150–1
cognitive aspects of the 'other' 79, 93–6
cognitive distress 292
cognitive function, people with decreased 285–9
collaborative partnerships 11, 13

colleagues in the health professions 267–9
    see also health professionals
colour, in cultural environments 112
comforting, encouraging *versus* discouraging 29–32
communication
    assertive 181–2
    augmentative and alternative (AAC) 95–6
    conflict and 176–84
    culturally appropriate 185–98
    definition 3–7
    ethical 138–48
    with indigenous peoples 200–12, 214
    and misunderstandings 215–24
    non-judgemental 172
    non-verbal 154–64
    'other'-centred 130–7
    overall goal, for health professionals 9–14
    remote 225–35
    specific goals, for health professionals 16–23,
        24–35
        comforting, encouraging *versus* discouraging
            29–32
        confronting unhelpful attitudes or beliefs 32–3
        gathering information 24–9
        providing information 20–2
        verbal introductions 17–20
    stereotypes, and judgements 166–74
    with the whole person 121–8
    see also effective communication; principles for
        effective communication; strategies for
        communicating
Communication Bill of Rights 238
communication skills, personal, self-awareness of
    65–6
communication styles
    expectations of 219
    of indigenous peoples 205, 209
communicative behaviours
    personality typology and resultant 72, 73
    preferences for managing information and
        resultant 70–1
communicators, rights of 238
concentration, as cognitive ability 93
confidentiality 143–5
    and demonstrating respect 84
conflict and communication 176–84
    patterns of relating during conflict 179–81
confronting unhelpful attitudes or beliefs 32–3
consent 142–3
consequences, understanding, as cognitive ability 93
context
    and culturally appropriate communication 187
    relevance of, to determine meaning 218
    of words, effect on meaning 5
control, individual 14
    see also empowerment of individuals; power
        imbalance; rights of communicators
critical care *see* life-limiting illness, people
    experiencing

cultural assumptions *see* cultural expectations/
    assumptions
cultural differences 187
    anticipation of difficulties concerning 193–4
    concerning illness, indigenous peoples 207
    understanding and learning about 193, 207
cultural environments 111–13
    colour 112
    personal space 111
    time 112–13
cultural expectations/assumptions 190–1, 220
    and demonstrating respect 83
    and effective listening 132–3
    and indigenous peoples 208
cultural identity 201–2
cultural/language background of individuals
    and effective communication 7
    information gathering 26
cultural norms, expectations governed by 220
cultural safety for indigenous peoples 202–8
cultural/social experiences and background of the
    'other' 79
cultural understanding 193
culturally appropriate communication 185–98
    definition 186
    factors affecting 187–90
    strategies for demonstrating 192–4
culturally safe communication with indigenous
    peoples
    barriers to 210–11
    factors contributing to 208–10
cultures
    definition 185–6
    of disease or ill-health 196
    of individual health professions 196

databases 229
deafness *see* hearing impairment, people experiencing a
death 290
decreased cognitive function, people with 285–9
defenses (defense mechanisms) 48–51
dementia *see* decreased cognitive function, people
    with
dependency boundaries, and therapeutic
    relationships 145
differences
    personal commitment to understanding 192–3
    respect regardless of 139–40
    see also cultural differences; educational differences;
        language differences
disasters *see* emergency, people experiencing an
discouragement/encouragement 29–32
discussion points
    about groups in the health professions 282–3
    about people experiencing a hearing impairment
        299
    about people experiencing a mental illness
        295–6
    about people experiencing domestic abuse 313

about single parents to children requiring
    assistance 274–5
procedures for 239
disease/ill-health, culture of 196
disengagement 133, 135
disorders of individuals, and effective communication
    7
distractions/interruptions, avoiding 106–7
distressed people 245–7, 291–2
documents, preparation of 228–9
domestic abuse, people experiencing 311–14
dress 102–3

educational differences, indigenous peoples 206–7
effective communication 3–4
    factors contributing to 5
        external to sender 5–6
        within the receivers or 'audience' 6–7
        within the sender 6
    mutual understanding and 4–5
    see also communication; principles for effective
        communication; strategies for communicating
effective listening 14, 130–4
effective listening skills, self-awareness of 66–7
effective speaking skills, self-awareness of 69–70
elderly people see older people
Elders, of indigenous peoples 208
emails, use of 231–2
emergency, people experiencing an 307–10
emotional aspects of the 'other' 79, 84–92
emotional competence of health professionals 147
emotional distress 291
emotional environments 108–11
    emotional responses to environmental demands
        109–11
    formal versus informal environments 108–9
emotions 11
    of adolescents 257
    of carers 264
    causes of misunderstandings 218
    of children 254
    of colleagues in the health professions 267–8
    during conflict 177–8
    and effective communication 7
    of members of groups in the health professions
        280–1
    negative
        responding to 30–1
        towards another 178–9
    of older people 260–1
    of parents to children requiring assistance 271
    of people experiencing a hearing impairment 298
    of people experiencing a life-limiting illness and
        their families 291–2
    of people experiencing a mental illness 294
    of people experiencing a visual impairment 302
    of people experiencing an emergency 307
    of people experiencing domestic abuse 312
    people experiencing strong 241–51

of people speaking a different language to the
    health professional 315
of people with decreased cognitive function 287
positive 14
of single parents to children requiring assistance
    273
of students in the health professions 276
empathy 11–12
    and emotional aspects of the 'other' 86–9
emphasis on words 6, 160
empowerment of individuals 11
    see also control, individual; power imbalance; rights
        of communicators
encouragement/discouragement 29–32
environmental context of words, effect on meaning 5
environments
    awareness of different 101–17
        cultural 111–13
        emotional 108–11
        physical 102–8
        sexual 113–14
        social 114–15
        spiritual 115
    introducing unfamiliar 18–19
    and non-verbal communication 155
equality in relationships 172
ethical codes of behaviour/conduct 147, 150–1
ethical communication 138–48
ethical responsibility, and protection of information
    144
ethnocentricity 188–90
expectations
    clarification of 141
    of communication styles 219
    cultural see cultural expectations/assumptions
    of events or procedures 219–20
    stereotypical, related to roles of health
        professionals 168–70
experiences of individuals, and meanings of words
    5–6
explaining, information provision 20
exposure to different cultures 193
external factors, and effective listening 131–2
extremely distressed people 245–7
eye contact 157

facial expressions 156–7
families
    as part of social environments 114
    of people experiencing a life-limiting illness 290–3
family, notion of, indigenous peoples 205
family/person-centred goals and practice 10–11, 14,
    89
fear see extremely distressed people
formal/informal environments 108–9
formatting of documents 229
foster-parents see parents to children requiring
    assistance
friends, as part of social environments 114

friendship boundaries, and therapeutic relationships 145
frustration *see* extremely distressed people
furniture placement 104–5

gender of health professionals, and indigenous peoples 207
gestures 157–8
glossary 316–21
gossip, protecting the 'other' from 145
grief 290
   see also extremely distressed people
group growth, stages of 280
group sessions 281
groups in the health professions 279–83
guardians *see* carers for people seeking assistance

health beliefs and behaviours 187
health professionals
   attitudes/behaviours expected/not expected of 267
   characteristics/abilities suited to 60–1
   emotions and thoughts of 144
   introducing roles of 18
   and physical environments 104
   stereotypical expectations of 168–70
   values of 59–60
   see also colleagues in the health professions; groups in the health professions; students in the health professions
health professions
   boundaries of roles of 145
   choice of career in 59
   cultures of 196
health services
   expectations of 219–20
   types of groups offered in 279–80
hearing impairment, people experiencing a 297–300, 305
history, and indigenous peoples 204–5
holistic care 122–5
   see also whole person
holistic communication 125–7
   see also whole person
honesty 140–1
humour, and self-awareness 72, 74

ICF (International Classification of Functioning) 9–10
ideas of individuals, and effective communication 7
illness
   cultural differences concerning, indigenous peoples 207
   culture of 196
imbalance of power *see* power imbalance
immature defenses 49, 50
indigenous peoples
   communication with 200–12, 214
   creating cultural safety for 202–8
   culturally safe communication with

   barriers to 210–11
   factors contributing to 208– 210
   principles of practice when working with 202–11
individual values 58–9
informal/formal environments 108–9
information
   to assist in relating to the 'other' 80
   inappropriate 211
   preferences for managing and responding to 70–1
   shared, protection of 143–4
   and signed agreements 142
information gathering 24–9
information processing, and indigenous peoples 209
information provision 20–2
informed consent 142–3, 152–3
institutions, as part of social environments 115
instructing 20
intellectual disability *see* decreased cognitive function, people with
interest groups, as part of social environments 114
internal factors, and effective listening 131–2
International Classification of Functioning (ICF) 9–10
internet, use of 231–3
interpretation 194
interpreters 194–5, 208–9
interruptions/distractions, avoiding 106–7
interviewing 25
introductions, verbal *see* verbal introductions

journals on life-limiting illnesses 304
judgements, stereotypical 166–74

kinship obligations, indigenous peoples 206
knowledge/understanding of individuals, and effective communication 6–7

language
   and culturally appropriate communication 187
   and effective listening 132
language/cultural background of individuals
   and effective communication 7
   information gathering 26
language differences
   indigenous peoples 206–7
   people speaking a different language to the health professional 315–17
learning styles *see* preferences for managing and responding to information
legal guardians *see* parents to children requiring assistance
letters (documents), preparation of 228–9
life circumstances, differences in, indigenous peoples 206
life-limiting illness, people experiencing 290–3, 304
lifespan, people in particular stages of the 252–62
listeners, preparing, information provision 20–1

listening
  active 131, 133, 134
  barriers to 67–9, 131–2
  effective 14, 130–4
  and indigenous peoples 209, 211
  preparation for 132–3
listening skills, effective, self-awareness of 66–7
loss 290
lunar calendars 112

Maoris see indigenous peoples
mature defenses 49, 50
medical records, preparation of 228–9
mental illnesses, people experiencing 294–6
mental retardation see decreased cognitive function,
    people with
misunderstandings
  causes of 217–20
  communication that produces 215–16
  factors that increase 216–17
  resolving 221–3
  strategies to avoid 220–1
mutual understanding 10–12
  effective communication and 4–5
  factors affecting 216–17
Myers–Briggs Type Indicator 72

names, using, and demonstrating respect 83
needs
  conflict between values and 63–4
  and effective communication 7
  personal unconscious 61–3
negative attitudes/emotions
  responding to 30–1
  towards another 178–9
neighbours, as part of social environments 114
neurotic defenses 49, 50
non-English-speaking background (NESB) see
    language differences
non-judgemental communication 172
non-native speakers (NNS) see language differences
non-verbal communication 154–64
  and indigenous peoples 209–11

older people 260–2
open communication, and indigenous peoples 209
'other' 78–99
  cognitive aspects of 79, 93–6
  definition 79–80
  emotional aspects of 79, 84–92
  information to assist in relating to 80
  physical aspects of 78, 84
  and respect 81–4
  sexual aspects of 79, 92–3
  social/cultural experiences and background of
      79
  social needs of 96
  spiritual needs of 79, 96–8
  as a whole person 78–9

'other'-centred communication 130–7
over-identification 146–7

palliative care 290
pamphlets, inappropriate 211
paralinguistic features of the voice 160–2
parents to children requiring assistance 270–2
    see also single parents to children requiring
      assistance
passive responses during conflict 180
pauses in speaking 160–1
people experiencing strong emotions 241–51
  aggression 242–4
  extreme distress 245–7
  reluctance to engage in communication 248–51
people in particular contexts 306–17
  experiencing an emergency 307–10
  experiencing domestic abuse 311–14
  speaking a different language to the health
      professional 315–17
people in particular roles 263–83
  as carers for people seeking assistance 264–6
  as colleagues in the health professions 267–9
  groups in the health professions 279–83
  as parents to children requiring assistance 270–2
  as single parents to children requiring assistance
      273–5
  as students in the health professions 276–8
people in particular stages of the lifespan 252–62
  adolescents 256–9
  children 253–5
  older people 260–2
people with particular conditions 284–305
  decreased cognitive function 285–9
  hearing impairment 297–300
  life-limiting illness 290–3, 304
  mental illness 294–6
  visual impairment 301–4
perfectionism as a value 64–5
person/family-centred goals and practice 10–11, 14,
    89
personal communication skills, self-awareness of
    65–6
personal space 111
personal unconscious needs 61–3
personality typology and resultant communicative
    behaviours 72–3
pets, as part of social environments 114
physical abilities 108
physical appearance, dress 102–3
physical aspects of the 'other' 78, 84
physical comfort 104–5
physical distress 291
physical environments
  avoiding distractions and interruptions 106–7
  familiarity with, and usual procedures
    health professionals 104
    people seeking assistance 103–4
  physical ability of the person 108

↳   physical appearance, dress 102–3
    rooms 104–6
    temperature 107–8
pitch of voice 159
positive emotional responses 14
power imbalance
    and indigenous peoples 207
    overcoming 172
    see also control, individual; empowerment of
        individuals; rights of communicators
preferences for managing and responding to
        information 70–1
prejudice, and stereotypical judgements 167, 170–1
principles for effective communication
    with adolescents 257
    with aggressive people 243
    with carers 265
    with children 254
    with colleagues in the health professions 268
    with extremely distressed people 245
    within groups in the health professions 282
    with older people 261
    with parents to children requiring assistance 271
    with people experiencing a hearing impairment
        298
    with people experiencing a life-limiting illness and
        their families 292
    with people experiencing a mental illness 295
    with people experiencing a visual impairment 302
    with people experiencing an emergency 308
    with people experiencing domestic abuse 312
    with people reluctant to engage in communication
        249
    with people speaking a different language to the
        health professional 316
    with people with decreased cognitive function 287
    with single parents to children requiring assistance
        274
    with students in the health professions 277
privacy 142
professional chat rooms 233
professional jargon, and effective communication 7
'professional' manner, and indigenous peoples 208
prosodic features of the voice 158–60
psychological distress 291
psychotic defenses 49, 50

questioning
    and indigenous peoples 209
    information gathering 25–9
questions
    clarifying 28
    closed 26
    'leading' 28
    open 27
    probing 27–8

rapport 13
rate of speaking 159–60

reactions to healthcare people and environment, by
        indigenous peoples 206
receivers of messages/information *see* audiences
reflection 39–52
    achieving self-awareness 41
    definition 39–41
    models of 45–8
    reasons for 42–5
    upon barriers to experiencing, accepting and
        resolving emotions 48–51
relationships
    equality in 172
    therapeutic, boundaries of 145–6
reluctance to engage in communication 248–51
remote communication 225–35
    characteristics of, for health professionals 226–7
    principles governing professional 228–33
reports, written, preparation of 228–9
respect 11
    definition 81
    demonstrating 82–4
    purpose and benefit of 81
    regardless of differences 139–40
rights of communicators 238
    see also control, individual; empowerment of
        individuals; power imbalance
role-models *see* parents to children requiring
        assistance
role playing
    adolescents 258–9
    aggressive behaviour 244
    assertive communication 182
    carers 265–6
    children 255
    colleagues in the health professions 268–9
    confronting unhelpful attitudes or beliefs 33
    emotional and empathic responses 111
    encouraging responses 31
    extremely distressed people 246–7
    family/person-centred goals and practice 89
    older people 261–2
    parents to children requiring assistance 272
    people experiencing a life-limiting illness 293
    people experiencing a visual impairment 303–4
    people experiencing an emergency 309
    people speaking a different language to the health
        professional 316–7
    people with decreased cognitive function 288
    procedures for 239
    reluctance to engage in communication 250
    students in the health professions 277–8
rooms 104–6

SAAFETY (listening skills) 132–3
scenarios *see* discussion points; role playing
seasonal calendars 112
self-awareness 41, 55–76
    as an essential tool 55–6
    and barriers to listening 67–9

beginning the journey of 56–8
of beliefs and attitudes 192
benefits of achieving 56
and characteristics/abilities suited to health
    professionals 60–1
and choice to become a health professional 59
and conflict between values and needs 63–4
and culturally appropriate communication 192
and humour 72, 74
and individual values 58–9
and perfectionism as a value 64–5
of personal communication skills 65–6
and personal unconscious needs 61–3
and personality typology and resultant
    communicative behaviours 72–3
and preferences for managing information and
    resultant communicative behaviours 70–1
of skills for effective listening 66–7
of skills for effective speaking 69–70
and values of a health professional 59–60
self-disclosure 146
self-respect 139–40
senders of messages 6
sequential interpretation 194
sexual aspects of the 'other' 79, 92–3
sexual environments 113–14
shared information, protection of 143–4
sign languages 299–300
signed agreements 142
silence
    and emotional aspects of the 'other' 91–2
    and indigenous peoples 210
simultaneous interpretation 194
single parents to children requiring assistance 273–5
    see also parents to children requiring assistance
situational context of words, effect on meaning 5
small group activity
    groups in the health professions 279
    people in particular roles 263
    people with particular conditions 284–5
    stages of the lifespan 252
    strong emotions 241
social/cultural experiences and background of the
    'other' 79
social distress 292
social environments 114–15
social needs of the 'other' 96
SOLER (listening skills) 133, 134
space (body language) 158
speakers of languages other than English (LOTE) see
    language differences
speaking skills, effective, self-awareness of 69–70
spiritual distress 292
spiritual environments 115
spiritual needs of the 'other' 79, 96–8
spirituality, concepts of, indigenous peoples 206
sporting teams, as part of social environments 114
stereotypical judgements
    and communication 166–74

developing attitudes that avoid 170–1
    and indigenous peoples 202, 210
    reasons to avoid 167–8
    relating to roles 168–70
stimuli
    for aggression 242–3
    for extreme distress 245
    for reluctance to engage in communication
        248–9
story-telling, and indigenous peoples 209
strategies for communicating
    with adolescents 258
    with carers 265
    with children 254
    with colleagues in the health professions 268
    with extremely distressed people 246
    as leaders of groups in the health professions 282
    with older people 261
    with parents to children requiring assistance 271–2
    with people experiencing a hearing impairment
        298
    with people experiencing a life-limiting illness and
        their families 292
    with people experiencing a mental illness 295
    with people experiencing a visual impairment 303
    with people experiencing an emergency 308
    with people experiencing domestic abuse 313
    with people reluctant to engage in communication
        249
    with people speaking a different language to the
        health professional 316
    with people with decreased cognitive function
        287–8
    with single parents to children requiring assistance
        274
    with students in the health professions 277
strong emotions, people experiencing 241–51
students in the health professions 276–8
styles of communication see communication styles
suprasegmentals 230
    paralinguistic features of the voice 160–2
    prosodic features of the voice 158–60
susceptibility
    to behaving aggressively 242
    to experiencing a hearing impairment 297
    to experiencing a mental illness 294
    to experiencing a visual impairment 302
    to experiencing an emergency 307
    to experiencing difficulties at health services
        adolescents 256–7
        children 253
        older people 260
        parents to children requiring assistance 270
        people with decreased cognitive function 287
    to reluctance to engage in communication 248
sympathy 86

telephones, strategies for using 230
temperature, physical environments 107–8

terminal illness *see* life-limiting illness, people experiencing
terms relating to indigenous peoples, correct use of 200–1
the 'other' *see* 'other'
therapeutic relationships 13
   boundaries of 145–6
thoughts of individuals, and effective communication 7
time, concept of, in cultural environments 112–13
time investment
   to establish trust with indigenous peoples 209
   to understand cultural differences 193, 207
time limits, and therapeutic relationships 145
timing information provision 21
tone of voice 161–2
Torres Strait Islanders *see* indigenous peoples
touch, and emotional aspects of the 'other' 90–1
traditional methods of managing illness, indigenous peoples 207
training in understanding cultural differences 207
transliteration 194
trauma *see* emergency, people experiencing an
treatment rooms 106
trust 12–13
24-hour schedules 112

unconscious needs, personal 61–3
understanding
   of consequences, as cognitive ability 93
   and effective communication 6–7, 210–11
   see also cultural understanding; misunderstandings; mutual understanding
unhelpful attitudes/beliefs, confronting 32–3

validation, and emotional aspects of the 'other' 84–6
values
   concerning caring, and indigenous peoples 207
   conflict between needs and 63–4
   of health professionals 59–60
   individual 58–9
   perfectionism as a value 64–5
verbal introductions 17–20
   introducing the unfamiliar environment 18–19
   introducing yourself and your role 18
video/teleconferencing 231
violent behaviour *see* aggressive behaviour
visual impairment, people experiencing a 301–5
voice
   paralinguistic features of the 160–2
   prosodic features of the 158–60
volume of voice 158–9

waiting rooms 105
websites
   codes of conduct for health professions 150–1
   hearing and visual impairment 305
   indigenous peoples 214
   life-limiting illness 304
wellbeing, concept of, indigenous peoples 207
whole person
   communication with 121–8
   definition 121–2
   see also holistic care; holistic communication
words
   context of, affect on meaning 5
   emphasis on, by senders of messages 6
   meanings of 210
written reports, preparation of 228–9